Foreword to the First Edition

The health of populations is related to features of society and its social and economic organization. This crucial fact provides the basis for effective policy-making to improve population health. While there is, understandably, much concern regarding the appropriate provision and financing of health services as well as ensuring that the nature of the services provided is based on the best evidence of effectiveness, health is a matter that goes beyond the provision of health services. Policies pursued by many branches of government and by the private sector, both nationally and locally, exert a powerful influence on health—and this book shows the direction in which we should be going. Just as decisions about health services should be based on the best evidence available, so should policies related to the social determinants of health.

Researchers associated with the International Centre for Health and Society at University College London have accumulated a wealth of knowledge on the social determinants of health. The World Health Organization Regional Office for Europe's Centre for Urban Health was concerned to package that knowledge in a way that is useful to policy-makers. The result was *Social determinants of health: the solid facts* (Wilkinson and Marmot 1998). This accumulation of evidence was also fundamental to the *Independent inquiry into inequalities in health* which I was commissioned to chair by the Government in Britain (Acheson *et al.* 1998). Indeed, many of the authors of this book were closely involved in the presentation of evidence that underpinned the formulation of recommendations for policy development that resulted from the Inquiry.

This book results from the welcome efforts of members of the International Centre for Health and Society and their collaborators to summarize their research evidence around themes useful to policy-makers. Policy-making will always involve a multiplicity of influences. The research summarized here shows that important among those influences must be the evidence on the social determinants of health.

Sir Donald Acheson
Chairman, International Centre for
Health and Society
University College London

References

Acheson, D. *Independent Inquiry into Inequalities in Health*. The Stationary Office, London.

Wilkinson, R. and Marmot, M. (ed.) (1998). *Social determinants of health: the solid facts*, World Health Organization, Copenhagen.

Acknowledgements

Special thanks are due to Ruth Bell and Patricia Crowley who have co-ordinated the efforts of the many contributors, keeping us up to the mark and providing the central point of contact between the editors, authors, Oxford University Press, and for the WHO Regional Office for Europe's Centre for Urban Health. Patricia Crowley took the main responsibility for the first edition and Ruth Bell for this revised and expanded second edition of *The Social Determinants of Health*. Their tenacity and kindly chivvying have been essential to keeping the project on schedule.

M.M.
R.G.W.

Social determinants of health

Social determinants of health

SECOND EDITION

Edited by

Michael Marmot

Department of Epidemiology and Public Health
University College London, UK

and

Richard G. Wilkinson

Department of Epidemiology and Public Health
University of Nottingham Medical School, Nottingham, UK

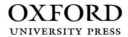

OXFORD
UNIVERSITY PRESS

OXFORD
UNIVERSITY PRESS

Great Clarendon Street, Oxford OX2 6DP

Oxford University Press is a department of the University of Oxford.
It furthers the University's objective of excellence in research, scholarship,
and education by publishing worldwide in

Oxford New York

Auckland Cape Town Dar es Salaam Hong Kong Karachi
Kuala Lumpur Madrid Melbourne Mexico City Nairobi
New Delhi Shanghai Taipei Toronto

With offices in

Argentina Austria Brazil Chile Czech Republic France Greece
Guatemala Hungary Italy Japan Poland Portugal Singapore
South Korea Switzerland Thailand Turkey Ukraine Vietnam

Oxford is a registered trade mark of Oxford University Press
in the UK and in certain other countries

Published in the United States
by Oxford University Press Inc., New York

First edition published in 1998 by the World Health Organization, Copenhagen
Second edition published 2006
Reprinted 2006, 2007, 2008, (twice)

British Library Cataloguing in Publication Data
Data available

Library of Congress Cataloging in Publication Data
Data available

Typeset by Newgen Imaging Systems (P) Ltd., Chennai, India
Printed in Great Britain
on acid-free paper by
Ashford Colour Press Ltd, Gosport, Hampshire

ISBN   978–0–19–856589–5 (Pbk.)

10 9 8 7

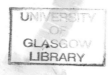

Contents

List of contributors

Mel Bartley
Department of Epidemiology and
Public Health,
University College London,
London, UK

David Blane
Division of Epidemiology,
Public Health and Primary Care,
Department of Primary Care and
Social Medicine, Imperial College,
London, UK

Elizabeth Breeze
Department of Epidemiology and
Public Health,
University College London,
London, UK

Eric Brunner
Department of Epidemiology and
Public Health,
University College London,
London, UK

Suzie Butterworth
MRC National Survey of Health and
Development,
Department of Epidemiology and
Public Health,
University College London,
London, UK

Jackie A. Cassell
Department of Primary Care and
Population Sciences,
University College London,
London, UK

George Davey Smith
Department of Social Medicine,
University of Bristol,
Bristol, UK

Danny Dorling
Department of Geography,
University of Sheffield,
Sheffield, UK

Jane Ferrie
Department of Epidemiology and
Public Health,
University College London,
London, UK

Alissa Goodman
Institute of Fiscal Studies,
London, UK

Martin J. Jarvis
ICRF Health Behaviour Unit,
Department of Epidemiology and
Public Health,
University College London,
London, UK

Anne M. Johnson
Department of Primary Care and
Population Sciences,
University College London,
London, UK

Michael Marmot
Department of Epidemiology and
Public Health,
University College London,
London, UK

Mark McCarthy
Department of Epidemiology and
Public Health,
University College London,
London, UK

Anne McMunn
Department of Epidemiology and
Public Health,
University College London,
London, UK

Catherine H. Mercer
Centre for Sexual Health and
HIV Research,
University College London,
London, UK

Scott M. Montgomery
Clinical Epidemiology Unit,
Department of Medicine,
Karolinska Hospital,
Karolinska Institute,
Stockholm, Sweden

James Y. Nazroo
Department of Epidemiology and
Public Health,
University College London,
London, UK

Zoe Oldfield
Institute of Fiscal Studies,
London, UK

Aileen Robertson
Suhr's University College,
Copenhagen, Denmark

Mary Shaw
Department of Social Medicine,
University of Bristol,
Bristol, UK

Aubrey Sheiham
Department of Epidemiology and
Public Health,
University College London,
London, UK

Johannes Siegrist
Department of Medical Sociology,
Medical Faculty,
University of Duesseldorf,
Duesseldorf, Germany

Mai Stafford
Department of Epidemiology and
Public Health,
University College London,
London, UK

Stephen A. Stansfeld
Centre for Psychiatry,
Barts and the London,
Queen Mary's School of Medicine
and Dentistry,
London, UK

Tores Theorell
Division of Psychosocial Factors
and Health,
Department of Public Health Science,
Karolinska Institute,
Stockholm, Sweden

Michael Wadsworth
MRC National Survey of Health and
Development,
Department of Epidemiology and
Public Health,
University College London,
London, UK

Jane Wardle
ICRF Health Behaviour Unit,
Department of Epidemiology and
Public Health,
University College London,
London, UK

Richard G. Wilkinson
Department of Epidemiology and
Public Health,
University of Nottingham
Medical School,
Nottingham, UK

David R. Williams
Department of Sociology,
Epidemiology, and The Survey
Research Center,
Institute for Social Research,
University of Michigan,
Michigan, USA

Chapter 1

Introduction

Michael Marmot

In the Scottish city of Glasgow, people living in the most deprived districts have life expectancy 12 years shorter than those living in the most affluent (NHS Health Scotland 2004). In some American cities, the differences are even greater. Among countries, too, the differences in life expectancy are large, even within Europe. Life expectancy for men in Russia is 58.4 years—a full 20 years less than in Sweden and Iceland (WHO 2005). To understand the causes of differences such as these and, more importantly, to do something about them, requires a focus on the social determinants of health.

Academic research has made substantial progress in understanding the 'social determinants of health'. But how is this to be translated into action to change inequalities in health within and between countries? It was to advance this translation from research to action, that the Centre for Urban Health at the WHO Regional Office for Europe approached us, at the International Centre for Health and Society at University College London. They asked us to summarize work on the social determinants of health in ten messages that could provide a guide for policy makers and public alike. Members of the International Centre for Health and Society, represented in this book, developed the ten brief messages that were first published as *The solid facts* (Wilkinson and Marmot 1998). An important consideration was that each message should be firmly supported by evidence. The first edition of this book grew directly out of that process. Each of the chapters in the book presented a summary of relevant research giving the evidence underlying the message.

The solid facts was a success. It was translated into more than 20 European languages and used in the policy process in many countries. We were therefore requested to produce a second edition (Wilkinson and Marmot 2003). In the 12 months after it was published in Autumn 2003, the second edition was downloaded from the web 218,000 times. It clearly reached an audience. This, the second edition of *Social determinants of health*, updates the evidence to support the ten facts included in the second edition of *The solid facts*. In addition, there are new chapters on ethnic inequalities in health, inequalities in health at older ages, neighbourhoods, housing and health, and sexual behaviours as well as the social determinants of transmission of sexually transmitted infections.

1.1 **The health gradient**

British statistics have shown, for as long as one has cared to look, that health follows a social gradient: the higher the social position, the better the health. I became aware of this gradient only when I started to analyse data from the first Whitehall study of British civil servants (Marmot *et al.* 1978). There had been a curious disjunction between the fact of the social gradient and the belief that the major killer in developed countries, coronary heart disease, affected most those of high status. The view appeared to be that there were diseases of the rich (heart disease and cancer) and diseases of the poor. Mortality for all causes reflected a balance of the two. We now know that this is inaccurate on two counts. First, in rich countries, most diseases affect people of lower position more than those of higher. In this sense, the diseases of affluence are few— breast cancer has been a notable exception to the pattern of low social position, high risk. Second, it is not only the poor who suffer. The Whitehall studies, for example, showed that in civil servants who are not poor, the lower the employment grade, the higher the risk of most causes of death.

This social gradient in health is a remarkably widespread phenomenon (Marmot 2004). It changes both the scientific questions and the policies that are needed to address the problem. Poverty, in its various guises, is a bad thing (Gordon and Townsend 2000). One of its nastier effects is that on health. But the social gradient in health is not confined to those in poverty. It runs from top to bottom of society, with less good standards of health at every step down the social hierarchy. Even comfortably off people somewhere in the middle tend to have poorer health than those above them. To understand the causes of this gradient, we have to examine the circumstances in which people live and work—the social determinants of health. But this book is not simply about the social gradient in health. Rather, the social gradient has shown us how sensitive health is to social and economic factors, and so enabled us to identify the determinants of health among the population as a whole.

1.2 **The causes of the causes**

Much of the epidemiology seeks to identify individual risk factors for disease. Smokers have higher risk of several diseases than those who have never smoked; raised plasma cholesterol or blood pressure are associated with increased risk of cardiovascular disease; newer risk factors such as C Reactive protein have been identified, and some call for their use in screening to identify individuals at high risk of subsequent disease who may be suitable for special intervention.

The approach we take is different. First, among risk factors, we distinguish those that are behaviours from those that are biological markers. A biological marker such as cholesterol or blood pressure may be useful if treatment to lower their levels reduces risk of subsequent disease. But it is important to seek the determinants of these biological markers if we are to find effective ways of improving public health. This leads—in the case of cholesterol and blood pressure—to consideration of diet, obesity, and alcohol. From a public health viewpoint, it is perhaps more useful to think of the behaviour (diet) as the cause of the disease rather than labelling plasma cholesterol (the biological effect of the diet) as causal.

Second, we go further to examine the causes of these causes. It is not an accident that people consume diets high in saturated fat and salt. It represents the nature of the food supply, culture, affordability, and availability, among other influences. These are the causes of the causes. For example, given that smoking is such an important cause of premature disease and death, we need to understand the social determinants of smoking. In particular, in many rich countries now, there is a social gradient in smoking: the lower the socio-economic position, the higher the rate of smoking.

One pathway, then, by which social circumstances affect health is through the influence on behaviours known to relate to disease risk. There are others.

1.3 Psychosocial and material conditions

In Britain, to take a typical example, infant mortality at the beginning of the 20th century was over 100/1000 live births (Rowntree 2001) At the beginning of the 21st century, it is around 5–6/1000 live births. Among one of the most deprived groups—single mothers registered as the only parent—it is under 10/1000 live births. There is no difficulty in understanding how material conditions could contribute to an infant mortality of 100/1000: dirty water, lack of calories, poor quality or absent medical care, with great risk of infection. These gross effects of material deprivation are, thankfully, now uncommon in the richer countries of the world.

Big social inequalities in health still exist but are now largely the result of differences in adult mortality. In the United States, for example, black men in deprived areas have 20 years' shorter life expectancy than richer white men. The major contributors to this excess mortality are violent deaths, HIV/AIDS, and cardiovascular disease. Poverty of material conditions does not provide a ready biological explanation for these causes of shortened lives. We need a richer understanding of how the social environment affects health. In so far as material deprivation can be seen to cause homicide or risky sexual behaviour or drug use, its effects are likely to be through psychological pathways. To be clear, we have had pathways linking material circumstances to disease via exposure to cold, infections, malnutrition. More recently, these have been supplemented by behaviours such as smoking, diet, and physical activity. The psychosocial approach emphasizes subjective experience and emotions that produce acute and chronic stress which, in turn, affect biology and, hence, physical and mental illness. Our growing understanding of psychological factors points to ways that the social environment can have a powerful influence on health. All three types of pathways—material, behavioural, and psychosocial—should be within our focus.

1.4 **Policy implications**

The solid facts sets out conclusions on social determinants, aimed at policy makers. Its intention was to lead to change. This book sets out the evidence leading to the conclusions summarized in *The solid facts*. It is based on the findings of many different kinds of study. Some have used prospective methods and have collected data from tens of thousands of people over decades, sometimes from birth, to see patterns of health and ill health as they emerged. Others have used cross-sectional methods and have studied individuals, neighbourhoods, and countries. Evidence from these sources has been supplemented by findings from intervention studies and, occasionally, from so-called 'natural experiments'. From time to time, interpretations have been influenced by studies of other primate species. But where, one might ask, is the evidence from randomized controlled trials that surely should precede recommendations if effectiveness and safety are to be assured? The answer is that these are, largely, lacking. A lack of trials to support recommendations is not unique to the social determinants area. It has been common in public health—probably more the rule than the exception. James Lind is rightly acknowledged as an exceptional public health figure because as early as the 18th century he conducted controlled investigations to show citrus fruit cured scurvy. By contrast, John Snow's determination in the 19th century that ingestion of contaminated water led to cholera, relied on careful observation and the exercise of reasoned judgement rather than his uncontrolled experiment of removing the handle of the Broad Street pump.

The judgements, based on evidence, that health would be improved by a nurturing environment for children, better education, a socially supportive environment for adults, better psychosocial working conditions, employment rather than unemployment, and improved infrastructure of communities, relies on observation more than experiment. We would argue, however, that the Hippocratic principle of 'first, do no harm' is honoured by such recommendations. More, they are likely to have benefits other than those for health. Childhood interventions aimed at breaking the link between deprivation and poor educational performance had, in the long-term follow-up of the Perry pre-school project, positive effects on crime and unemployment of the individuals enrolled. High social capital and friendship are goods in themselves, quite apart from the evidence showing their benefit for health. Increased accessibility of public transport may be good for health; it will also have beneficial effects on the environment. Increased participation in management in the workplace may well increase productivity quite apart from the positive effects of control at work on health (Conyon and Freeman 2001).

An explicit intention of *The solid facts* and this book is to give definition to the social determinants of health—to unpick the social environment—in order to be more precise about areas of policy making. Because this is an area of scientific enquiry, we do not imagine that we have final answers to questions about the most important aspects of the social environment. The authors are, however, convinced by epidemiological observations of differences in disease rates within and between countries, by rapid time changes in rates of disease and social inequalities, and by the changing rates of disease in migrants that the social environment is of crucial importance. Good social policy will pay attention to these social determinants at the same time as further research will do much to clarify the nature of their relationships to health. Yes, as we academics are fond of saying, we need more research. But we also need more social action on the basis of the knowledge we have.

References

Conyon, M.J. and Freeman, R.B. (2001). Shared modes of compensation and firm performance: UK evidence. *NBER Working Paper* 8448.

Gordon, D. and Townsend, P. (2000). *Breadline Europe: the measurement of poverty*. The Policy Press, Bristol.

Marmot, M. (2004). *Status syndrome*. Bloomsbury, London.

Marmot, M.G., Rose, G., Shipley, M., and Hamilton, P.J.S. (1978). Employment grade and coronary heart disease in British civil servants. *Journal of Epidemiology and Community Health* 32, 244–9.

NHS Health Scotland. (2004). Public Health Institute for Scotland, www.phis.org.uk

Rowntree, B.S. (2001). Poverty: a study of town life (1901). In: *Poverty, inequality and health in Britain, 1800–2000: a reader* (ed. G. Davey Smith, G.D. Dorling, and M. Shaw). The Policy Press, Bristol.

Wilkinson, R. and Marmot, M. (eds) (1998). *Social determinants of health: the solid facts*. World Health Organization, Copenhagen.

Wilkinson, R. and Marmot, M. (eds) (2003). *The solid facts* (2nd edn). World Health Organization, Copenhagen.

World Health Organization. (2005). The World Health Report 2005. World Health Organization, Geneva.

Chapter 2

Social organization, stress, and health

Eric Brunner and Michael Marmot

2.1 Introduction

Two major health problems illustrate the social determinants of health: the social gradient in disease, and the striking differences in life expectancy between the countries of western Europe and those of central and eastern Europe that have emerged over the last 30 years. In relation to the social gradient, observed in the Whitehall studies of British civil servants (Marmot *et al.* 1984, 1991), we argued that it is significant that it runs right across the social hierarchy from the top employment grades to the bottom. The fact that civil servants in the second grade from the top have worse health than those at the top shows that we are dealing not only with the effects of absolute deprivation. Rather, position in the hierarchy is important. This suggests some concept of relative rather than absolute deprivation. This is a psychosocial concept. What this might mean is discussed in other chapters of this book (in particular, Chapters 6, 8, and 16). Is it plausible that circumstances in which people live and work, that differ according to where they are in the hierarchy, could powerfully influence health by acting through psychological pathways?

Similarly, the evidence from central and eastern Europe (Bobak and Marmot 1996) is consistent with the hypothesis that psychosocial factors, including financial insecurity and hopelessness, play an important role in accounting for the worse health of those countries compared to the more favoured countries of the 'West' (see Fig. 2.1). Is it again plausible that these factors might be crucial and, if so, how do they operate to cause disease?

This chapter takes up the issue of biological plausibility (Brunner 1997). There are, in fact, two broad issues here. First, is it plausible that the organization of work, degree of social isolation, and sense of control over life, could affect the likelihood of developing and dying from chronic diseases such as diabetes and cardiovascular disease? The answer is an emphatic 'yes'. As we shall discuss, a variety of biological pathways can plausibly change the risk of developing major disease. The second issue is more complicated—do any of the plausible biological pathways actually operate; that is, not could they cause disease, but do they? The evidence on this is incomplete and is an

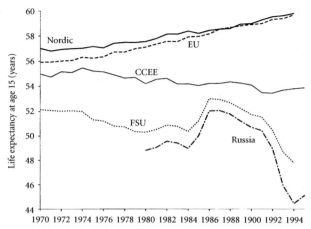

Fig. 2.1 Life expectancy trends in the EU, Nordic countries, and countries of the former USSR and central and eastern Europe, 1970–95. The powerful impact of social organization on health is seen over the period of transition from the centrally planned to the free market economy in central and eastern Europe. (CCEE, Countries of Central and Eastern Europe; EU, European Union; FSU, former Soviet Union.) (Source: WHO Health for All data.)

important topic for current and future research, but it is sufficiently suggestive to point to hypotheses for testing.

The issue of biological plausibility is, of course, important as a contribution to discussion of whether the variety of associations observed in this book represent causation. To take one example—does low socio-economic status lead to poor health, or does poor health lead to low socio-economic status? This is variously described as health selection, reverse causation, or, for economists, endogeneity. There are various ways of designing studies or analysing data to address this question. One contribution is to set out a plausible model of how socio-economic status could influence health and then test the various stages of the model. We set out an example of such a model in this chapter. Part of the model describes how factors in the environment, acting through the central nervous system, could influence biology to cause ill health.

2.2 **The personal and the social**

In the past, the debate about stress and health has seen stress as a property of individuals. This has led to the view that what is stress for one person is stimulation for another. The approach we take is different. We relate the biological response of the individual to the social environment acting upon him or her. The response will clearly be influenced by previous experience and perhaps genetic make-up, but there is sufficient regularity of the response to suggest that the right approach is to understand how the social environment impacts on biology to cause disease.

Selye's approach calls the response of the organism, 'stress' (Selye 1956). Others have used an engineering analogy, in which external demands are considered to be the stressor and the biological response may or may not (depending on the resilience of the subject) have undesirable consequences. What is clearly known is the physiology of the fight-or-flight response. What has been more difficult to tie down is how the fight-or-flight response relates to chronic stress and, later on, to disease. The model elaborated by Sapolsky is that the fight-or-flight response is adaptive in acute stress but may be maladaptive in chronic stress in today's urban environment (Sapolsky 1993). Thus, for example, the average life span of African–American men in Harlem, despite much higher material living standards, is shorter than that of men in Bangladesh.

Psychosocial factors and their influences on health are active areas of research (Brunner *et al.* 2004). There is now enough evidence to suggest that this is an important field for those concerned with improving public health in both economically developed and developing countries. Plausible mechanisms linking psychosocial factors to health are described in the first half of this chapter. We then look to the evidence from both human and animal literature to illustrate the ways in which social organization can influence our biology and, therefore, the health of individuals and populations.

2.3 Biological pathways in a social context

Biological processes must be involved in the connection between social structure and health. But, perhaps even more than health, biology is thought of as an individual rather than a social attribute. Individuals develop some disturbance of their biology. They become sick so they go to see the doctor. The doctor treats individuals, except perhaps when there is an outbreak of infectious disease, or when a vaccination programme is undertaken. The individual, clinical view of health determinants is vitally important. It underlies medical training and biomedical science, and provides the framework for the treatment, cure, and amelioration of disease.

We can extend the conceptual framework to provide a public health view in which the emphasis is on prevention rather than cure. Figure 2.2 is an example of such a framework, in which factors operating beyond the level of the individual, as well as individual characteristics, are recognized. Thus, social structure (top left of the diagram) influences well-being and health (bottom right). The influences of social structure operate via three main pathways. Material circumstances are related to health directly, and via the social and work environment. These in turn shape psychological factors and health-related behaviours. Early life experiences, cultural, and genetic factors also exert influences on health. Figure 2.2 is a generalization. A specific diagram for each disease category could be constructed, given the evidence. Further, the balance of influences on health depends on geographical location and historical circumstances of the population in question. For example, coronary heart disease is considerably more common in northern Europe than in the south of the continent, and, within the

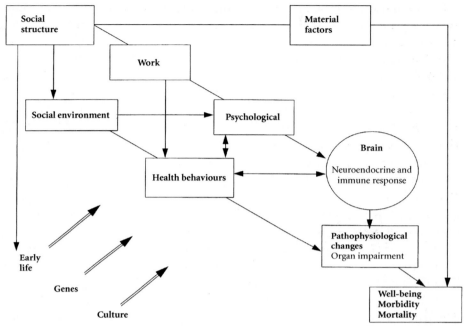

Fig. 2.2 Social determinants of health. The model links social structure to health and disease via material, psychosocial, and behavioural pathways. Genetic, early life, and cultural factors are further important influences on population health.

UK and France, similar north–south gradients exist. It should be noted, however, that there is no evidence to suggest that lack of sunshine or northern latitude *per se* are risk factors for heart disease.

The left-hand side of Fig. 2.2 adds social causes to our picture of the determinants of health. The social and cultural environment, and organization of work, are among the upstream factors that have re-emerged in thinking about public health policy (Blane *et al.* 1996), partly as a response to the weaknesses of the education behaviour change model which dominated the field between the 1960s and the 1980s. Moving towards the right of Fig. 2.2, we encounter the psychological and biological dimensions. These downstream factors are the proximal causes of disease which tend to be the main focus of medical attention. These factors are the intermediates on the pathway from social position to well-being or disease in individuals. Put another way, there can be no doubt that the effects of social organization on population health are mediated by psychological and biological processes. The two big questions, outlined in the introduction, are, first, what are the processes involved and, secondly, given the plausibility of stress pathways, what is the importance of 'stress biology' in comparison with behavioural explanations which place factors such as smoking, exercise, and diet at centre stage?

The plausibility question is answered illustratively below. Even if the reader is initially sceptical about the pubic health importance of direct stress pathways operating independently of health-related behaviours, the social patterning of health-damaging habits, such as smoking, suggests that psychological and biological processes are, at least indirectly, important in understanding health differences within and between populations.

2.3.1 The fight-or-flight response

Humans evolved to rise rapidly to the challenge of external, potentially lethal, but short-term threats. Such threats may be physical, psychological, or biological, and often are a combination of all three. From a physiological point of view, the fight-or-flight response is similar in all mammals, whether man, woman, mouse, or lion. Sensory information is the trigger for a set of nerve and hormone signals which prepare the brain and body to respond to the emergency. The resulting physiological changes can be the key to survival in the face of a predator's attack or physical injury. For the mouse, and particularly the lion, such stressors are brief and fairly unusual, and the accompanying disturbances to the body's internal status quo are, likewise, uncommon events. For humans, the contemporary environment is radically different. Physical and biological emergencies are comparatively rare but, instead, life is filled with psychological demands and challenges which may activate the fight-or-flight response too hard and too often.

The mechanism of the fight-or-flight response involves two main pathways which together co-ordinate an array of metabolic and physiological changes. Because these rely on parts of the nervous system and several hormonal or endocrine transmitters, they are known collectively as neuroendocrine pathways. Both are signal pathways that originate in the brain, where the threat is perceived and evaluated and the resulting signal is initiated. The first pathway comes into action very rapidly, utilizing the sympathetic (as opposed to the parasympathetic) branch of the autonomic nervous system. The hormonal products of the pathway are noradrenaline, released at nerve endings, and adrenaline, secreted into the bloodstream by the medulla (or middle part) of the adrenal glands. This system is the sympatho-adrenal pathway. One effect of this involuntary reaction is known to us all—the unpleasant tightening of the gut we feel in response to a sudden shock. The second pathway comes into operation over minutes and hours instead of milliseconds. Its key components are three hormone-secreting glands (the hypothalamus and pituitary, respectively in and just below the brain, and the adrenal glands, located on the kidneys)—hence the name of the second pathway, the hypothalamic–pituitary–adrenal axis. The adrenal glands secrete the important hormone, cortisol, among other steroid hormones.

The sympatho-adrenal pathway

The almost instantaneous release of noradrenaline from sympathetic nerve endings and adrenaline from the adrenal medulla evokes responses throughout the body

Table 2.1 Effects of circulating adrenaline and sympathetic nerve activity in the fight-or-flight response

- Accelerate heart rate
- Increase metabolic rate
- Increase blood pressure
- Increase sensory vigilance
- Dilate pupils
- Dilate airways
- Constrict blood vessels in skin and gut
- Dilate blood vessels in skeletal muscles
- Inhibit salivation
- Increase sweat secretion

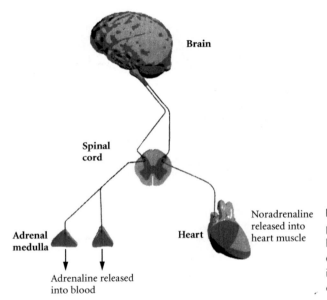

Brain

Spinal cord

Adrenal medulla

Heart

Adrenaline released into blood

Noradrenaline released into heart muscle

Fig. 2.3 Sympatho-adrenal pathway and the heart. The heart rate is influenced directly by sympathetic nerve impulses and indirectly by the circulating adrenaline level.

(Table 2.1). The effects are due, in varying degrees, to the presence of sympathetic nerves in the target organs, and to increased secretion of adrenaline into the circulation. One important target organ is the heart (Fig. 2.3) which is controlled, directly, by nerves of the autonomic nervous system and, indirectly, by the level of adrenaline in the blood. The combined effects of sympatho-adrenal activation on the mind and body are psychological arousal and energy mobilization, and inhibition of functions which are irrelevant to immediate survival, such as digestion and growth. The precise nature of the activation varies according to the stressor and its duration, but its function is essentially to prepare for, or to maintain, physical exertion. The sympatho-adrenal pathway can be switched off rapidly. Even the circulating adrenaline has short-lived effects because its half-life is just a few minutes.

There is much evidence of wide variations between individuals in the size and duration of responses. These variations appear to be partly constitutional and partly due to social and individual differences in psychological coping resources. The impact of these variations on the development of chronic disease is uncertain.

The hypothalamic–pituitary–adrenal axis

The second, slow component of the stress response is the hypothalamic–pituitary–adrenal (HPA) axis. This pathway results in cortisol release into the bloodstream (Fig. 2.4) from the adrenal glands. The hormonal cascade starts in the brain with the release of corticotrophin releasing factor (CRF) into small vessels that carry it the few millimetres from the hypothalamus to the pituitary gland. Here, specialized cells respond to the presence of CRF by secreting the second hormone, adrenocorticotrophic hormone (ACTH) into the circulation. Within a few minutes, the level of ACTH in the adrenal cortex is sufficiently raised to stimulate cortisol release. As Fig. 2.4 shows, there are several feedback loops which regulate the activity of the HPA axis. The control system, involving each of the three hormones, provides sensitive

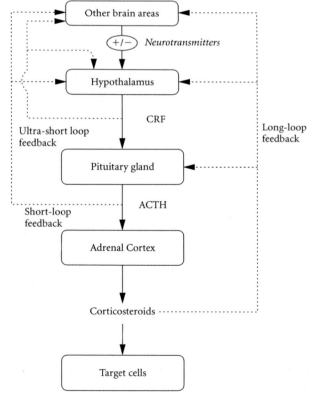

Fig. 2.4 The hypothalamic–pituitary–adrenal axis. The diagram shows how stimuli in the brain influence metabolic and immune functions in other parts of the body. The dotted lines show feedback controls which regulate release of cortisol and other corticosteroids from the adrenal cortex. (CRF, corticotrophin releasing factor; ACTH, adrenocorticotrophic hormone.) (Redrawn from Brown 1994.)

mechanisms for adjustment of the circulating cortisol level during everyday life and in stress situations.

Cortisol and other related glucocorticoid hormones have both metabolic and psychological effects. They play a key role in the maintenance and control of resting and stress-related metabolic functions. As antagonists of the hormone, insulin, they mobilize energy reserves by raising blood glucose and promoting fatty acid release from fat tissues. During an emergency, this is a desirable effect, but in the physically inactive situation, the superfluous availability of energy tends to increase output into the blood of cholesterol-carrying particles from the liver. The brain is also a target for glucocorticoids, which promote vigilance in the short term. However, a prolonged high level of cortisol, such as occurs in Cushing's syndrome, can provoke paranoia or depression. Some depressed patients respond to the drug, metyrapone, which inhibits the production of cortisol within the adrenal gland (Checkley 1996), while in others, alterations of HPA axis functioning appear to override the effect of the drug and cortisol output from the adrenal continues at a high level.

2.3.2 Acute and chronic stress

The neuroendocrine pathways outlined above, which generate the fight-or-flight response, are valuable properties of human biology because they provide the means to survive in the face of environmental challenge. From an evolutionary perspective, it is easy to see that systems which gave survival advantage during the past million years, and have therefore been inherited by modern *Homo sapiens*, may not be without a downside for the health of the present-day city dweller. The material and social environment has changed beyond recognition over the past 10,000 years since agriculture began, and in the past 200 years, successive waves of industrial development have altered living conditions at a great pace. Yet our underlying biology is essentially the same as it was in ancient Babylon.

What, then, is the effect of living in social isolation on a shabby housing estate? Of growing up with parents who have no work and little self-respect? Of being a low-paid office worker surrounded by high-income executives? In advanced industrialized countries such groups of individuals will usually have adequate material circumstances, food, and clean water. Financial strain, lack of social support, and monotonous work may, however, produce a low level of psychosocial stress as a feature of daily life. Modern populations are largely free of the risks of fatal infectious disease, but not of the more subtle exposures which may repeatedly and frequently activate the fight-or-flight response over a period of decades. The increased risks of diabetes and cardiovascular disease among those lower down the social hierarchy fit this interpretation very well.

This is not to argue for stress counselling rather than poverty alleviation and social reform. The point is to dispel a common misconception that 'stress' is predominantly a health risk for senior managers, stockbrokers, and others in positions of corporate and public responsibility. Acute stress in such contexts provides challenges which often will be exciting, stimulating and, after the event, emotionally and intellectually satisfying. As Siegrist and his group have shown, high effort linked to high reward is generally health promoting (Siegrist 1996). In contrast, ill health is associated with prolonged exposure to psychological demands when possibilities to control the situation are perceived to be limited and chances of reward are small (Bosma *et al.* 1997). How might such repeated activation of the fight-or-flight response relate to the development of chronic disease?

2.3.3 The limits of stress reactivity

A principle of animal physiology is that an organism requires a stable internal environment in order to live successfully. Claude Bernard saw this to be true almost 150 years ago when he wrote '*La fixité du milieu interieur est la condition de la vie libre*'. Constant temperature, carbon dioxide concentration, and osmotic pressure are essential for the well-being of cells, tissues, and organs and, therefore, for the integrity of the whole organism. At the same time, blood sugar, other circulating nutrients and waste products, blood pressure, and heart rate are also controlled, but the controls have wider margins. Variability in these factors is a fact of life, and the maintenance of a constant internal environment (termed homeostasis) is about balancing necessary variation against the need for physiological stability (Cannon 1929). Neuroendocrine regulation, based on complex and interlocking positive and negative feedback mechanisms, is central to this function.

The nature and size of the biological response to psychological demands can influence health in several ways. A particular type of response may be directly responsible for disease or may increase vulnerability to certain illnesses, such as colds or flu. The pattern of reactivity may disrupt existing disease processes, acting as a trigger for acute events such as heart attack.

There is good evidence for the disruptive effect of stressors, such as life events, on existing medical conditions, including diabetes and rheumatoid arthritis, and for the precipitation of myocardial infarction by emotional trauma. But although a habitual pattern of high blood pressure reactivity has been seen to be a likely cause of hypertension, it has proved difficult to demonstrate that heightened blood pressure reactions are more common in those who go on to develop disease than in those who do not.

An explanation for these findings may be found by considering the ways in which blood pressure may depart from and return to its baseline level. Figure 2.5 depicts three types of reactivity pattern which might apply to adrenaline and cortisol and other stress hormones, as well as to blood pressure. Time is on the horizontal axis, measured in minutes for adrenaline and blood pressure, and hours in the case of cortisol. Blood pressure level (or hormone concentration) is on the vertical axis. In Fig. 2.5(a), the stimulus produces a sharp reaction with a fast return to baseline; in Fig. 2.5(b), the initial reaction is similar but the return to baseline is delayed, and there is a prolonged departure from the resting level; in Fig. 2.5(c), there is a blunted

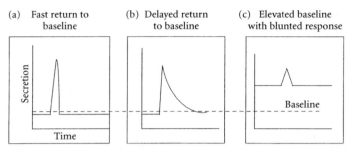

Fig. 2.5 Stress reactivity patterns. Idealized representations of neuroendocrine and metabolic reactivity: (a) fast return to baseline: reactivity is responsive and flexible; (b) delayed return to baseline: reactivity is responsive with slow recovery; (c) elevated baseline with blunted response: weak reactivity and abnormal resting level.

response and an elevated baseline. Other combinations of baseline and stimulated levels are also feasible, such as blunted response with a low basal level. The optimal reactivity pattern for each physiological system may be different.

For the blood pressure response to a psychological challenge, it may be that a large reaction is not harmful, provided there is a fast return to baseline, as in Fig. 2.5(a). If, however, such a response is provoked too frequently, the reactivity pattern may become like that shown in Fig. 2.5(b) or (c), and elevated blood pressure might follow. This example illustrates how feedback controls within the neuroendocrine system may be reset to a new level by environmental factors (Steptoe and Marmot 2002; Steptoe *et al.* 2002)

The allostatic load hypothesis (McEwen 1998) links the psychosocial environment to physical disease via neuroendocrine pathways. Allostatic load, or stress-induced damage, is considered relevant in cardiovascular disease, cancer, infection, and cognitive decline, and has been described as a sign of accelerated ageing. The concept of allostasis—the ability to achieve stability through change—extends the idea of homeostasis to include processes leading to disease. The price of adaptation to external and internal stress may be wear and tear on the organism, the result of chronic over- or underactivity of allostatic systems to produce allostatic load. For instance, the physiological system controlling blood glucose may be pushed towards diabetes. Allostatic load was investigated in a longitudinal study of older Americans (Seeman *et al.* 1997), where it was defined by measures of five established cardiovascular risk factors, plus urinary adrenaline and cortisol, and serum dehydroepiandrosterone sulphate (an adrenal androgen). Subjects with lower baseline allostatic load scores had better physical and mental functioning. Over the follow-up period, the same group showed less decline in functioning and were less likely to develop cardiovascular disease.

The general description of stress reactivity in this section leads to many questions about individual and social differences in response to the same stimulus, which may or may not threaten homeostasis. This topic will be taken up later in the chapter.

2.3.4 **The blood clotting system**

Blood flow is vital for the transport of gases, nutrients, and waste materials to and from body tissues. It is also important that physical injury does not result in massive blood loss, and the clotting (haemostatic) system provides the mechanism to prevent such a disaster. The sensitivity of this system to a variety of triggers suggests that it may be an important stress pathway in heart disease.

The change of blood from the liquid to the solid state involves a series of chemical reactions in which more than a dozen blood proteins take part. When the first protein is activated, it in turn activates the second protein, and so on. At the end of this cascade, the thrombin molecule catalyses the splitting of fibrinogen into fibrin. The fibrin molecules so produced condense to form threads which intermesh, trapping red blood cells and platelets, and very quickly a blood clot is formed. Major abnormalities of the haemostatic system are life-threatening; in haemophilia, for example, loss of blood after injury results from a defective clotting mechanism. An increased tendency for the blood to clot even in the absence of injury is very dangerous, and may be provoked in susceptible individuals by hormones such as those found in oral contraceptives.

The clotting system is, like other physiological systems, influenced by environmental stressors. The fight-or-flight response produces, via the increase in circulating adrenaline, increased 'stickiness' in platelets. The blood tends to become more concentrated and viscous at the same time, and stress-related hormones can increase the output of fibrinogen from the liver. It is plausible that, over decades, such small changes may add to the formation of arterial plaques and, therefore, increase risks of heart disease and stroke (Vrijkotte *et al.* 1999; von Kanel *et al.* 2001)

2.3.5 **Infection, inflammation, and immunity**

Infectious disease continues to contribute to ill health, particularly among poorer groups, in developed as well as in developing countries. Standards of housing and sanitation, vaccination, and other infectious disease control programmes are crucial to reducing this public health burden. Recent research suggests that infection and immunity may also be important in two poorly recognized ways. First, as a contributory cause of diseases not previously considered to be due to infection (Vallance *et al.* 1997) and, secondly, because chronic stress may alter susceptibility to infection and its severity. Though the evidence is incomplete, immunity has been implicated in a variety of conditions, such as peptic ulcer, gastric, cervical and other cancers, and coronary heart disease. The brain is able to influence immune function. Nerves of the autonomic nervous system are found in all relevant tissues (bone marrow, thymus, spleen, and lymph nodes) and hormones, including cortisol, have large effects on the immune system.

It is now evident that long-term, but low-level inflammatory processes resulting from undetected infection alter circulating levels of hormones and proteins in ways which increase the risk of heart disease by damaging the walls of blood vessels and promoting the development of atherosclerosis. Modification of these processes by stress is possible. In the absence of infection, the stress of space flight produced a rise in urinary output of interleukin-6 (Stein and Schluter 1994)—a cytokine that regulates immune and inflammatory responses. Experimental stress in the laboratory has been shown to initiate rapid changes in cytokines (Brydon *et al.* 2004). Blood interleukin-6

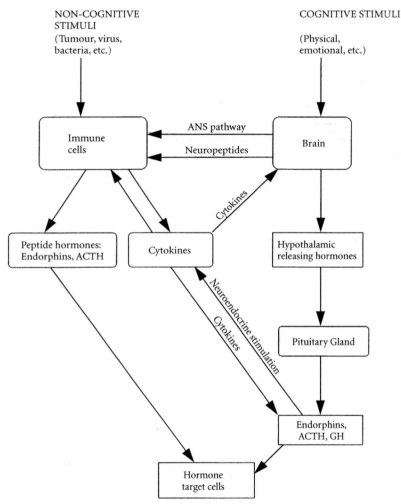

Fig. 2.6 Communications between brain, hypothalamic–pituitary–adrenal axis, and immune system. The brain perceives cognitive stimuli which can influence immune function via neuropeptides, the autonomic nervous system (ANS), and the HPA axis. The immune system responds to non-cognitive stimuli (infection and tumour growth) by secreting cytokines (immune messengers) and peptide hormones which act on the brain and neuroendocrine system. The immune system thus has a sensory function. (Redrawn from Brown 1994.)

levels rose in the two hours after psychological stress tasks, with rapid return to baseline in higher social status individuals, and slower decline in lower status individuals.

2.3.6 Integration

The endocrine, immune, haemostatic, and nervous systems are often studied as distinct and separate entities. This simplification has been useful, and probably essential, because it allows laboratory scientists to focus on the details of their chosen mechanism. In this way, each discipline has come to understand the complexity of the relevant pathways, each with its set of feedforward and feedback controls. The reality, of course, is that there are not clear boundaries between these systems.

Figure 2.6 shows, schematically, some of the interconnections between the neural, endocrine, and immune systems. The diagram shows how the brain and then the HPA axis are able to respond to non-cognitive stimuli and, conversely, how the immune system has the capacity to respond to perception and emotion. The brain (central nervous system) cannot itself detect the presence of infection. One of the functions of the immune system is, therefore, to act as a sensory system, making the brain aware of infection by means of messengers of the immune system, the cytokines, which enter the brain via the bloodstream. Immune function responds to cognitive stimuli via the autonomic nervous system and the release of hormones from the hypothalamus and pituitary gland. In animals, isolation rearing, crowding, low dominance status, and social stress influence the effectiveness of defences against infection.

This brief account has emphasized the roles of the autonomic nervous system and the HPA axis in the stress response. However, it is important to recognize that there are at least 15 neurotransmitter substances which convey sensory and cognitive information in the human nervous system. Among these, serotonin appears to be important in depression and hostility, and both psychological states have been linked with increased heart disease risk in a variety of studies (Williams 2002), and serotonin responsivity has been shown to vary by socio-economic status. (Manuck *et al.* 2004). In animal studies, learned helplessness (the tendency to passivity in the face of repeated experimental stress) is associated with a reduced level of serotonin receptors in the hippocampus, an area of the brain which responds to cortisol (Checkley 1996).

2.4 Human studies and epidemiological evidence

The sections above have illustrated some of the major biological pathways that plausibly change risk of developing major disease according to social and psychological circumstances. Central to these processes is the concept of disturbance of homeostatic equilibrium and, thus, increased risk of ill health. We now turn to the second question posed at the beginning of the chapter: what is the evidence that these pathways do actually operate to produce or accelerate disease? Throughout this book there are numerous examples of the ways in which aspects of social organization are correlated with measures of health and disease. Here, the aim is to examine some of the evidence for the biological pathways which intervene. The research findings are divided into two groups: those based on human subjects (discussed here), and those based on observational and experimental studies of animals (discussed later).

2.4.1 Psychological effect on growth

Psychogenic dwarfism is a rare syndrome associated with severe childhood deprivation. Psychosocial growth retardation of a less dramatic nature appears to have been documented in Widdowson's study of orphaned children in post-war Germany (Widdowson 1951). Under identical food rationing regimes, those who lived in the 'Bienenhaus' orphanage, initially under the control of the stern and forbidding Fräulein Schwarz, gained less weight and grew more slowly than children cared for by the affectionate Fräulein Grün at the 'Vogelnest' orphanage. By chance, Schwarz replaced Grün during the study and the growth rates reversed, despite the provision of extra food at 'Vogelnest'. This controlled cross-over study provides evidence that adverse psychosocial circumstances in childhood can influence growth (although it is not clear whether this was the result of upset appetite and eating, or a direct psychosocial effect). Separately, there is evidence that attained height is a marker of health capital, or constitution, which is a protective factor for adult disease. Long-term effects on health may be produced by early deprivation, even among children born in the British welfare system of the 1950s (Montgomery et al. 1997; Power et al. 1998).

2.4.2 Social patterning of coronary risk factors in adults

Measures of social and economic status, including occupation, are extremely powerful predictors of premature heart disease. Employment grade proved, on its own, to be more powerful than the combination of classic risk factors including smoking, serum cholesterol, and blood pressure, in a follow-up study of 17,000 British civil servants (Marmot et al. 1984). This important observation prompted a new, long-term study to investigate the possible psychosocial causes of heart disease and other important health problems. Biology is given special attention in the Whitehall II study, in order to clarify the mechanisms involved.

At the baseline of the Whitehall II study in 1985–88 (Marmot et al. 1991), there was a stepwise relationship between civil service employment grade (1992 salary range £7400–£87,600) and the prevalence of several health-related psychosocial factors: low control and lack of variety at work, lack of social contact with friends, distressing life events, difficulty paying bills, hostility, and health locus of control. These relationships were seen before employment security in the British civil service was reduced in the late 1980s (Ferrie et al. 1995) and it is likely that their prevalence is now higher, particularly within the lower grades of staff.

Biochemical and physiological risk factors were studied in detail at the second medical examination of Whitehall II subjects in 1991–93 (Brunner et al. 1997). We found that

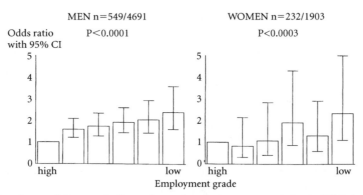

Fig. 2.7 Prevalence of the metabolic syndrome by employment grade in the Whitehall II study. Odds ratios and 95 per cent confidence interval (CI) adjusted for age and, in women, menopausal status. P values are for trend test across grades. (From Brunner *et al.* 1997.)

a particular pattern of risk factors was associated with lower occupational status (Fig. 2.7). The 'metabolic syndrome' pattern predicts diabetes and coronary disease in many populations, including South Asian migrants to the UK (McKeigue *et al.* 1991). It is a very common disorder. In the USA, some 47 million people are estimated to have metabolic syndrome (Ford *et al.* 2002).

As the grade hierarchy is descended, a progressively larger proportion of subjects exhibits adverse levels of components of the metabolic syndrome (Fig. 2.8; moving from left to right in each block of histograms). The top four panels of Fig. 2.8 (a–d) are components reflecting adverse homeostatic alterations in carbohydrate and lipid metabolism, and Fig. 2.8(e) shows that abdominal obesity (a fat pattern particularly associated with coronary risk) is also strongly associated with low status. Figure 2.8(f) shows that the blood clotting protein, fibrinogen, also shows a strong inverse social gradient (Brunner *et al.* 1996).

The findings for blood glucose are particularly interesting because they are based on a metabolic challenge rather than a measurement of fasting or baseline level. Subjects in the fasting state were given 75 g of glucose as a drink and, 2 hours later, the level of blood glucose was measured. The results (Fig. 2.8a) show that the lower the position in the civil service, the greater was the probability that a subject had difficulty in clearing the glucose into body tissues for storage or energy functions and returning to the baseline state. This finding corresponds to the condition shown in Fig. 2.5(b) or perhaps in Fig. 2.5(c). It illustrates that the ability to mount a hormonal response to the glucose challenge, and thus to maintain homeostasis, in some way depends on occupational status.

Chronic stress may be involved in development of the metabolic syndrome cluster of risk factors, which includes raised blood glucose (Bjorntorp 1991; Brunner 1997; McEwen 1998). A detailed study, based on Whitehall II participants, simultaneously

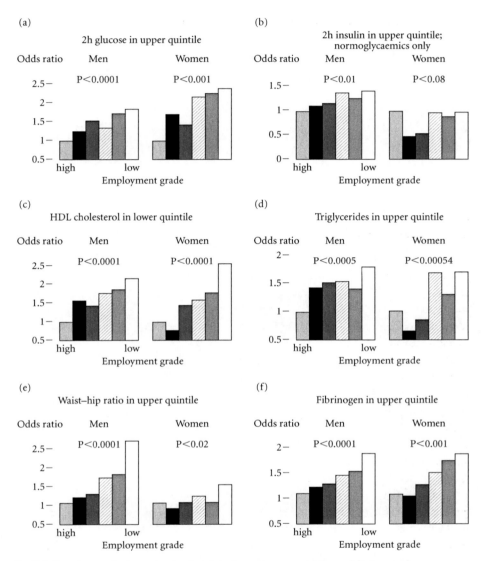

Fig. 2.8 Prevalence of adverse levels of metabolic syndrome variables and fibrinogen by employment grade in the Whitehall II study. Odds ratios and 95 per cent confidence interval for occupying top quintile (except HDL cholesterol: bottom quintile). Adjusted for age and, in women, menopausal status. P values are for trend test across grades. (From Brunner *et al.* 1997.)

links major neuroendocrine stress axes, low level inflammation, and autonomic activity of the heart (see section 2.3) with the metabolic syndrome (Brunner *et al.* 2002) Output of cortisol and adrenaline in 24-hour urine samples was raised among metabolic syndrome cases. The altered HPA and autonomic activity among cases suggests stress-related changes in biology may contribute to increased risk of cardiovascular disease. The evidence is not complete, however. A cross-sectional study does not demonstrate the causal sequence (Fig. 2.9) and it could be that neuro-endocrine changes accompany, rather than precede, the development of metabolic syndrome.

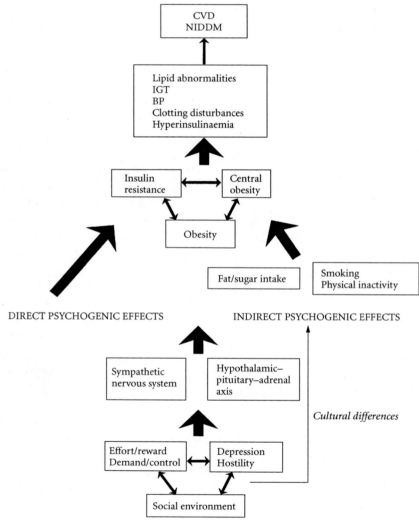

Fig. 2.9 Psychosocial and biological pathways in cardiovascular disease (CVD) and non-insulin-dependent diabetes (NIDDM). Hypothesized research model. (IGT, impaired glucose tolerance; BP, blood pressure.)

2.4.3 **Socio-economic status and cortisol secretion in two cities**

Middle-aged men in Lithuania and Sweden had similar coronary heart disease mortality rates in 1978. Subsequently, rates rose in Lithuania and fell in Sweden, so that by 1994 coronary mortality was fourfold higher in Lithuania. The divergence in life expectancy, in addition to coronary disease rates, between the countries of eastern and western Europe around the time of the collapse of the Soviet system illustrated the importance of socio-economic factors in health (Bobak and Marmot 1996). Differences in the psychosocial environment may play a part.

Kristenson *et al.* and co-workers examined the possible causes for the differences in coronary heart disease incidence between Lithuania and Sweden, and between men of high and low socio-economic status in each country (Kristenson *et al.* 1997, 1998). Random samples of 150 50-year-old men participated in each of two cities: Linköping in southern Sweden (population 130,000) and Vilnius (600,000). Response rates were 82 and 76 per cent, respectively. The conventional risk factors (smoking, serum cholesterol, and blood pressure) did not provide a good explanation for national differences in risk, as was the case in the Whitehall study (Marmot *et al.* 1984). Substantial differences in blood levels of antioxidant vitamins were found, suggesting that dietary differences were important. Psychosocial factors followed precisely the predicted pattern. Vilnius men reported more social isolation, more job strain, and more depression than those in Linköping. The low-income groups in both cities likewise reported higher levels of isolation and vital exhaustion and greater difficulties coping than those on higher incomes.

Here then is evidence from a cross-cultural study, conducted in 1993–95, that certain dietary and psychosocial factors are important in explaining the differences in coronary risk both between Swedes and Lithuanians, and between those with financial insecurity and their relatively well-off neighbours. Quality of life and perceived health showed a large differential (one standard deviation) in favour of Linköping. Although depression was more common in Vilnius, the mean hostility score in Linköping was substantially higher than that in Vilnius. It may be that those living in Vilnius had a sense of defeat and a lack of confidence in their post-Soviet society.

The contrasting psychosocial environments in Linköping and Vilnius translate into different patterns of the HPA axis stress response. Subjects took a standardized laboratory stress test involving anger recall, mental arithmetic, and immersion of one hand in iced water. Subjects attended the test the morning after an overnight fast in order to standardize the biological measurements. Attending the clinic, and fasting, can be considered to be additional stressors, but since all men did the same it does not detract from the findings. Figure 2.10 shows that both the high- and low-income groups of Swedish men had what is considered to be an adaptive response to the experimental challenge: low baseline followed by a rise and fall in blood cortisol. The difference in

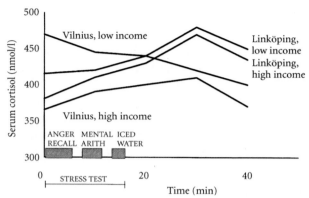

Fig. 2.10 Serum cortisol responses to a standardized stress test in Vilnius, Lithuania, and Linköping, Sweden, by income group. Low income: group with lowest 25 per cent of income. High income: group with highest 25 per cent of income. (Redrawn from Kristenson *et al.* 1998.)

findings with the Vilnius subjects is striking. The high-income group exhibited a low baseline level like the Swedes, but a relatively blunted response. However, the low-income group showed a very different response from the other groups. There was a much higher baseline level of blood cortisol and a failure to respond to the challenge, corresponding to the condition shown in Fig. 2.5(c).

The implications of these results, if confirmed in other studies, are dramatic. They highlight the significance of quality of life, in terms of the social and working environment, as key determinants of population health. The demonstration of a biological mechanism, involving altered functioning of the main neuroendocrine stress pathway, is evidence that the psychosocial hypothesis is not only plausible, but that it is a significant social policy consideration. In a subsample of Whitehall II men (but not women), those in lower employment grades had higher salivary cortisol levels during the day than their higher status counterparts, providing some evidence that social rank alters cortisol secretion (Steptoe *et al* 2003).

An outstanding question is whether the apparently adverse cortisol responses are indeed responsible for future ill health or are merely markers of psychological state. Related to this is the issue of reversibility, since a stress response pattern which becomes fixed early in life would have specific policy implications. Barker's group has demonstrated, for example, that lower birthweight is associated with higher morning plasma cortisol level among 59–70-year-old men (Phillips *et al.* 1998). Their findings give evidence that plasma cortisol levels within the normal range are among the determinants of blood pressure and glucose tolerance. However, in this group of men, fetal programming of the HPA axis was more important than the effect of current socio-economic position, suggesting that interventions after infancy may be ineffective. Nevertheless, it seems likely that both fetal growth and experiences during the life course will turn out to be of importance in shaping neuroendocrine function in later life.

2.5 Animal models

Animal studies provide some added dimensions to our understanding of the connections between social organization, stress, and health. Referring to our general model in Fig. 2.2, it is clear that direct analogies are to be avoided. The human social environment is immensely and uniquely complex. From a psychological perspective, the faculties of abstract thought, emotion, and memory appear largely to be limited to our own species. However, many animals live within hierarchical social structures and mammalian biology is potentially comparable across species. An added value of such studies is that, unless required to by man, animals do not smoke, drink coffee or alcohol, take drugs, or sit in front of a computer all day. This truism means that we do not have the problem of separating these behavioural effects from purely psychosocial processes which may influence disease risks.

2.5.1 Genes, constitution, and destiny

With due attention to relevance, animal studies can tell us about the plausible links between psychosocial factors, biology, and health. Their value is not confined to the social gradient in health (see section 2.5.2), and is also a way to understand effects such as the interaction between genetic predisposition to disease and environmental factors. Our first example may provide a caution to those who view genetic susceptibility, in the absence of medical intervention, as an irreversible destiny.

The genetically 'spontaneously hypertensive rat' (SHR) is an animal model often used in the study of hypertension. An experiment in cross-fostering (Cierpial and McCarthy 1987) shows the importance of early environment in expressing this characteristic. When pups of SHR rats were cross-fostered with Kyoto–Wistar mothers, they did not develop hypertension as they matured. This 'pure' genetic characteristic did not manifest itself as the phenotype of hypertension in the absence of the appropriate environmental stimulus.

Another example of the impact of nurture on nature comes from Suomi's elegant long-term studies of rhesus monkeys (*Macaca mulatta*) (Suomi 1997). Some 20 per cent of any troop are 'high reactors' who are more likely than others to exhibit depressive responses to maternal separation, along with greater and prolonged activation of the HPA axis, more dramatic sympatho-adrenal arousal, and immunosuppression. These responses remain quite stable throughout development. The pattern of arousal appears to be determined genetically, but it can be reproduced in other non-susceptible animals by raising them without their mothers (suggesting that non-genetic inter-generational transmission may be an alternative explanation). Interestingly, the high reactors tend to end up at the bottom of the social hierarchy.

The genetic, or at least constitutional, high-reactor destiny can be interrupted by changing the environment. When reared with especially nurturing mothers, such animals showed no signs of the usual behavioural disorder. Instead, they showed signs of precocious behavioural development and rose to the top of the hierarchy as adults. Females adopted the maternal style typical of their especially nurturing mothers. Further evidence from the same research group (Suomi 1997) suggests that the consequences of experimental social isolation can be modified with timely intervention, and that long-term effects are most likely to be seen under stress conditions in adult life.

2.5.2 Social dominance among wild baboons

Determinants of circulating levels of the protective high-density lipoproteins (HDL), which promote 'reverse transport' of cholesterol away from the arterial wall, appear to be important in explaining the social differential in coronary risk. We have seen above that the HDL cholesterol level in civil servants is strongly related to employment grade, and is a component of the cluster of factors making up the metabolic syndrome (Fig. 2.8). To our surprise, the same pattern of blood fat levels was found in the social hierarchy of wild male baboons (Sapolsky and Mott 1987).

The neuroscientist Sapolsky has been studying the behaviour and physiology of wild baboon troops in the Serengeti for many years. He argues that the animals are ideal subjects for investigating psychosocial factors. Food is plentiful, predators are scarce, and infant mortality is low. Only some four hours per day are required for foraging, leaving the animals, who live in groups of 50–100, plenty of time to engage in social activity. Attainment and maintenance of social rank is a preoccupation which determines access to a variety of resources. On the basis of these behaviours, Sapolsky classified males of the troop into dominants and subordinates. Blood samples obtained following anaesthesia under controlled conditions showed, just as in Whitehall II men, that total and low-density lipoprotein cholesterol were similar by rank position, and that HDL levels were higher in the dominant compared to the subordinate males, again mirroring findings in civil servants. Subordinate baboons were found to have higher resting cortisol levels, and levels of the hormone were inversely correlated with HDL.

Do these parallels reflect the common psychosocial effects of position within the two primate hierarchies? That the baboons are non-smokers and non-drinkers is consistent with a psychosocial explanation, since smoking is known to lower, and alcohol consumption to raise, HDL levels. Production of the more favourable physiological profile in dominant baboons might be the direct consequence of their assertions of supremacy and consequent feelings of well-being, or alternatively the result of easier access to the best available food. Equally, these observational data are compatible with the view that the fittest attain the highest rank. However, studies utilizing captive macaque monkeys suggest that this is not the case (Shively and Clarkson 1994). Initial rank in small groups of females fed an atherogenic diet was altered experimentally by switching animals between groups. The effects of manipulating social status were dramatic. Dominants who became subordinate had a five-fold excess of coronary plaques compared with animals who remained dominant, while subordinates who became dominant had a two-fold excess of atherosclerotic changes compared to those remaining subordinate. Experimental manipulation of social status in male macaques also produced injury to the endothelial lining of coronary arteries. (Strawn *et al.* 1991) Half of the monkeys were treated with metoprolol (a β-adrenergic blocking agent) to reduce activation of the sympathetic nervous system during the experiment. Compared with untreated monkeys, this group had reduced damage in coronary arteries. In these animals, the adverse effects of an atherogenic diet depended partly on the level of arousal of the sympathetic nervous system in response to social stress.

2.6 **Conclusions**

Disturbance of usual homeostatic equilibrium by the repeated activation of the fight-or-flight response may be responsible for social differences in neuroendocrine, physiological, and metabolic variables which are the precursors of ill health and disease. Social and individual differences in the response to social and environmental stressors appear to be determined by many factors, including birthweight and conditioned hypo- or hyper-responsiveness. It seems likely that the optimal stress response in relation to health in the long term is associated with living and working environments typical of the materially advantaged. This optimal response can be characterized as one with a rapid return to a resting level and, thus, a high resistance to stress-related disorder (Fig. 2.11). The level of demands does not in itself pose a risk to health, provided that the individual has adequate coping resources and the opportunity to control his or her environment.

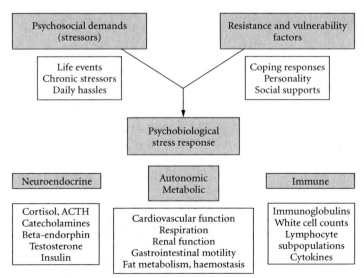

Fig. 2.11 The psychobiological stress response. Resistance and vulnerability factors influence the response to psychosocial stressors. The major hormonal, metabolic, and immune elements of the response are shown. (From Steptoe 1998.)

The causal role of psychosocial factors in coronary heart disease has been reviewed recently (Kuper *et al.* 2002). The evidence from longitudinal studies involving more than 500 healthy subjects was strongest for social isolation, depression, and psychosocial work characteristics, including low control.

2.7 Summary

Stress has short-term effects on the human body and mind. The effects are positive if the situation is right, but everyone has his or her limits. We are now beginning to recognize that people's social and psychological circumstances can seriously damage their health in the long term. Chronic anxiety, insecurity, low self-esteem, social isolation, and lack of control over work appear to undermine mental and physical health.

The power of psychosocial factors to affect health makes biological sense. The human body has evolved to respond automatically to emergencies. This stress response activates a cascade of stress hormones which affect the cardiovascular and immune systems. The rapid reaction of our hormones and nervous system prepares the individual to deal with a brief physical threat: the heart rate rises, blood is diverted to muscles, anxiety and alertness increase. This response is highly adaptive: it may save life in the short term. But if the biological stress response is activated too often and for too long, there may be multiple health costs. These include depression, increased susceptibility to infection, diabetes, high blood pressure, and accumulation of cholesterol in blood vessel walls, with the attendant risks of heart attack and stroke.

These health problems increase progressively down the social strata in industrialized countries. Clustering and accumulation of psychosocial disadvantage, perhaps beginning with a poor emotional environment in early childhood, is a neglected area of public health prevention and social policy. This is an area of active research.

Acknowledgements

Dr Brunner's and Professor Marmot's research is supported by the Medical Research Council and the British Heart Foundation.

References

Bjorntorp, P. (1991). Visceral fat accumulation: the missing link between psychosocial factors and cardiovascular disease? *J. Int. Med.* **230**, 195–201.

Blane, D., Brunner, E.J., and Wilkinson, R. (1996). The evolution of public health policy: an anglocentric view of the last fifty years. In: *Health and social organization: towards a health policy for the the 21st century* (ed. D. Blane, E. Brunner, and R.G. Wilkinson), pp. 120. Routledge, London.

Bobak, M. and Marmot, M.G. (1996). East–West mortality divide and its potential explanations: proposed research agenda. *BMJ* **312**, 421–5.

Bosma, H., Marmot, M.G., Hemingway, H., Nicholson, A., Brunner, E.J., and Stansfeld, S. (1997). Low job control and risk of coronary heart disease in the Whitehall II (prospective cohort) study. *BMJ* **314**, 558–65.

Brown, R.E. (1994). *An introduction to neuroendocrinology.* Cambridge University Press, Cambridge.

Brunner, E.J. (1997). Stress and the biology of inequality. *BMJ* **314**, 1472–6.

Brunner, E.J., Davey Smith, G., Marmot, M.G., Canner, R., Beksinska, M., and O'Brien, J. (1996). Childhood social circumstances and psychosocial and behavioural factors as determinants of plasma fibrinogen. *Lancet* **347**, 1008–13.

Brunner, E.J., Hemingway, H., Walker, B.R., Page, M., Clarke, P., Juneja, M., *et al.* (2002). Adrenocortical, autonomic, and inflammatory causes of the metabolic syndrome: nested case-control study. *Circulation* **106**, 2659–65.

Brunner, E.J., Kivimaki, M., Siegrist, J., Theorell, T., Luukkonen, R., Riihimaki, H. *et al.* (2004). Is the effect of work stress on cardiovascular morality confounded by socioeconomic factors in the Valmet study? *J. Epidemiol. Community Health* **58**; 1010–20.

Brunner, E.J., Marmot, M.G., Nanchahal, K., *et al.* (1997). Social inequality in coronary risk: central obesity and the metabolic syndrome. Evidence from the Whitehall II study. *Diabetologia* **40**, 1341–9.

Brydon, L., Edwards, S., Mohamed–Ali,V., and Steptoe, A. (2004). Socioeconomic status and stress-induced increases in interleukin-6. *Brain Behav. Immun.* **18**, 281–90.

Cannon,W.B. (1929). Organization for physiological homeostasis. *Physiol. Reviews* **9**, 399–431.

Checkley, S. (1996). The neuroendocrinology of depression and chronic stress. *Br. Med. Bull.* **52**, 597–617.

Cierpial, M.A. and McCarthy, R. (1987). Hypertension in SHR rats: contribution of maternal environment. *Am. J. Physiol.* **253**, H980–4.

Ferrie, J.E., Shipley, M.J., Marmot, M.G., Stansfeld, S., and Davey Smith, G. (1995). Health effects of anticipation of job change and non-employment: longitudinal data from the Whitehall II study. *BMJ* **311**, 1264–9.

Ford, E.S. Giles, W.H., and Dietz, W.H. (2002). Prevalence of the metabolic syndrome among US adults. Findings from the Third National Health and Nutrition Examination Survey. *JAMA* **287**, 356–59.

Kristenson, M., Kucinskiene, Z., Bergdahl, B., and Orth–Gomer, K. (2001). Risk factors for coronary heart disease in different socioeconomic groups of Lithuania and Sweden: the Livicordia study. *Scand.J.Public Health* **29**, 140–50.

Kristenson, M., Orth-Gomer, K., Kucinskiene, Z., Bergdahl B., Calkauskas, H., Balinkyiene, I. *et al.* (1998). Attenuated cortisol response to a standardised stress test in Lithuanian vs. Swedish men. *Int. J. Behav. Med.* **5**, 17–30.

Kristenson, M., Zieden, B., Kucinskiene, Z., *et al.* (1997). Antioxidant state and mortality from coronary heart disease in Lithuanian and Swedish men: concomitant cross sectional study of men aged 50. *BMJ* **314**, 629–33.

Kuper, H., Marmot, M., and Hemingway, H. (2002). Systematic review of prospective cohort studies of psychosocial factors in the etiology and prognosis of coronary heart disease. *Seminars in Vascular Medicine* **2**, 267–314.

McEwen, B.S. (1998). Protective and damaging effects of stress mediators. *N. Engl. J. Med.* **338**, 171–9.

McKeigue, P.M., Shah, B., and Marmot, M.G. (1991). Relation of central obesity and insulin resistance with high diabetes prevalence and cardiovascular risk in South Asians. *Lancet* **337**, 382–6.

Manuck, S.B., Flory, J.D., Ferrell, R.E., and Muldoon, M.F. (2004). Socioeconomic status covaries with central nervous system serotonergic responsivity as a function of allelic variation in the serotonin transporter gene-linked polymorphic region. *Psychoneuroendocrinology* **29**, 651–68.

Marmot, M.G., Davey Smith, G., Stansfeld, S.A., *et al.* (1991). Health inequalities among British civil servants: the Whitehall II study. *Lancet* **337**, 1387–93.

Marmot, M.G., Shipley, M.J., and Rose, G. (1984). Inequalities in death—specific explanations of a general pattern. *Lancet* **i**, 1003–6.

Montgomery, S., Bartley, M., and Wilkinson, R.G. (1997). Family conflict and slow growth. *Arch. Dis. Child.* **77**, 326–30.

Phillips, D.I.W., Barker, J.P., Fall, C.H.D., *et al.* (1998). Elevated plasma cortisol concentrations: a link between low birth weight and insulin resistance syndrome? *J. Clin. Endocrinol. Metab.* **83**, 757–60.

Power, C., Matthews, S., and Manor, O. (1998). Inequalities in self-rated health: explanations from different stages of life. *Lancet* **351**, 1009–14.

Sapolsky, R.M. (1993). Endocrinology alfresco: psychoendocrine studies of wild baboons. *Recent Prog. Horm. Res.* **48**, 437–68.

Sapolsky, R.M. and Mott, G.E. (1987). Social subordinance in wild baboons is associated with suppressed high density lipoprotein–cholesterol concentrations: the possible role of chronic social stress. *Endocrinology* **121**, 1605–10.

Seeman, T.E., Singer, B.H., Rowe, J.W., Horwitz, R.I., and McEwen, B.S. (1997). Price of adaptation—allostatic load and its health consequences. *Arch. Intern. Med.* **157**, 2259–68.

Selye, H. (1956). *Stress of life*. McGraw–Hill, New York.

Shively, C.A. and Clarkson, T.B. (1994). Social status and coronary artery atherosclerosis in female monkeys. *Art. Thromb.* **14**, 721–6.

Siegrist, J. (1996). Adverse health effects of high-effort/low-reward conditions. *J. Occup. Health Psychol.* **1**, 27–41.

Stein, T.P. and Schluter, M.D. (1994). Excretion of IL-6 by astronauts during spaceflight. *Am. J. Physiol.* **266**, E448–E552.

Steptoe, A. and Marmot, M. (2002). The role of psychobiological pathways in socio-economic inequalities in cardiovascular disease risk. *Eur. Heart .J.* **23**, 13–25.

Steptoe, A., Feldman, P.J., Kunz, S., Owen, N., Willemsen, G., Marmot, M. (2002). Stress responsivity and socioeconomic status. A mechanism for increased cardiovascular risk? *Eur. Heart J.* **23**, 1757–63.

Steptoe, A., Kunz, S., Owen, N., Feldman, P.J., Willemsen, G., Kirschbaum, C., *et al.* (2003). Socioeconomic status and stress related biological responses over the working day. *Psychosom. Med.* **65**, 461–70.

Strawn, W.B., Bondjers, G., Kaplan, J.R., Manuck, S.B., Schwenke, D., Hansson, G., *et al.* (1991). Endothelial dysfunction in response to psychosocial stress in monkeys. *Circulation* **68**, 1270–79.

Suomi, S.J. (1997). Early determinants of behaviour: evidence from primate studies. *Br. Med. Bull.* **53**, 170–84.

Vallance, P., Collier, J., and Bhagat, K. (1997). Infection, inflammation, and infarction: does acute endothelial dysfunction provide a link? *Lancet* **349**, 1391–2.

Von Kanel, R., Mills, P.J., Fainman, C., and Dimsdale, J.E. (2001). Effects of psychological stress and psychiatric disorders on blood coagulation and fibrinolysis: A biobehavioral pathway to coronary artery disease. *Psychosom. Med.* **63**, 531–44.

Vrijkotte, T.G.M., van Doornen, L.J.P., and De Geus, E.J.C. (1999). Work stress and metabolic and hemostatic risk factors. *Psychosom. Med.* **61**, 796–805.

Widdowson, E.M. (1951). Mental contentment and physical growth. *Lancet* **i**, 1316–18.

Williams, R. (2002). Hostility, psychosocial risk factors, changes in brain serotonergic function, and heart disease. In: *Stress and the Heart: Psychosocial Pathways to Coronary Heart Disease* (ed. S.A. Stansfeld and M. Marmot), pp. 86–100. BMJ Books, London.

Chapter 3

Early life

Michael Wadsworth and Suzie Butterworth

3.1 Introduction

Poverty and social inequality adversely affect children's health and development in all countries, regardless of medical knowledge and the availability of health care, and regardless of cultural context (Williams *et al.* 1994; Helman 1994; Wilkinson 1996; Keating and Hertzman 1999; World Bank 2003). Yet it is commonly acknowledged that child health is of the greatest importance for the future health of a nation, since today's children grow up to become the next generation of parents and workers, and because health in early life is the basis of health in adult life. Early life health has lifelong effects that result from the interaction of biological development and social and environmental circumstances. The concomitants of good health in childhood are educational receptivity, good parenting, and good maternal health and education. Therefore, investment in physical and mental health and education of mothers and children has beneficial effects on the future health of a nation, as well as on the functioning and well-being of its citizens.

The purpose of this chapter is to outline knowledge of the social and biological processes that determine physical and mental health in early life, and the reasons put forward for their association with adult health. Conclusions are drawn about policies to improve health in early life.

3.2 Physical growth and health in early life

Growth before birth has been argued to be vital to health in subsequent childhood and adult life because 'Many tissues and organs are formed with regard to cell numbers at or shortly after birth. Most of postnatal growth is a consequence of the enlargement of pre-existing cells rather than the accretion of additional cells'. (Hales 1997). The original hypothesis about this unique period of opportunity for vital organ and tissue development has been called the biological programming hypothesis, because it asserts that 'the fetus responds to under-nutrition with permanent changes in physiology, metabolism and structure' (Barker 1998, p. 10) which lead to raised illness risk in later life. Malnutrition at critical phases of development before birth 'may permanently reduce the number of cells in particular organs' (Widdowson and McCance 1975; McCance and Widdowson 1974).

The concept of biological programming rests on knowledge about and evidence of growth before and after birth, and Barker's original propositions about biological programming, together with a mass of more recent work, shows the importance of growth in early life to health and function throughout life (Kuh and Ben Shlomo 2004). A wide range of adult life health outcomes is associated with poor growth in early life, including: cardiovascular and respiratory function (Barker 1998; Dezateux and Stocks 1997; Cheung et al. 2000); cognitive function (Richards et al. 2002); chronic obstructive pulmonary disease (Barker 1998); schizophrenia (Jones and Done in press); psychological function and susceptibility to stress (Nilsson et al. 2001; Cheung 2002; Jones and Done in press); coronary heart disease and diabetes (Davey Smith et al. 2001); serum cholesterol early in adulthood (Miura et al. 2001); atopic disease (Steffensen et al. 2000); and breast cancer (de Stavola et al. 2004).

Low weight at birth is a consequence of poor delivery of nutrients and oxygen to the fetus (Barker 1998), a delivery which is related to the mother's health and environment, and her access to appropriate foods and exposure to risk factors during the pregnancy (e.g. smoking, exercise, diet, alcohol consumption, atmospheric pollution, experience of infections) (Brooke et al. 1989; Hall and Peckham 1997; Bobak et al. 2000). Birth weight is therefore likely to be associated with the mother's health before pregnancy (Kramer et al. 2002), as well as with genetic factors (Perry and Lumey 2004). It has also been argued that the mother's health and opportunity for growth as a child and adolescent is related to the fetal growth of her offspring through her development of risk of hypertension and of raised body mass (Perry and Lumey 2004).

The socially mediated factors that adversely affect growth before birth and in infancy include poverty, maternal smoking, excess alcohol intake, drug misuse, and poor and deficient diet of mothers and babies. Factors that affect the mother's health in pregnancy affect the child not only prenatally but also in the immediate postnatal environment and in infancy. Maternal smoking and dietary knowledge and dietary availability affect the infant during the vital period of prepubertal growth. Increasingly, there is evidence that poor growth at this stage in life, together with poor socio-economic circumstances, is associated with long-term risk to adult health (Hardy et al. 2000; Eriksson et al. 2003), for example through overweight (Fig. 3.1). Additionally, poor infant feeding may have further adverse affects, for example on cognitive development and on respiratory health (Oddy et al. 2003; Shaheen 1997).

How may poor growth and health in early life affect health in the long term, that is, in adult life? First, it may be because growth and developmental processes unique to early life are not optimally achieved, thus leaving the child vulnerable to later insults. In addition to the importance of prenatal growth (Barker 1998), evidence has grown for the importance of growth during infancy (Erikkson et al. 2003; Hardy et al. 2000). That may be because some aspects of physical development continue into infancy. But it may also be because some developmental processes are contingent on interaction of the

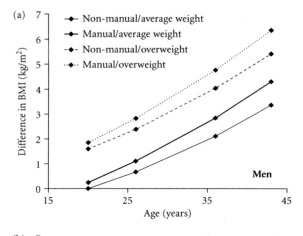

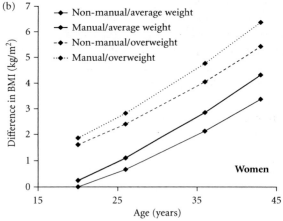

Fig. 3.1 Estimated differences in body mass index (BMI) compared to men and women at age 20 years, with relative weight of 100 at 14 years and with non-manual social class of origin. Source: Hardy *et al.* (2000), with permission from Macmillan Publishers Ltd.

development of the organ, for example the eye (Gregory 1998), with the environment. Keating and Hertzman (1999) described such interaction as 'biological embedding . . . during which the experiences of the organism will be encoded, especially in the neural system' (p. 12). Montgomery *et al.* (1997) argued that an adverse emotional environment in early life reduces height growth because of its impact on the glucocorticoid-hippocampal hypothalamic pathway. More recently, Boyce and Keating (2004) have suggested that:

> All of the basic pathways involved in human emotion, volition, movement, and thought are already in place at birth, awaiting the experiential input that will propel latent pathways into the neural substrates of individual personalities, predispositions, talents and failings. Over the course of the next several postnatal months, this rich neural network is progressively 'pruned', selectively eliminating neurones (through apoptosis, or programmed cell death) and synapses from the less utilised pathways and circuits. It appears that this process of neural elimination is as essential to the emergence of normal intelligence, behaviour, and mental functioning, as is the stage of neuronal proliferation that precedes it within fetal life. (p. 421)

The interaction between the social environment and the child's physical endowment at birth may be the key to understanding the associations between social circumstances and physical health and development in early life. A similar interaction has also been suggested to explain comparable processes at post-developmental ages. For instance, chronic stress exposure may, through chronic arousal of the sympatho-adrenal and the hypothalamic-pituitary-adrenal systems, increase the risk of specific ill health (Brunner 2000; Welberg and Seckl 2001).

The second type of explanation offered for the association of poor growth in early life with adult ill health is concerned with the adverse effects of the accumulation and interaction of risk—a process initiated by the relationship of poor growth with poor socio-economic circumstances. For example, poor early life socio-economic circumstances are associated with a raised likelihood of subsequent poor educational attainment, poor health-related habits (e.g. smoking), poor diet in adulthood, low income (Lynch et al. 1997), and overweight and obesity (Mustillo et al. 2003; Preston et al. 1998; Martikainen and Valkonen 1996; Montgomery et al. 1996).

The third type of explanation suggests that some adverse circumstances in early life, such as an infectious illness, require an additional adverse adult challenge, such as obesity or infection, to push the organism, made vulnerable by adverse early life exposures or development, into ill health (Martyn 1997; Leon et al. 1996).

Arguably, these three explanations are not incompatible and are likely to be interrelated. Furthermore, it has been proposed that, in some illnesses, poor growth in early life may be of genetic origin—a genetic effect that also predisposes to a later specific disease outcome. That has been put forward as an explanation for the association of low birth weight with adult diabetes and vascular disease (Hattersley and Tooke 1999).

The adverse effects of poor growth in early life may not be inevitable if, after infancy, the accumulation of risk does not continue, either in socio-economic or biological form, or if there is a protective effect of improvement in socio-economic circumstances in childhood. Parental upward social mobility has been shown to be associated with height growth and cognitive function scores that are better than those in children who began in the same social circumstances and remain in them (Douglas 1964; Kuh and Wadsworth 1989), and higher socio-economic status of parents is associated with better infant catch-up growth after poor birth weight (Teranishi et al. 2001). These associations may, in part, be explained by nutrition. There is much evidence that nutrition cannot only promote growth but also be protective against childhood illness that comprises adverse long-term risk, such as infant pulmonary disease (Strachan and Sheikh 2004), and of cognitive function (Morely and Lucas 1997; Gibson and Green 2002). Higher levels of parental educational attainment and socio-economic circumstances also help children to catch up faster in cognitive performance compared with children who do not have those advantages (Fig. 3.2; Feinstein 2003). The mechanisms involved here are not clear, but may include elements as diverse as nutrition and parental intellectual stimulation. In due course, the child's own higher educational

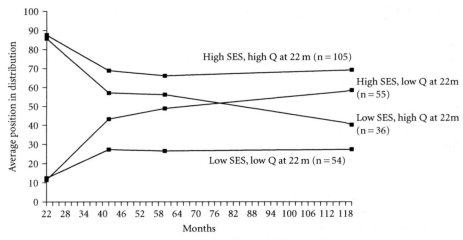

Fig. 3.2 Average rank of test scores at 22, 42, 60, and 120 months by socio-economic status (SES) of parents and early rank position. Source: Feinstein (2003), with permission from Blackwell Publishing.

attainment is, to an extent, protective against adult cognitive decline (Richards and Sacker 2003).

Clearly, poor socio-economic environment in early life increases risks to health through the interaction of adverse environmental influences with developmental processes. A poor environment is associated with poor maternal diet, smoking, alcohol abuse, and raised risk of infection in the mother during the prenatal period, and also with poor growth of the child in the postnatal period. Poor maternal educational attainment and low literacy will further increase risk and help to perpetuate their effects. In countries experiencing war and civil unrest or large-scale epidemics, all these kinds of risks are greatly increased.

3.3 **Temperament and behaviour in early life**

The early life adverse influences of poor social circumstances that act on physical and cognitive development in the long term, affect also temperament and behaviour.

There is a great deal of evidence that maltreatment in childhood, in the form of emotionally inconsistent, disturbing and, in particular, abusive and punitive parenting, are risks for later antisocial behaviour problems, conduct disorders, and antisocial personality (Rutter *et al.* 1998). There is further evidence that early age at maltreatment increases the risk of these adverse outcomes (Keiley *et al.* 2001). Emotional disturbance in the family is a long-term risk for mental health, particularly depression in women (Maughan 2002). Adverse childhood emotional circumstances because of poor relationships between parents are raised risks for suicidal thoughts and suicidal behaviour in adolescence and early adulthood (Fergusson *et al.* 2000). Poor maternal education, combined with teenage motherhood, is associated with raised risk of oppositional problems and aggression (Nagin and Tremblay 2001), poor educational attainment in the child, raised risk of substance abuse, mental health problems, and antisocial behaviour (Fergusson and Woodward 1999). Low parental self-esteem may be a raised risk for child abuse (Stratton and Swaffer 1988). The childhood experience of an extremely stressful environment, for example in the form of domestic violence, is associated with raised risk to brain development (Koenen *et al.* 2003; Tucker *et al.* 1997). Early signs of poorly controlled temperament and behaviour are associated with adult problems of mental health and behaviour, including depression, social isolation, and substance dependence, with consequential adverse effects on work and personal relationships (Moffitt *et al.* 2002).

The likelihood of adverse behavioural and mental health outcomes following maltreatment and emotionally disturbing experience in childhood is greatly increased by concurrent poor socio-economic circumstances in childhood. Poor mothering and poor physical care, overcrowding, welfare dependence, and family emotional instability are risks for adult depressive disorder, particularly for depression in women in early adulthood (Sadowski *et al.* 1999), and a cumulative process is associated also with suicidal ideation and behaviour in late adolescence and early adulthood (Fergusson *et al.* 2000). Poor educational attainment is a likely corollary of problems of behaviour and temperament in childhood and that, in turn, is a raised risk for adult low self-esteem, low economic capability, and poor personal relations, all of which are associated with adult behavioural difficulties (Nagin and Tremblay 2001). Poor educational attainment is also an increased risk following the experience of parental separation (Ely *et al.* 1999).

The cumulative effect of adverse emotional experiences, together with poor socio-economic circumstances in childhood, is evidently a considerable risk in childhood. Explanations for the apparently long-term effects of such childhood risk have been sought in psychological, psychosocial, social, and biological models.

Psychological explanations suggest that childhood psychological and physical insults may damage emotional regulation, attachment security, quality of relationships with others, and concept of self-worth. Psychological explanations include the concept of a sensitive period, at ages 6 to 8 months, when children 'must develop their core attachment to their parents'; and between ages 12 and 13 months is a sensitive stage for intellectual and linguistic development (Sylva 1997). Disruption of these processes at sensitive periods, as well as at later times in childhood, may be a long-term source of risk because the child acquires a maladaptive response style which affects learning and response to others (van Os and Jones 1999).

Psychosocial explanations propose that response style to adverse experience may reduce the child's self-esteem (Sweeting and West 1995) and self-control (Pulkkinen and Hamalainen 1995), and have consequent risks to social attainment and status at later ages in terms, for example, of education and employment, personal relationships, and coping with adverse life events (Rodgers 1994). At puberty, the observed increase in depression and anxiety in girls is greater than in boys, perhaps because as social and sexual roles develop during adolescence, self-evaluation tends to be lower in those who have suffered emotional damage earlier in life (Maughan 2002). That, in turn, may initiate social vulnerability that is manifest in such risks as a raised likelihood of early pregnancy, with consequent raised risk of poor interpersonal relations and lower educational attainment, lower occupational prospects, and greater risk of depressive illness (Maughan and Lindelow 1997). Bartley (2004) suggests that children who successfully develop 'an inner security and the ability to form and maintain relationships' (p. 19) may be better able to maintain their identity in societies where traditional social ties of religion, family, and caste are weakening.

Social explanations suggest that poor emotional self-management, low educational attainment, and a higher risk of unemployment have adverse effects on own socioeconomic attainment, self-esteem, and life chances (Caspi *et al.* 1991; Tremblay *et al.* 1995; Montgomery *et al.* 1996; Nagin and Tremblay 2001).

Biological explanations include the possible adaptation of emotional response style to deal with unbearable emotional pressure experienced during the developmental period, since adaptation may be detectable in later psychophysiological responses to stress (Wadsworth 1976) and in the adult immune response (Surtees *et al.* 2003). These are further examples of 'biological embedding' of social experience. There are also explanations concerned with the adverse effect of chronically high levels of stress acting through high glucocorticoid levels and their effects on the hypothalamic-pituitary-adrenal system, with adverse long-term consequences for mental and physical function, as already described (Brunner 2000; Montgomery *et al.* 1997; Richards *et al.* 2002; Heim *et al.* 2000). There may also be protective genetic effects (Caspi *et al.* 2002) and raised risks associated with the interaction of genetic and environmental factors (Jaffee *et al.* 2003).

In the development of mental health and temperament, as in physical health, it seems likely that in all but the most extremely damaging environments it is not inevitable that adverse consequences will occur in adulthood. The cumulative effect model of causation may operate only in the presence of familial and/or psychophysiological transmission of vulnerability to stressful life experiences (van Os and Jones 1999), or only when additional adult stressful experience occurs (Rodgers 1994). There are protective effects from good relationships in childhood. For example, a high level of parental interest in the child's education is protective against the adverse effects of parental separation on educational outcomes (Wadsworth and MacLean 1986). Experience of positive family interaction and stimulation is associated with better educational attainment (Sylva 1997). In Britain, a study of resilience to childhood stressful situations, and to physical and sexual abuse, showed the long-term value and effectiveness of having a close relationship with a stable adult as a protection against depression in adult life, reducing depression in women who had experienced abusive childhoods from 42 per cent among those who had no support of this kind to 19 per cent in those who had received support (Bifulco and Moran 1998).

Werner (1995, p. 161) shows that protective factors for children living in poverty or in psychologically stressful family circumstances in the Kauai longitudinal study, and in others, may be characterized in three ways. First are the protective factors that are characteristics of the individual. Werner describes these individuals as engaging to others: 'they have good communication and problem-solving skills, including the ability to recruit substitute care givers . . . they have faith that their own actions can make a positive difference in their lives'. Secondly, these resilient children also had family relations or friends who provided affectional ties that 'encouraged trust, autonomy, and initiative'. Thirdly, such children also had relationships with others in the community who provided positive role models and reinforced and rewarded 'competencies of resilient children'.

The developing child's adaptation to the social environment is likely to be a process of accommodation of temperament and physical capability to the demands of the context (Scarr and Weinberg 1983; Jones *et al.* 1994). Although much of the research evidence on the adverse effects of emotional insults on physical growth and on temperament and behaviour is derived from studies of parental discord, in global terms it is likely that the social upheaval of war and of such epidemics as HIV/AIDS have a powerful impact on children's mental health and temperament. The consequences, at the societal level, of poor mental health in childhood, particularly poor mental health associated with war and epidemics, have not yet, to our knowledge, been systematically and extensively investigated.

3.4 **The societal context**

Increasing societal affluence is associated with positive health changes. A study of the height of Norwegian military conscripts between 1921 and 1962 showed a consistent secular increase (Udjus 1964, quoted by Tanner *et al.* 1982). The majority of that increase was in leg length, the component of height that develops particularly strongly in early life. This change was attributed to dietary and health improvements. Similar findings were reported from Japan (Tanner *et al.* 1982). In Britain, the greater social equality and the increase in the mean of height growth achieved in cohorts born since the end of the Second World War (Fig. 3.3) may also be the result of improved nutrition and of improved health care, and reduction in infectious illness. This postwar increase in height growth is likely also to be associated with the observed inter-cohort and inter-generation increase in scores on cognitive function tests (Wadsworth *et al.* 2003; Feinstein 2003). However, increasing nutritional choice and greater spending power tend also to be associated with greater risk of overweight and obesity in childhood (Wadsworth *et al.* 2003), and with raised risk of diabetes and other cardiovascular risks (Eriksson *et al.* 2003).

At times when unemployment risk is high, there is raised risk to physical and mental health in adults (Montgomery *et al.* 1996). Because unemployment is more likely

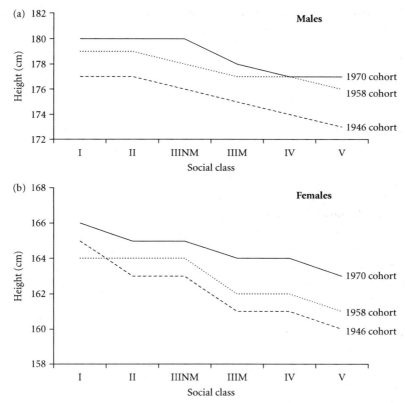

Fig. 3.3 Mean adult height in relation to father's social class across the population of three British national birth cohort studies. Source: Wadsworth *et al.* (2003).

among those with low educational attainment and least skill, and because in many countries employment defines status, experience of unemployment tends to bring not only low income but also social isolation and reduced self-esteem. Arguably, the social gradient in health among those in employment owes something to these attributes of self-esteem and status. Unemployment of parents impacts on children. Studies of the psychological effects of periods of mass unemployment show the adverse effects on temperament and subsequent child rearing among those who had this experience (Elder *et al.* 1984). Graham (1984, p. 18) observed that:

> Family poverty is inextricably linked to employment policy and the policies for income maintenance for those not in paid employment. Since families outside the labour market are particularly vulnerable to poverty, employment remains the most effective guarantee against both poverty and the ill health with which it is associated.

The apparent effects of parental separation and divorce have already been described, and the rising rates of these salient events in the lives of children and parents are likely to be associated with increased health and behaviour problems. In 2002, Britain had the third highest rate of divorce in Europe, at 2.7 per thousand population, compared with the average for countries in the European Community of 1.9 per thousand; in 2002, two in three children of divorcing parents in Britain were aged under 10 years (Summerfield and Babb 2004). As traditional family ties have weakened in high- income countries, so too have traditional social networks (Wilkinson 1996; Bartley 2004), and those changes may reduce opportunities for the kinds of social support that have been shown to promote resilience in children (Werner 1995; Bifulco and Moran 1998).

Similarly, another form of fundamental change and disruption of life, namely migration, can bring associated health risks. This has been shown among migrants from the Tokelau Islands (Beaglehole *et al.* 1979), from Japan (Marmot *et al.* 1975), and from southern Asia (McKeigue *et al.* 1992). Explanations have been given in terms of genetic differences, social differences, dietary and psychological change, and the effect of 'cultural bereavement' (Eisenbruch 1988; Helman 1994). In terms of growth and development in early life, poor nutrition in the pre- and postnatal period prepares the body's system and organs to deal with that low level of nutrition (Barker 1998). Subsequent migration to a richer society then greatly increases the risks to health associated with obesity and with glucose intolerance (McKeigue *et al.* 1992).

The economic demands of war and of HIV/AIDS epidemics impose heavy burdens on the lives of mothers and children by siphoning resources away from health, by enforced migration, and by food shortages. The Food and Agricultural Organisation (2003) observes, of HIV/AIDS epidemics, that:

> Hunger accelerates both the spread of the virus and the course of the disease. Hungry people are driven to adopt risky strategies to survive. Frequently they are forced to migrate, often to urban slums where HIV infection rates are high. In desperation, women and children barter sex for money and food, exposing themselves to the risk of infection. (p.11)

The relationship between undernourishment and mortality is evident (Table 3.1), but the reduction in the proportion of the population undernourished in developing countries between 1995–1997 and 1999–2001 was only 1 per cent, from 18 to 17 per cent. A less well-recognized, and less well-measured concomitant of social disorganization on the scale associated with war, extensive epidemics, and famine, is the serious psychological damage that is undoubtedly inflicted on children, together with the cessation of educational opportunities and the positive effects of a stable family life. Poverty, within countries, brings a similar risk of psychiatric morbidity (Costello *et al.* 1996).

In many countries, the education of women lags seriously behind that of men, although progress is being made. In Britain, it was not until the 1970s that women entered universities in a proportion equal to that of men. Thus, the consequent health-related value to children of increasing access to educational opportunities for their mothers would not have been seen until after that time, and the health value in terms of pre-motherhood health and growth would not have been seen until the generation

Table 3.1 Poverty, child mortality, and child nutritional status in developing countries and countries in transition, classified by category of prevalence of undernourishment

Category of prevalence of undernourishment (% in population 1999–2001)	Poverty (% population below the poverty line 1990–2000)		Child mortality (Under-5 mortality rate 2001 per 1000 births)	Child nutritional status (% underweight children under 5 years 1995–2001)
	Rural	Urban		
>2.5	14–28	20–30	5–27	1–20
2.5–4	15–47	7–25	12–41	1–14
3–19	5–68	2–49	9–197	4–48
20–34	10–82	12–57	19–265	5–52
35 & more	33–83	8–62	35–316	3–49

Source: Food and Agricultural Organisation (2003).

born to those mothers. In countries rated as low in human development, the ratio of literate females to males at ages 15–24 years rose from 70 to 81 women per 100 men, and the gender ratio in primary education rose from 86 to 92 girls per 100 boys in developing countries between 1990 and 1999–2000 (United Nations 2003). Nevertheless, in developing countries, 60 per cent of women aged 15–24 years are literate compared with 80 per cent of men of the same age; two thirds of the world's illiterate persons are women (United Nations 2003).

A further important influence of social context that varies over historical time, as well as between countries, is that of custom and fashion. Deeply ingrained customs in family life and in the division of labour can impact strongly on the health of mothers and children. Some of the most striking examples are found in programmes designed to introduce new methods of contraception. Barroso and Correa (1995) note that whereas contraceptive programme planners make assumptions about choice and rationality, in practice, 'conception is linked to sex—a meeting place for reason, passion, desire, ecstasy, cultural norm, religion, God and the devil, as well as the pleasure of taking risks so typical of games of chance'. Williams et al. (1994) observe that 'in Lesotho, sexual intercourse is taboo while the woman is breast feeding, so migrant male workers bring home formula cans to their wives, who can then bottle feed their babies and have sex' (p. 29).

Customs that commonly prohibit female inheritance or even ownership of land and resources, as well as the opportunity of more than the most elementary education, also keep levels of women's health low through the effects of poverty, lack of civil rights, and low self-esteem. Women in some developing countries work a particularly arduous form of 'double day', combining their customary agricultural or industrial labour with the care of the family (Pearce 1995). Although in many countries, women now form an increasing part of the labour force, 'labour laws seldom provide adequate protection against discrimination, or protect rights to employment and to social security during illness and pregnancy' (Watkins 1995, p. 27).

Fashion in health-related habits affects health in early life. It was, for example, neither fashionable nor customary for women to smoke until the late 1920s in Britain, when women in the upper social classes established the habit as fashionable. The habit spread to other social classes, accelerated by the acceptance of smoking as a relaxant during the Second World War, and has subsequently become a habit more frequent in women in socially disadvantaged circumstances and those with young children (Graham 1984), and is high in men and women living in poverty (Flint and Novotny 1997). There are similarly relevant fashion changes in physical exercise, which is currently becoming increasingly fashionable in Britain, and in the consumption of alcohol, which is growing rapidly, particularly among young women. Why the view of what is fashionable changes, and what drives the individual acceptance or rejection of what is fashionable, are important questions which are only now beginning to be studied (Lindbladh *et al.* 1997). Giddens' (1991) concept of self identity has usefully been operationalized by Schooling (2001) to show that the individual's health- related behaviour is influenced by the interaction between the public and the private image of that activity. For example, when the social or public image of smoking is one of a mildly rebellious, machismo activity, those who wish to present that image will tend to smoke. On the other hand, when smoking is seen as an unpleasant habit with a serious health risk, those who wish to present their public image as healthy and responsible are less likely to smoke.

Most international comparisons of societal effects on health use data on income (in some form) and on spending on education, welfare, and health to distinguish nations according to their degree of concern for health and welfare. Graham (2002) shows that international comparisons of health risks in early life should take account of welfare arrangements, and gives the example of the Nordic countries, where welfare benefits are designed to protect the income of those with young children. Bartley (2003) describes the value of characterizing countries by other forms of welfare arrangements, such as the proportion of elderly who live with their children, as a way of describing societal arrangements that relate to health outcomes.

3.5 **Policy implications**

The need for policies to improve physical health in early life has been recognized internationally. Less well recognized is the need to improve mental health in early life. Endowing the child with good health and educational opportunities is an investment for the life of the child, as well as for the well-being and improvement of society (World Health Organisation 2002). In asking how policy can be developed to improve children's health, it is relevant first to see the scale of the problem revealed by comparison of health indicators in differing socio-economic environments.

Indicators of health in early life show great differences between groups of countries ranked by the World Bank (2003) as having low, middle, and high income. Although improvement over the two decades up to 2001 is evident, there are differences in the extent of change according to national income level. Life expectancy was 21 years less in low-income countries compared with those of high income in 1980, and was still 19 years less in 2001 (Table 3.2). Similarly, although there was improvement in infant mortality over the same period, it was much less in low-income countries (27%) than in the high-income countries (58%) (Table 3.2). Mortality under age five years, over the same period, also lagged considerably in the low-income countries (Table 3.2). The large inter-country differences in adolescent fertility rates, and the high prevalence of low weight at birth in the low-income countries (Table 3.2), also show the scale of the difficulties that policies have to tackle.

Risk factors, such as smoking, are greater in high-income countries, and others, such as HIV/AIDS, are higher in the low-income countries (Table 3.3). HIV prevalence in women aged 15–24 years was, in 2001, as high as 39.5 per thousand women in Swaziland and 33.0 per thousand women in Zimbabwe. HIV caused 10.4 million children aged under 15 years to be orphaned, and there were two million war-related child deaths in the period 1992–2002 (Boyce and Keating 2004).

Low-income countries spent proportionately less in 2000 on health (2.8 per cent of GDP) and education (1.1 per cent of GDP), compared with high-income countries (5.3 per cent and 6.0 per cent of GDP, respectively) (Table 3.3). As a recent United Nations report notes: 'Educated girls and women . . . have fewer children, seek medical attention sooner for themselves and their children and provide better care and nutrition for their children' (United Nations 2003). Improvements in educational opportunities for women are likely to be related to the proportion of women in ministerial appointments, and there are still considerable inter-country differences, as well as low

Table 3.2 Early life health and survival, and fertility in young women, in relation to national income group

		Low-income countries	Middle-income countries	High-income countries
Life expectancy at birth (yrs)	1980	53	66	74
	2001	59	70	78
Yrs of increase in life expectancy		6 yrs	4 yrs	4 yrs
Infant mortality per 1000 births	1980	109	55	12
	2001	80	31	5
% reduction in infant mortality		27%	44%	58%
Under-5s mortality per 1000 live births	1980	171	80	15
	2001	121	38	7
% reduction in under-5s mortality		29%	53%	53%
Fertility per 1000 women aged 15–19 yrs	2002	104	40	24
% of babies of low birthweight	1992–2000	27	8	7

Source: World Bank (2003).

Table 3.3 Indicators of health and health risks in relation to national income

		Low-income countries	Middle-income countries	High-income countries
% GDP spent on health	2000	2.8	4.5	5.3
% GDP spent on education	2000	1.1	3.0	6.0
% women at ministerial level	1994	4	5	13
	1998	6	n/a	13
% population with access to an improved water source	1990	66	76	n/a
	2000	76	82	n/a
% population with access to improved sanitation facilities	1990	30	47	n/a
	2000	44	59	n/a
% population undernourished	1990–92	28	15	n/a
	1998–00	25	10	n/a
% pregnant women receiving prenatal care	1996	62	77	n/a
% of women with anaemia	1985–2000	65	44	n/a
% children under 1 yr immunized against measles	2001	60	86	90
% children under 1 yr immunized against diptheria, pertussis, and tetanus	2001	61	85	94

Source: World Bank (2003).

rates even in high-income countries (Table 3.3). The variation between these same groups of countries in spending on essential environmental services, and in success in preventing malnutrition, is considerable, and the prevalence of malnutrition was not greatly reduced during the period 1990–2000 (Table 3.3). The same United Nations report notes: 'Education, health, nutrition and water and sanitation complement each other, with investments in any one contributing to better outcomes in the others' (United Nations 2003). Inter-country differences in access even to minimal prenatal care, in the risk of anaemia, and in immunization achievements are also considerable (Table 3.3).

What can be done to improve physical health in early life? Where improvement has been achieved, it can usually be ascribed to a complex of effects, and is not the result of attempts at solving one aspect of the problem. The United Nations (UN 2003) gives examples of improvement in low-income countries, and within states or provinces of a country. For example, 'the state of Kerala, India, has health indicators similar to those of the United States—despite a *per capita* income 99 per cent lower and annual spending on health of just $28 a person.' Similarly, 'Cuba's *per capita* income is a small fraction of that in the United States, yet it has the same infant mortality rate and has kept HIV/AIDS under control' (p. 87). These kinds of successes are attributed to social equity in spending on health and education, and to gender equity in education, ownership rights, and occupational and earnings opportunities (UN 2003). Hanmer *et al.* (2003) illustrate the value of education as a means of translating economic progress into social development. In high-income countries, the improvements in women's education and health are likely to be part of the explanation for growth in children's height in the second half of the twentieth century (section 3.4 and Fig. 3.3), together with improvements in early life in nutrition, reduction in risk of infectious illness, and increasingly effective infant care programmes including growth monitoring.

Care of risks to health in early life requires, at the environmental level, provision of good sanitation, clean water, and good nutrition. At the individual level, dealing with known health risks in early life, such as low birth weight, poor growth in early life, and overweight and obesity is more complex. Assessment must be made of the likely value of treating the source of risk (Boyce and Keating 2004). Risk identified as appropriate for attempted prevention, or at least reduction, will require service provision and probably also training of health care professionals. For early life care, the effectiveness of linking maternity benefits to preventive care was well demonstrated to be effective, and part of the reason why, in the 1970s, Finnish early life health indicators were so much better than those in Britain, and why they had improved much more rapidly than the British indicators in the 20 years before that (Wynn and Wynn 1974). That is one way to raise awareness and change attitudes.

Caring for ill health in children involves providing appropriate services and educating parents in recognition of when help is needed. Access to health services and continuing training of health personnel is essential for the care of physical health in early life. Oluwole *et al.* (2000) reported that 'In Zambia health workers correctly managed less than 5 per cent of cases of diarroheal disease before training. After training they correctly managed 82 per cent of cases at three months follow-up and 60 per cent after one year.' In low-income countries generally, neonatal mortality is particularly in need of an effective programme, since that aspect of child mortality shows the least improvement compared with mortality at later ages (Table 3.2; Darmstadt *et al.* 2003). Parental education about children's health is essential to improve awareness of when medical care should be sought for illness, both physical and mental. By comparison, recognition and care of mental illness and emotional disturbance in childhood is much less well-developed.

Developing policies to reduce ill health and risks to health in early life is, therefore, complex. It is difficult to persuade governments that investment and change is needed, and a number of strategies are used. Chief among them are publications that show the extent of health risks and problems, and research projects that show the adverse outcomes of specific risks. Such projects may need to be repeated, even after sufficient scientific demonstration of association has been achieved, in order to raise awareness and, thus, to increase pressure for political action. It is now particularly necessary, for example, to raise awareness of mental health risks to children growing up in war zones and in AIDS/HIV epidemic areas as a necessary preliminary to the development of effective means of care. At present, even simple descriptive statistics about mental health in children, adolescents, and mothers are not produced on a regular basis.

Childhood mental health outcomes should be measured and reported in national and international statistics, comparable with the indicators of mortality and morbidity (Table 3.2).

Demonstration intervention projects are also of great value in persuading governments of the need for new policy development. Notable examples include Barker and colleagues' (1992) programme to provide support to new parents in poor socio-economic circumstances and programmes developed by Garber and Heber (1981) and by Achenbach and colleagues (1990) to improve cognitive function in children of low birth weight or in poor circumstances. One of the most striking interventions is the High/Scope Perry Pre-school Programme that was undertaken in the pre-school years with poor, urban, American children:

> . . . [it] enables children to better carry out the first school tasks that they encounter. This better performance is visible to everyone involved—the child, the teacher, the parents and other children. Realising they have the ability to achieve classroom success, children believe and act accordingly, thereby developing a stronger commitment to schooling. Teachers recognise better school performance and react to it with higher expectations. (Schweinhart *et al.* 1993, p. 18)

Children who experienced the programme were compared at age 27 years with others who had not had this experience but who came from similar social circumstances, and the results were striking. Programme children had significantly higher earnings, a higher percentage of home ownership, and higher levels of completed years of schooling, and a lower percentage received help from social services, and there were significantly fewer arrests. Unfortunately, health outcomes were not measured. Like the High/Scope Perry Project, most intervention studies show benefits across a range of outcomes including health, behaviour, and cognition. The risk with intervention projects is that effective results are often not immediately apparent. Reviews of such programmes are given by Schweinhart *et al.* (1993) and by Hertzman and Wiens (1996).

However, health intervention studies have, at best, an inconsistent track record, for example those targeted at nutrition in pregnancy (Rush *et al.* 1980; Barker 1994) and, more broadly, at smoking (Rose *et al.* 1983; Jarvis *et al.* 1984). By contrast, the educational intervention studies and intervention studies on the larger social scale have had much greater success, as outlined above. This may be because they target young children, who are arguably at their most susceptible and at a sensitive period for learning. But it is certainly also because most educational and social intervention programmes have taught, in childhood, a range of basic ways of coping (cognitive skills) and the reinforcement of self-esteem. In comparison, the health programmes have targeted adults, and endeavoured to teach that something was good for them, which in many cases may well have gone against the grain and the socially supported habit.

It may be concluded that three kinds of intervention would be valuable in the care of health in early life. The first would be designed to improve the wider social context, namely the improvement in opportunities, particularly educational, for girls. This could only be achieved through pressure for political change. The proverb quoted by

Bali (1995, p. 216) aptly summarizes the importance of such intervention for the health and development of children: 'If you plan for one year grow rice, if you plan for ten years grow trees, if you plan for 100 years educate women.'

The second kind of intervention, intended, as Barker (1998) recommends, to improve diet and growth in girls, is necessary but needs to be delivered in the least didactic way possible. Whereas in some countries this might take the form of teaching about diet from an early age, it might also be necessary, elsewhere, to supplement diet. The educational intervention studies show that effective teaching is usually greatly enhanced by parental involvement. Growth monitoring would also be necessary. This kind of intervention is difficult to achieve successfully, and certainly needs the support of the third kind of intervention which is concerned with the development of cognitive and coping skills, which can be taught successfully, as the educational intervention studies show. This intervention would, in effect, build a basis of future confidence and self-esteem, which would help individuals to take control of their health and to make positive choices in health.

3.6 Conclusions

Research, largely carried out in high-income countries but equally applicable in middle- and low- income countries, shows the vital role played by social circumstances in the development of health in early life, beginning with the mother's health in the prenatal years, as well as during pregnancy, and in infancy and childhood. The interaction of the child's development with the social environment during the years of developmental plasticity forms the basic endowment of physical and mental health for later life—the basis of the health pathways that will be continuously reformed by subsequent interactions throughout life. The extent that the period of developmental plasticity can be said to be deterministic must be tempered by the fact that the lifelong process of interaction is not predictable. Nevertheless, the effects of the interactions during the early life period set the scene for what follows, and form the basis of the individual's biological, psychological, and human capital.

The social factors shown to be most important during the early years are those that condition the mother and child's physical and emotional environment, and that are associated with physical growth and emotional support. Data that describe those aspects of the environment show that, for many children, the physical and emotional context of early life is not good, that education of women is gradually improving, but that progress towards improvement is, in general, slow (United Nations 2003; World Bank 2003). Descriptive monitoring data lacks sufficient detail about the exposure of children and their mothers to psychological sources of stress. The monitoring information is vital because it is the stimulus to action, as well as the marker of progress.

Policies to improve health and education in early life should have immediate and long-term benefits for health. Mehrotra (2000) summarizes the common elements demonstrated to be associated with successful health outcomes in low-income countries as:

> ... public provision of basic social services for all; investment in health and education early in the development process; public health and education expenditures well above their regional average; elimination of male-female differentials in social indicators, and enabling conditions which favoured the 'agency' role of women. (p.63)

These requirements are now well understood and are reflected in policies and in monitoring statistics. However, life course studies of development show that prolonged exposure to emotional stress in the early years has damaging effects on growth, mental health, and temperament, with important associated risks for educational receptivity and social behaviour, as well as mental and physical health. That risk has yet to be appropriately reflected in policy priorities and concerns and indicators of health.

It is still strongly the case that 'the primary determinants of disease are mainly economic and social, and therefore its remedies must also be economic and social. Medicine and politics cannot and should not be kept apart' (Rose 1992).

Acknowledgement

Professor Wadsworth's and Ms Butterworth's research is funded by the Medical Research Council.

References

Achenbach, T., Phares, V., Howell, C.T., Rauh, V., and Nurcombe, B. (1990). Seven year outcome of the Vermont intervention program for low birth-weight infants. *Child Dev.* **61**, 1672–81.

Bali, P. (1995). Health problems and needs of women in developing countries. In: *Health care of women and children in developing countries* (ed. H.M., Wallace, K. Giri, and C.V. Serrano) (2nd edn), pp. 209–17. Third Party Publishing, Oakland.

Barker, D.J.P. (1998). *Mothers and babies and health in later life* (2nd edn). Churchill Livingstone, Edinburgh.

Barker, D.J.P. (1994). *Mothers, babies, and disease in later life*. BMJ Publishing Group, London.

Barker, W., Anderson, R., and Chalmers, C. (1992). *Child protection; the impact of the child development programme*. Early Childhood Development Unit, Bristol.

Barroso, C. and Correa, S. (1995). Public servants, professionals and feminists: the politics of contraceptive research in Brazil. In: *Conceiving the New World order* (ed. R. Ginsburg and R. Rapp), pp. 292–306. University of California Press, Berkeley.

Bartley, M. (2003) Health inequality and societal institutions. *Soc. Theory. Hlth.* **1**, 108–29.

Bartley, M. (2004). *Health inequality*. Policy Press, Oxford.

Beaglehole, R., Eyles, E., and Prior, I. (1979). Blood pressure and migration in children. *Int. J. Epidemiol.* **8**, 5–10.

Bifulco, A. and Moran, P. (1998). *Wednesday's child*. Routledge, London.

Bobak, M., Richards, R., and Wadsworth, M.E.J. (2000). Air pollution and birth weight in Britain in 1946. *Epidemiology* **16**, 358–59.

Boyce, W.T. and Keating, D.P. (2004). Should we intervene to improve childhood circumstances? In: *A life course approach to chronic disease epidemiology* (ed. D. Kuh and Y. Ben–Shlomo), pp, 413–45. Oxford University Press, Oxford.

Brooke, O.G., Anderson, H.R., Bland, J.M., Peacock, J.L., and Stewart, C.M. (1989). Effects on birthweight of smoking, alcohol, caffeine, socioeconomic factors, and psychosocial stress. *Br. Med. J.* **298**, 795–801.

Brunner, J. (2000). Towards a new social biology. In: *Social epidemiology* (ed. L.F. Berkman and I. Kawachi), pp. 306–31. Oxford University Press.

Caspi, A., Elder, G.H., and Herbener, E.S. (1991). Childhood personality and the prediction of life-course patterns. In: *Straight and devious pathways from childhood to adulthood* (ed. L. Robins and M. Rutter), pp.13–35. Cambridge University Press, Cambridge.

Caspi, A., McClay, J., Moffitt, T.E., Mill, J., Martin, J., Craig, I.W., *et al.* (2002). Role of genotype in the cycle of violence in maltreated children. *Science* **297**, 851–4.

Cheung, Y.B. (2002). Early origins and adult correlates of psychosomatic distress. *Soc. Sci. Med.* **55**, 937–48.

Cheung, Y.B., Low, L., Osmond, C., Barker, D., and Karlberg, J. (2000). Fetal growth and early postnatal growth are related to blood pressure in adults. *Hypertension* **36**, 795–800.

Costello, E.J., Angold, A., Burns, B.J., Stangl, D.K., Tweed, D.L., Erkanli, A., *et al.* (1996). The Great Smoky Mountains study of youth. *Arch. Gen. Psychiat.* **53**, 1129–36.

Darmstadt, G.L., Lawn, J.E., and Costello, A. (2003). Advancing the state of the world's newborns. *Bul. WHO* **81**, 224–5.

Davey Smith, G., Greenwood, R., Gunnell, D., Sweetnam, P., Yarnell, J., and Elwood, P. (2001). Leg length, insulin resistance, and coronary heart disease risk. *J. Epidemiol.* **55**, 1–6.

de Stavola, B.L., dos Santos Silva, I., McCormack, V., Hardy, R.J., Kuh, D.J., and Wadsworth, M.E.J. (2004). Childhood growth and breast cancer. *Am. J. Epidemiol.* **159**, 671–2.

Dezateux, C. and Stocks, J. (1997). Lung development and early origins of childhood respiratory illness. In: *Fetal and early childhood environment* (ed. M.G. Marmot and M.E.J. Wadsworth). *Br. Med. Bull.* **53**, 40–57.

Douglas, J.W.B. (1964). *The home and the school.* MacGibbon and Kee, London.

Eisenbruch, M. (1988). The mental health of refugee children and their cultural development. *Int. Migration Rev.* **22**, 282–300.

Elder, G.H., Liker, J.R., and Cross, C.E. (1984). Parent–child behaviour in the Great Depression; life course and intergenerational influences. In: *Life-span development and behaviour* (ed. P.B. Baltes and O.G. Brim), pp. 109–57. Academic Press, New York.

Ely, M., Richards, M.P.M., Wadsworth, M.E.J., and Elliott, B.J. (1999). Secular changes in the association of parental divorce and children's educational attainment. *J. Soc. Policy* **28**, 437–55.

Eriksson, J.G., Forsen, T., Tuomilehto, J., Osmond, C., and Barker, D.J.P. (2003). Early adiposity rebound in childhood and risk of type 2 diabetes in adult life. *Diabetologia* **46**, 190–4.

Food and Agricultural Organisation (2003). *The state of food insecurity in the world 2003.* Food and Agricultural Organisation of the United Nations, Rome.

Feinstein, L. (2003). Inequality in the early cognitive development of British children in the 1970 cohort. *Economica* **70**, 73–98.

Fergusson, D.M. and Woodward, L.J. (1999). Maternal age and educational and psychosocial outcomes in early adulthood. *J. Child Psychol. Psychiat.* **40**, 479–89.

Fergusson, D.M., Woodward, L.J., and Horwood, L.J. (2000). Risk factors and life processes associated with the onset of suicidal behaviour during adolescence and early adulthood. *Psychol. Med.* **30**, 23–39.

Flint, A.J. and Novotny, T.E. (1997). Poverty status and cigarette smoking prevalence and cessation in the United States 1983–1993: the independent risk of being poor. *Tob. Control* **6**, 14–18.

Garber, H.L. and Heber, R. (1981). The efficacy of early intervention with family rehabilitation. In: *Psychosocial influences in retarded performance*, Vol. 2 (ed. M.J. Begab, R.C. Haywood, and H.L. Garber), pp. 71–88. University Park Press, Baltimore.

Gibson, E.L. and Green, M.W. (2002). Nutritional influences on cognitive function. *Nutr. Res. Rev.* 15, 169–206.

Giddens, A. (1991). *Modernity and self identity: self and society in the late modern age*. Polity Press, Oxford.

Graham, H. (1984). *Women, health and the family*. Harvester Press, Brighton.

Graham, H. (2002). Building an inter-disciplinary science of health inequalities; the example of life-course research. *Soc. Sci. Med.* 55, 2005–16.

Gregory, R.L. (1998). *Eye and brain*. Oxford University Press, Oxford.

Hales, C.N. (1997). Non-insulin-dependent diabetes mellitus. In: *Fetal and early childhood environment* (ed. M.G. Marmot and M.E.J. Wadsworth). *Br. Med. Bull.* 53, 109–22.

Hall, A.J. and Peckham, C.S. (1997). Infections in childhood and pregnancy as a cause of adult disease—methods and examples. In: *Fetal and early childhood environment* (ed. M.G. Marmot and M.E.J. Wadsworth). *Br. Med. Bull.* 53, 10–23.

Hanmer, L., Lensink, R., and White, H. (2003). Infant and child mortality in developing countries: analysing the data for robust determinants. *J. Dev. Studies*, 40, 101–18.

Hardy, R.J., Wadsworth, M.E.J., and Kuh, D. (2000). The influence of childhood weight and socioeconomic status on change in adult body mass index in a British national birth cohort. *Int. J. Obesity* 24, 725–34.

Hattersley, A.T. and Tooke, J.E. (1999). The fetal insulin hypothesis: an alternative explanation of the association of low birthweight with diabetes and vascular diesase. *Lancet* 353, 1789–92.

Heim, C., Newport, D.J., Heit, S., Graham, Y.P., Wilcox, M., Bonsall, R., *et al.* (2000). Pituitary-adrenal and autonomic responses to stress in women after sexual and physical abuse in childhood. *J. Am. Med. Assoc.* 284, 592–7.

Helman, C. (1994). *Culture, health and illness* (3rd edn). Butterworth Heinemann, London.

Hertzman, C. and Wiens, M. (1996). Child development and long-term outcomes: a population health perspective and summary of successful interventions. *Soc. Sci. Med.* 43, 1083–95.

Jaffee, S.R., Moffitt, T.E., Caspi, A., and Taylor, A. (2003). Life with (or without) father: the benefits of living with two biological parents depend on the father's antisocial behaviour. *Child Dev.* 74, 109–26.

Jarvis, M., West, R., Tunstall Pedoe, H., and Vessey, M. (1984). An evaluation of the intervention against smoking in the multiple risk factor intervention trial. *Prevent. Med.* 13, 501–9.

Jones, P. and Done. J. (1997). From birth to onset: a developmental perspective of schizophrenia in two national birth cohorts. In: *Neurodevelopment and adult psychopathology* (ed. M.S. Keshavan and R.M. Murray), pp. 119–36. Cambridge University Press, Cambridge.

Jones, P., Rodgers, B., Murray, R., and Marmot M. (1994). Child developmental risk factors for adult schizophrenia in the British 1946 birth cohort. *Lancet* 344, 1398–1402.

Keating, D.P. and Hertzman, C. (eds) (1999). *Developmental health and the wealth of nations*. The Guilford Press, New York.

Keiley, M.K., Howe, T.R., Dodge, K,A., Bates, J.E., and Pettit, G.S. (2001). The timing of child physical maltreatment. *Dev. Psychol.* 13, 891–912

Koenen, K.C., Moffitt, T.E., Caspi, A., Taylor, A., and Purcell, S. (2003). Domestic violence is associated with environmental suppression of IQ in young children. *Dev. Psychopathol.* 15, 297–311.

Kramer, M.S., Morin, I., Yang, H., Platt, R.W., Usher, R., and McNamara, H. (2002). Why are babies getting bigger? *J. Pediatrics* 141, 538–42.

Kuh, D. and Ben-Schlomo, Y. (eds) (2004). *A life course approach to chronic disease epidemiology*, 2nd edn. Oxford University Press, Oxford.

Kuh, D. and Wadsworth, M.E.J. (1989). Parental height, childhood environment and subsequent adult height in a national birth cohort. *Int. J. Epidemiol.* **18**, 663–8.

Leon, D.A., Koupilova, I., Lithell, H.O., Berglund, L., Mohsen, R., Vagero, D., *et al.* (1996). Failure to realise growth potential in utero and adult obesity in relation to blood pressure in 50 year old Swedish men. *BMJ* **312**, 401–6.

Lindbladh, E., Lyttkens, H., Hanson, B.S., and Ostergren, P.–O. (1997). The diffusion model and the social-hierarchical process of change. *Hlth. Promot. Int.* **12**, 323–30.

Lynch, J.W., Kaplan, G.A., and Shema, S.J. (1997). Cumulative impact of sustained economic hardship on physical, cognitive, psychological, and social functioning. *N Eng. J. Med.* **337**, 1889–95.

McCance, R.A. and Widdowson, E.M. (1974). The determinants of growth and form. *Proc. R. Soc. London (Biol.)* **185**, 1–17.

McKeigue, P.M., Pierpoint, T., Ferrie, J.E., and Marmot, M.G. (1992). Relationship of glucose intolerance and hyperinsulinaemia to body fat pattern in South Asians and Europeans. *Diabetologia* **35**, 785–91.

Marmot, M.G., Syme, S.L., and Kagan, A. (1975). Epidemiologic studies of CHD and stroke in Japanese men living in Japan, Hawaii and California; prevalence of coronary and hypertensive heart disease and associated risk factors. *Am. J. Epidemiol.* **102**, 514–25.

Martikainen, P.T. and Valkonen, T. (1996). Excess mortality of unemployed men and women during a period of rapidly increasing unemployment. *Lancet* **348**, 909–12.

Martyn, C.N. (1997). Infection in childhood and neurological diseases in adult life. In: *Fetal and early childhood environment* (ed. M.G. Marmot and M.E.J. Wadsworth). *Br. Med. Bull.* **53**, 24–39.

Maughan, B. (2002). Depression and psychological distress: a life course perspective. In: *A life course approach to women's health.* (ed. D. Kuh and R. Hardy), pp. 161–76. Oxford University Press, Oxford.

Maughan, B. and Lindelow, M. (1997). Secular change in psychosocial risks: the case of teenage motherhood. *Psychol. Med.* **27**, 1129–44.

Mehrotra, S. (2000). Health and education policies in high achieving countries: some lessons. In: *Development wih a human face* (ed. Mehrotra, S. and Jolly, R.), pp. 63–110. Oxford University Press, Oxford.

Miura, K., Nakagawa, H., Tabata, M., Morikawa, Y., Nishijo, M., and Kagamimori, S. (2001). Birth weight, childhood growth, and cardiovascular disease risk factors in Japanese aged 20 years. *Am. J. Epidemiol.* **153**, 783–9.

Moffitt, T.E., Caspi, A., Harrington, H., and Milne, B.J. (2002). Males on the life-course-persistent and adolescence-limited antisocial pathways: follow-up at age 26 years. *Develop. Psychopath.* **14**, 179–207.

Montgomery, S.M., Bartley, M.J., Cook, D.G., and Wadsworth, M.E.J. (1996). Health and social precursors of unemployment in young men in Great Britain. *J. Epidemiol. Comm. Hlth.* **50**, 415–22.

Montgomery, S.M., Bartley, M.J., and Wilkinson, R.J. (1997). Family conflict and slow growth. *Arch. Dis. Childhood* **77**, 326–30.

Morely, R. and Lucas, A. (1997). Nutrition and cognitive development. In: *Fetal and early childhood environment* (ed. M.G. Marmot and M.E.J. Wadsworth). *Br. Med. Bull.* **53**, 123–35.

Mustillo, S., Worthman, C., Erkanli, A., Keeler, G., Angold, A., and Costello, E.J. (2003). Obesity and psychiatric disorder: developmental trajectories. *Pediatrics* **111**, 851–9.

Nagin, D.S. and Tremblay, R.E. (2001). Parental and early childhood predictors of persistent physical aggression in boys from kindergarten to high school. *Arch. Gen. Psychiat.* **58**, 389–94.

Nilsson, P.M., Nyberg, P., and Ostergren, P.–O. (2001). Increased susceptibility to stress at a psychological assessment of stress tolerance is associated with impaired fetal growth. *Int. J. Epi.* **30**, 67–80.

Oddy, W., Kendall, G.E., Blair, E., de Klerk, N.H., Stanley, F., Landau, L.I., *et al.* (2003). Breast feeding and cognitive development in childhood: a prospective birth cohort study. *Paediat. Perinat. Epidemiol.* **17**, 81–90.

Oluwole, D., Mason, E., and Costello, A. (2000). Management of childhood illness in Africa. *BMJ* **320**, 594–5.

Pearce, T.O. (1995). The health of working women in developing countries. In: *Health care of women and children in developing countries* (2nd edn) (ed. H.M. Wallace, K. Giri, and C.V. Serrano), pp. 218–24. Third Party Publishing, Oakland.

Perry, I.J. and Lumey, L.H. (2004). Fetal growth and development: the role of nutrition and other factors. In: *A life course approach to chronic disease epidemiology* (ed. D. Kuh and Y. Ben–Shlomo) (2nd edn), pp. 240–59. Oxford University Press, Oxford.

Preston, S.H., Hill, M.E., and Drevenstedt, G.L. (1998). Childhood conditions that predict survival to advanced age among African Americans. *Soc. Sci. Med.* **47**, 1235–46.

Pulkkinen, L. and Hamalainen, M. (1995). Low self-control as a precursor to crime and accidents in a Finnish longitudinal study. *Crim. Behav. Mental Health* **5**, 424–38.

Richards, M. and Sacker, A. (2003). Lifetime antecedents of cognitive reserve. *J. Clin. Expmt. Neuropsychology* **25**, 614–24.

Richards, M., Hardy, R., Kuh, D., and Wadsworth, M.E.J. (2002). Birthweight, postnatal growth and cognitive function in a national UK birth cohort. *Int. J. Epidemiol.* **31**, 342–8.

Rodgers, B. (1994). Pathways between parental divorce and adult depression. *J. Child Psychol. Psychiat.* **35**, 1289–308.

Rose, G. (1992). *The strategy of preventive medicine.* Oxford University Press, Oxford.

Rose, G., Tunstall Pedoe, H.D., and Heller, R.F. (1983). UK heart disease prevention project: incidence and mortality results. *Lancet* **1** (8333), 1062–6.

Rush, D., Stein, Z. and Susser, M. (1980). A randomized controlled trial of prenatal nutritional supplementation in New York City. *Pediatrics* **65**, 683–97.

Rutter, M., Giller, H., and Hagell, A. (1998). *Antisocial behaviour by young people.* Cambridge University Press, Cambridge.

Sadowski, H., Ugarte, B., Kolvin, I., Kaplan, C., and Barnes, J. (1999). Early life family disadvantages and major depression in adulthood. *Br. J. Psychiat.* **174**, 112–20.

Scarr, S. and Weinberg, R.A. (1983). The Minnesota adoption studies: genetic differences and malleability. *Child Dev.* **54**, 260–7.

Schooling, C.M. (2001). *Health behaviour in a social and temporal context.* PhD thesis, University of London.

Schweinhart, L.J., Barnes, H.V., and Weikart, D.P. (1993). *Significant benefits: the High/Scope Perry Preschool Study through age 27 years.* High/Scope Press, Ypsilanti.

Shaheen, S. (1997). The beginnings of chronic airflow obstruction. In: *Fetal and early childhood environment* (ed. M.G. Marmot and M.E.J. Wadsworth). *Br. Med. Bull.* **53**, 58–70.

Steffensen, F.H., Sorensen, H.T., Gillman, M.W., *et al* (2000). Low birthweight and preterm delivery as risk factors for asthma and atopic dermatitis in young adult males, *Epidemiology* **11**, 18–88.

Strachan, D.P. and Sheikh, A. (2004). A life course approach to respiratory and allergic diseases. In: *A life course approach to chronic disease epidemiology* (2nd edn) (ed. D. Kuh and Y. Ben–Shlomo), pp. 240–59. Oxford University Press, Oxford.

Stratton, P. and Swaffer, R. (1988). Maternal causal beliefs for abused and handicapped children. *J. Reprod. Infant Psychol.* **6**, 201–16.

Summerfield , C. and Babb, P. (2004) *Social trends.* No. 34, p. 32. HMSO, London.

Surtees, P., Wainwright, N., Day, N, Brayne, C., Luben, R., and Khaw, K.–T. (2003). Adverse experience in childhood as a developmental risk factor for altered immune status in adulthood. *Int. J. Behav. Med.* **10**, 251–68.

Sweeting, H. and West, P. (1995). Family life and health in adolescence: a role for culture in the health inequalities debate? *Soc. Sci. Med.* **40**, 163–75.

Sylva, K. (1997). Critical periods in childhood learning. In: *Fetal and early childhood environment* (ed. M.G. Marmot and M.E.J. Wadsworth). *Br. Med. Bull.* **53**, 185–97.

Tanner, J.M., Hayashi, T., Preece, M.A., and Cameron, N. (1982). Increase in length of leg relative to trunk in Japanese children and adults from 1957 to 1977. *Ann. Hum. Biol.* **9**, 411–23.

Teranishi, H., Nakagawa, H., and Marmot, M. (2001). Social class difference in catch up growth in a national British cohort. *Arch. Dis. Child.* **84**, 218–21.

Tucker, J.S., Schwartz, J.E., Tomilnson–Keasey, C., Friedman, H.S., Criqui, M.H., Wingard, D.L., *et al.* (1997). Parental divorce: effects on individual behavior and longevity. *J. Personality Soc. Psychology* **73**, 381–91.

Tremblay, R.E., Boulerice, B., Jungner, M., and Arsenault, L. (1995). Does low self-control during childhood explain the association between delinquency and accidents in early adolescence? *Crim. Behav. Mental Health* **5**, 439–51.

Udjus L.G. (1964) *Anthropometrical changes in Norwegian men in the twentienth century.* Oslo University Press. Quoted in Tanner, J.M., Hayashi, T., Preece, M.A., and Cameron, N. (1982). Increase in length of leg relative to trunk in Japanese children and adults from 1957 to 1977. *Ann. Hum. Biol.* **9**, 411–23.

United Nations. (2003). *Human development report 2003.* United Nations, New York.

van Os, J. and Jones, P.B. (1999). Early risk factors and adult person–environment relationships in affective disorder. *Psychol. Med.* **29**, 1055–67.

Wadsworth, M.E.J. (1976). Delinquency, pulse rates and early emotional deprivation. *Brit. J. Criminol.* **16**, 245–56.

Wadsworth, M.E.J. and Maclean, M. (1986). Parents' divorce and children's life chances. *Child. Youth Services Rev.* **8**, 145–59.

Wadsworth, M.E.J, Butterworth, S.L., Montgomery, S.M., Ehlin, A., and Bartley, M.J. (2003). Health. In: *Changing Britain, changing lives.* (ed. E. Ferri, M.E.J. Wadsworth, and J.Bynner), pp. 207–36. Institute of Education Press, London.

Watkins, K. (1995). *The OXFAM Poverty Report.* OXFAM, Oxford.

Welberg, L.A.M. and Seckl, J.R. (2001). Prenatal stress, glucocorticoids and the programming of the brain. *J. Neuroendocrinology* **13**, 113–28.

Werner, E. (1995). Resilience in development. *Curr. Direct. Psychol. Sci.* **32**, 159–62.

Widdowson, E.M. and McCance, R.A. (1975). A review: new thought on growth. *Pediatr. Res.* **9**, 154–6.

Wilkinson, R.G. (1996). *Unhealthy societies.* Routledge, London.

Williams, C.D., Baumslag, N., and Jelliffe, D.B. (1994). *Maternal and child health* (3rd edn). Oxford University Press, Oxford.

World Bank (2003). *World devlopment indicators.* The World Bank, Washington.

World Health Organization (2002). *Healthy start in life; report on the global consultation on child and adolescent health and development.* World Health Organization, Geneva.

Wynn, M. and Wynn, A. (1974). *The protection of maternity and infancy.* Council for Children's Welfare, London.

Chapter 4

The life course, the social gradient, and health

David Blane

4.1 Introduction

The life-course perspective on health and its social determinants sees a person's biological status as a marker of their past social position and, through the structured nature of social processes, as liable to selective accumulation of future advantage or disadvantage. A person's past social experiences become written into the physiology and pathology of their body. The social is, literally, embodied; and the body records the past, whether as an ex-officer's duelling scars[1] or an ex-miner's emphysema. In turn, the duelling scar, as a mark of social distinction, predisposes to future advancement and social advantage, while the emphysema robs the employee of their ability to work and predisposes to future deprivation and social disadvantage. From a life-course perspective, the social distribution of health and disease results from these processes of accumulating advantage or disadvantage.

A number of scientific developments have contributed to an understanding of the usefulness of a life-course approach (Wadsworth 1997; Acheson *et al.* 1998; Berkman and Kawachi 2000; Dannefer 2003; Bartley, 2004). The chronic natural history of most of the prevalent causes of death in affluent societies has generated an interest in cumulative developmental stresses throughout life (Wilkinson 1996; van de Mheen *et al.* 1998; Kuh and Ben Shlomo 2004). The maturing of the British birth cohort studies has demonstrated how health in adulthood is influenced by circumstances in the earlier phases of life (Kuh *et al.* 2002; Power *et al.* 2002*a*; Langenberg *et al.* 2003; Power *et al.* 2003). A series of studies has demonstrated the long-term influence of childhood socio-economic circumstances on adult, particularly cardiovascular, health (Notkola *et al.* 1985; Gliksman *et al.* 1995; Brunner *et al.* 1999; Wamala *et al.* 2001; Lawlor *et al.* 2002). Research into the idea of biological programming has shown an association between intra-uterine and infant circumstances and the prevalent diseases of late

---

[1] The example of the duelling scars of the Officer Corps is simple to understand, but dated. A more contemporary illustration might refer to the stature (tall average height, large lung capacity, and so forth) of those born into the social elite; or to their bearing, which assumes compliance from others; or their accent, which shapes the mouth and acts as a sign of status.

middle age and older (Barker 1994; Marmot and Wadsworth 1997). And these developments, in turn, have stimulated an interest in the range of methodologies that can be used to study life-course influences on health (Caselli *et al.* 1991; Salhi *et al.* 1995; Belli 1998; Giele and Elder 1998; Belli 2000; Berney and Blane 2004).

4.2 **Social structure and the life course**

The life course may be regarded as combining biological and social elements which interact with each other. Individual biological development takes place within a social context which structures life chances so that advantages and disadvantages tend to cluster cross-sectionally and accumulate longitudinally. Exposure to one environmental hazard is likely to be combined with exposure to other hazards and these exposures are likely to accumulate over the course of life (Blane *et al.* 1997).

Cross-sectionally, advantage or disadvantage in one sphere of life is likely to be accompanied by similar advantage or disadvantage in other spheres. A person whose working environment is free of hazards is likely to reside in good-quality housing, to live in an area of little air pollution, and to have an income that permits a varied diet. In contrast, someone who is exposed to physicochemical and psychosocial hazards during work is at greater risk of occupying damp and inadequately heated accommodation, of being exposed to industrial and traffic exhaust atmospheric pollution in their area of residence, and of earning an income that restricts dietary choice.

Social organization also structures advantage and disadvantage longitudinally. Advantage or disadvantage in one phase of the life course is likely to have been preceded by, and to be succeeded by, similar advantage or disadvantage in the other phases of life. A child raised in an affluent home is likely to succeed educationally, which will favour entry to the more privileged sectors of the labour market, where an occupational pension scheme will provide financial security in old age. At the other extreme, a child from a disadvantaged home is likely to achieve few educational qualifications and, leaving school at the minimum age, to enter the unskilled labour market where low pay and hazardous work combine with no occupational pension, which ensures reliance on welfare payments in old age.

4.3 **Health and the life course**

These social processes interact with health in a number of ways. The relationship may be direct and disease-specific. For example, periconceptual intake of folic acid influences strongly the risk of fetal neural tube defects (MRC Vitamin Study Research Group 1991) and the sharp social gradient in these defects most plausibly arises from low incomes and the consequent restriction of dietary choice (Smithells *et al.* 1976). More general relationships are also possible. For instance, parental social class is a predictor of birth weight (Drever and Whitehead 1997) and, as noted, birth weight is associated with a range of health outcomes in later life. Part of this association may be due to 'biological programming' (Barker 1994); marginally incomplete fetal development, of which low birth weight is a non-specific marker, may, later in life, manifest as specific types of organ failure such as respiratory disease, diabetes, or hypertension. The life-course perspective adds to this approach by pointing out that any effects of biological programming will be interwoven with the effects of such ongoing social processes as accumulation, mobility, and protection.

4.3.1 Social accumulation

The underlying dynamic of the ongoing process of social accumulation is the continuity of social circumstances from parental social class to social conditions during childhood and adolescence and, eventually, to adult socio-economic position[2]. The aspect of this process that appears to be most important to health is not any one factor which has a major long-term influence on health, but a number of comparatively minor factors which become linked into a chain of disadvantage. To continue the example of birth weight, parental social class influences birth weight (Drever and Whitehead 1997); and adult health is influenced, independently of any biological programming or long-term effect of marginally incomplete fetal development, by social conditions during childhood and adolescence as well as during adulthood (Kuh and Ben Shlomo 2004). Birth weight, in consequence, may act as a marker of both biological programming and social conditions in later life.

Data on the male members of the 1958 British birth cohort demonstrate the 'social conditions in later life' part of this relationship (Bartley *et al.* 1994). Birth weight, divided into those weighing above and below six pounds (2721g) at birth, was examined in relation to a range of social data collected when the cohort members were aged 7, 11, 16, and 23 years. These analyses found that the low birth-weight babies were more likely to spend their childhood in less affluent families and poor-quality residential accommodation. For example, at age 7 years, 43 per cent of low birth- weight babies, compared with 35 per cent of those weighing 2721g or more, had fathers in clerical or manual social classes and lived in overcrowded homes; in contrast, 17 per cent of low birth- weight babies, but 22 per cent of those born weighing 2721g or above,

---

[2] There are two circumstances where such continuity may appear to be lacking. The first occurs when a person moves between social classes, either inter-generationally or intra-generationally; such movement is examined in section 4.3.2. The second circumstance occurs when the socio-economic system evolves, as is happening presently with the transition from an industrial to a service economy. The continuity of disadvantage in this case will involve a change in its nature and possible consequences. Take, for example, the former assembly line worker in a car plant who, after the factory is automated, finds re-employment as a home deliveryman, servicing mail order companies. The monotony, job strain, and repetitive musculoskeletal stress of the former occupation will have been replaced by the hazards of casual labour (low wages, no sickness or holiday pay, no job security, long and unsocial hours of work), as will the potential health consequences. Social disadvantage, nevertheless, characterizes both employment situations.

had fathers in professional social classes I and II. This association was observed throughout childhood; $P = 0.01, 0.01$, and 0.13 at ages 7, 11, and 16 years, respectively. When not having access to, or sole use of, a set of household amenities (inside toilet, hot water supply, bathroom) was substituted in the analysis for residential overcrowding, virtually identical results were obtained.

The relationship between birth weight and later socio-economic circumstances was graded in a stepwise fashion across the whole birth-weight distribution, and did not reflect simply the existence of an exceptionally disadvantaged low birth-weight group. In these same analyses, dividing the birth- weight distribution into fifths produced a graded relationship with the proportion of cohort members who subsequently lived in inadequate housing at all three ages during childhood and adolescence (ages 7, 11, and 16 years); overall test of association $P = 0.0009$ (Table 4.1). The proportion of cohort members who had experienced financial hardship at least once (either in their parents' home, between birth and 16 years, or as young adults at age 23 years) also showed a graded relationship across the birth-weight distribution; test for trend: $P = <0.001$ (Bartley *et al.* 1994). Broadly similar relationships were also found among the female members of the 1958 cohort (Power *et al.* 1996).

As well as the plausible short-term effects on health of straitened circumstances and an inadequate home, these types of disadvantage may have less obvious longer-term effects. The 1958 British birth cohort study allows the same example to be pursued further. A series of analyses investigated the predictors of unemployment, operationalized as those who had experienced more than one year of unemployment between the ages of 22 and 32 years, among young men (Montgomery *et al.* 1996). Height at age seven years proved a powerful predictor of the subsequent risk of unemployment (Table 4.2). When the distribution of height at age seven was divided into fifths, the relationship of

Table 4.1 Birth weight and subsequent social circumstances in male members of the 1958 British birth cohort study; percentage of each fifth of the birth-weight distribution who later experienced housing inadequacy and financial difficulties (N = 4321)

Birth weight (fifths)	Housing inadequacy[a]	Financial difficulties[b]
Highest: >136oz (>3800g)	18.1	31.6
Fourth: 125–135oz (3500–3800g)	20.4	33.7
Third: 116–124oz (3260–3500g)	20.4	35.0
Second: 106–115oz (3000–3260g)	22.0	36.3
Lowest: <105oz (<2890g)	26.6	39.2

Source: Bartley *et al.* (1994); adapted from Tables III and IV.

[a] Housing inadequacy: overcrowding and/or either no use or shared use of basic household amenities (inside toilet, hot water supply, bathroom) at each of ages 7, 11, and 16 years.

[b] Financial difficulties: one or more of the following—father in social class V at birth; parents reported family financial problems at subject's age 7 years; in receipt of free school meals at subject's age 11 or 16 years; in receipt of supplementary or unemployment benefit at age 23 years.

Table 4.2 Childhood height and subsequent social experience in male members of the 1958 British birth cohort; relative odds of each fifth of the childhood-height distribution experiencing later unemployment during early adulthood (N = 2256)

Height at age seven	Relative odds of unemployment[a]	
	Unadjusted	Adjusted[b]
Shortest	2.9	2.41
Second	2.02	1.81
Third	1.3	1.23
Fourth	1.19	1.2
Tallest	1	1

Source: Montgomery *et al.* (1996); adapted from Table 2.

[a] Unemployment: more than one year of unemployment between ages 22 and 32 years.

[b] Adjusted for parental height; social class at birth; residential crowding and region at age seven; social adjustment at age 11; and educational qualifications and height at age 23.

later unemployment across the distribution of childhood height was graded in a step-wise manner, with the chances of later unemployment in the shortest fifth of children being nearly three times (relative odds 2.90; 95 per cent confidence interval (CI) 1.84–4.57) that of the tallest fifth. Adjustment for a series of possible confounders such as social class at birth, educational qualifications, and parental height, had little effect; the relative odds reduced from 2.90 to 2.41 (95% CI 1.43–4.04) and the graded relationship across the whole distribution remained. Adult height was a weaker predictor of unemployment risk than height at age seven; and adjustment for possible confounders removed the association between adult height and unemployment risk.

Height at age seven in these results was interpreted as a measure of delayed growth during childhood, caused by the socio-economic and psychosocial adversity entailed in factors such as poor nutrition and disrupted sleep patterns (Montgomery *et al.* 1997). Poor nutrition and disrupted sleep relate directly to the financial hardship, domestic conflict, and crowded residential accommodation which have been discussed earlier. When put together, these analyses of the 1958 British birth cohort suggest a plausible chain: parental disadvantage and low birth weight; some, or all of, financial hardship leading to poor nutrition, crowded residential accommodation producing disrupted sleep patterns, and the consequent delayed growth during childhood; and the social circumstances which delay childhood growth predispose to labour market disadvantage, as indexed by prolonged or frequent spells of unemployment. Slow childhood growth may identify a particularly disadvantaged subgroup within each social class, who obtain lower educational qualifications and grades than their social class peers. These educational disadvantages subsequently weaken their labour market position which, in turn, exposes them to the health hazards of unemployment and casual employment in the poorly regulated secondary labour market. It is probably unusual for any of these factors on their own to have a major impact on health, but an effect on health becomes plausible when these factors are assembled into an accumulating chain of disadvantage[3].

The Boyd Orr cohort allows these processes to be followed into the older age groups. The following examples are based on a random sample of the full Boyd Orr cohort (see section 4.4.4 below), stratified by socio-economic conditions during childhood (Blane *et al.* 1999*c*). Sample members, when children, had been examined during 1937–39. They were re-examined in their early old age, during 1997–98, when information was collected about past exposure to a range of occupational and residential hazards to health. These hazard exposures were quantified as lifetime combined hazard exposure scores, which summed the number of years of exposure to each of six hazards (occupational fumes and dusts, physically arduous work, low job control, atmospheric pollution in area of residence, residential damp, inadequate nutrition). Social disadvantage during childhood, as indicated by low household *per capita* expenditure on food, predicted forward to the number of years up to early old age when subjects had been exposed to an occupational or residential hazard to health (Table 4.3). Those who

Table 4.3 Childhood food expenditure group and lifetime combined hazard exposure scores; household *per capita* food expenditure in 1937–39; combined hazard exposure scores accumulated by early old age in 1997–98; male and female members of a stratified random sample of the Boyd Orr cohort (N = 292)

1937–39 food expenditure group	Lifetime combined hazard exposure scores[a]		
	Mean	SD	N
Group 6 (> 11 shillings/head/week)[b]	21.0	27.2	23
Group 5 (9–11 shillings/head/week)	30.9	26.2	33
Group 4 (7–9 shillings/head/week)	37.6	33.6	52
Group 3 (5–7 shillings/head/week)	48.7	33.3	76
Group 2 (3–5 shillings/head/week)	49.0	38.4	93
Group 1 (< 3 shillings/head/week)	79.8	32.8	15

Source: previously unpublished data.

[a] Sum of number of years exposed to each of: occupational fumes and dusts, physically arduous work, low job control, atmospheric pollution in area of residence, residential damp, inadequate nutrition.

[b] 1939 values.

SD = standard deviation.

-----

[3] This *chain of disadvantage* (accumulation model) needs to be distinguished from the *pathway model* of life-course processes, which suggests that a person's pathway through childhood and adolescence is important to their health mainly because it determines their adult social position; and that it is primarily their adult social position which influences their health. Distinguishing, empirically, between the accumulation and pathways models is difficult (Hallqvist *et al.* 2004) but evidence in favour of the former comes from the literature on biological programming and suboptimal infant and child development, from the biological plausibility of the health consequences of socio-economic adversity during childhood, adolescence, and early adulthood, and from the long natural history of the prevalent chronic diseases.

in 1937–39 were children of households with the lowest *per capita* food expenditure had lifetime combined hazard exposure scores by early old age in 1997–98 which were approximately four times those in the highest food expenditure group. The relationship was graded in an approximately stepwise fashion between these extreme groups.

In the same way that disadvantage in childhood predicted forward to disadvantage during the subsequent stages of life, so disadvantage during early old age predicted back to the amount of disadvantage which had accumulated during the preceding years (Berney *et al.* 2000). Whether disadvantage in early old age was judged in terms of housing tenure, receipt of welfare benefits, or social class, among the men and women of this stratified random sample of the Boyd Orr cohort, the mean lifetime combined hazard exposure scores of the disadvantaged category was higher than the mean score of the advantaged category at conventional levels of statistical significance (Table 4.4).

When the Boyd Orr cohort results from the two extremes of life are put together, they illustrate a process of cumulative advantage or disadvantage which stretches across the whole life course. Although specific types of disadvantage are attached to each of low food expenditure during childhood, high lifetime combined hazard exposure scores, and receipt of welfare benefits during early old age, each measure also indicates more generalized disadvantage. When interpreted in this latter sense, the Boyd Orr cohort results demonstrate the continuity of general disadvantage across the life course—as well as vice versa, the social accumulation of advantage.

Table 4.4 Socio-economic position in early old age and lifetime combined hazard scores; socio-economic position in 1997–98; combined hazard exposure scores accumulated by early old age in 1997–98; male (N = 137) and female (N = 154) members of a stratified random sample of the Boyd Orr cohort

Socio-economic position in early old age	Mean lifetime combined hazard exposure score[a]	
	Men	**Women**
Housing tenure		
Owner occupier	82.3 (47.0;115)[b]	49.5 (38.1;115)
Non-owner occupier	126.6 (39.0;22)**	74.9 (42.5;38)*
Welfare benefits		
No welfare benefits	81.3 (45.8;105)	49.2 (36.9;116)
In receipt of welfare benefits	116.6 (48.0;32)**	76.7 (44.4;38)**
Social class		
Non-manual social class	60.0 (36.6;68)	44.4 (34.9;96)
Manual social class	118.1 (40.7;70)**	75.1 (41.7;58)**

Source: Berney *et al.* (2000), adapted from Table 4.

[a] Sum of number of years exposed to each of: occupational fumes and dusts, physically arduous work, low job control, atmospheric pollution in area of residence, residential damp, inadequate nutrition.

[b] Values in parentheses are standard deviation and number of subjects (sd;N).

* $p < 0.01$; ** < 0.001

4.3.2 **Social mobility**

Social mobility provides a further mechanism by which health and social factors can accumulate across the life course. Parental socio-economic position influences many aspects of childhood which, in turn, influence the chances and direction of social mobility into a different social class where further advantage or disadvantage accumulates. This process has been explored in the male members of the West of Scotland Collaborative Study (Blane *et al.* 1999a). In this data set, adult height, the chances of having left full-time education at the statutory minimum age, and the number of siblings in the family of origin were all independently associated ($P < 0.0001$) with father's occupational class during the study subject's childhood. Those from working-class homes were more likely than those from middle-class homes to have been brought up in a large family, to have left school early, and to have stopped growing at a short final height.

Each of these factors is subject to a range of influences; for example, height is influenced by parental height, education by the quality of local schools, and number of siblings by parental religion. Collectively, however, these factors represent the clustering of various dimensions of advantage and disadvantage during childhood: adult height indexes childhood health and growth; education indexes the cultural environment; and number of siblings, the material conditions of the family of origin. In the West of Scotland Collaborative Study, each of these factors was also associated independently ($P < 0.001$) with the chances and direction of social mobility. They were also associated independently ($P < 0.0001$) with the subject's own social class during adulthood; and, in each case, an increase in the size of the regression coefficients showed that the association with adult class was stronger than with father's class. Height, years of education, and number of siblings are measures of, and result from, childhood advantage or disadvantage. They also indicate the chances and direction of social mobility, so that their association with other types of social advantage or disadvantage strengthens as the life course unfolds.

The effect of these life-course selective processes, somewhat counter-intuitively, tends to constrain rather than widen adult inequalities[4]. The contribution of social mobility to the size of social inequalities can be observed in a social mobility matrix by comparing the size of inequalities among the socially stable (on the matrix diagonal) with the size of inequalities in the whole population, which consists of both the socially stable and the socially mobile (on the matrix bottom row). If the former is larger than the latter, the effect of social mobility has been to constrain the size of the inequalities. Such constraint can be illustrated with data from the West of Scotland Collaborative

---

[4] Whether or not *gradient constraint* occurs is an empirical issue, which may well vary with stage of the life course, country, and dimension of health examined. To date, however, it has been found in a sufficient number of data sets that it becomes reasonable to think in terms of a general tendency.

Table 4.5 Inter-generational social mobility matrix; mean height (cm); male members of the West of Scotland Collaborative Study (n = 5645)

Father's social class	Own social class				
	I & II	IIIN	IIIM	IV & V	ALL
I & II	176.9	174.7	172.3	172.8	176.0
IIIN	175.7	172.8	173.6	172.3	174.4
IIIM	174.7	173.4	171.5	170.3	172.5
IV & V	174.4	172.5	170.6	170.5	171.4
ALL	175.5	173.2	171.3	170.6	

Source: Blane et al. (1999a), adapted from Table 2.

Study, in relation to social class differences in mean height. In Table 4.5, the difference in mean heights among the socially stable (I & II—176.9 cm; IV & V—170.5 cm; difference = 6.4 cm) is greater than among the total population (I & II—175.5 cm; IV & V—170.6 cm; difference = 4.9 cm), so the net effect of social mobility has been to constrain the size of social inequalities in height.

This phenomenon was described first by Bartley and Plewis, in relation to limiting long-term illness (1997). Subsequently, broadly consistent results have been found in other data sets (Elstad 2001; Power et al. 2002b; Elstad 2003; Chandola et al. 2003; Cambois 2004) and for many types of social inequality, including years of education and number of siblings (Blane et al. 1999a), premature death (Blane et al. 1999b), health-related behaviours (Karvonen et al. 1999), and physiological and clinical status and cause-specific mortality (Hart et al. 1998).

The constraining effect occurs because although the upwardly mobile tend to be more advantaged than those they leave behind (socially stable in their class of origin), they tend to be less advantaged than those they join (socially stable in class of destination). Similarly, the downwardly mobile tend to be disadvantaged in comparison with those they leave, but more advantaged than those they join. In Table 4.5, for example, those who are upwardly mobile from social class IIIN are taller than the socially stable in their class of origin (175.7 cm v 172.8 cm) but shorter than the socially stable in their class of destination (175.7 cm v 176.9 cm). This relationship may not be found in every cell of a social mobility matrix, but a gradient-constraining effect will result whenever this relationship occurs in the majority of cells or in the cells containing the majority of socially mobile individuals. One consequence of this process of gradient constraint may be to counterbalance the life-course accumulation of advantage or disadvantage which, if unrestrained, might tend to widen inequalities across the life course.

Data which demonstrate this phenomenon are far from new. Some 40 years ago, for example, Morris' famous study of coronary heart disease in London busmen demonstrated that the measured physique of the upwardly mobile bus conductors who became bus drivers was midway between the measured physique of the direct-entry bus drivers, who can be regarded as socially stable members of class IIIM, and the measured physique of those who remained bus conductors and, hence, can be regarded as socially stable members of class IV (Heady *et al.* 1961). In the past, those interpreting such data have tended to concentrate on the half of the picture which shows that the upwardly mobile are more advantaged than those they leave behind and, on this basis, to conclude that social mobility tends to widen social inequalities. The innovation has been to see the whole picture, including the half which shows that the upwardly mobile are less advantaged than those they join, and to realize that the overall effect of these processes may not be to widen inequalities but to constrain their growth.

4.3.3 Social protection

Social protection provides a third mechanism by which health and social advantage or disadvantage interact over the life course. Previous socio-economic circumstances condition the impact of new disadvantage, minimizing its impact among the advantaged and amplifying its effect among the disadvantaged; and the importance of this conditioning effect increases as the wider external environment becomes more hazardous. Analyses of General Household Survey data have illustrated this mechanism (Bartley and Owen 1996).

In the General Household Survey, men of working age who report a limiting long-standing illness are more likely than those who report good health to be unemployed or economically inactive. The likelihood that chronic ill health will be associated with exclusion from employment varies with socio-economic position (Fig. 4.1). Employment rates among the chronically ill in the advantaged socio-economic groups are higher than among those with similarly poor health in the less advantaged socio-economic groups.

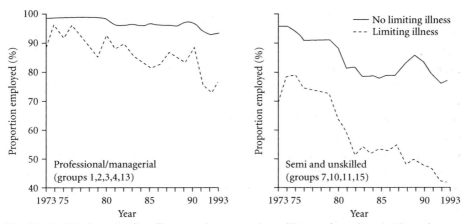

Fig. 4.1 Limiting longstanding illness, socio-economic position, and employment in male General Household Survey subjects, 1973–93. (From Bartley and Owen 1996; adapted from Figure 2.)

When chronic disease develops, the previous level of general social advantage, as indexed by socio-economic group, can be interpreted as either, in the case of professionals and managers, protecting against the further disadvantage of labour market exclusion or, in the case of semi- and unskilled manual workers, as adding the further disadvantage of unemployment to the pre-existing disadvantages of chronic disease and the standard of living obtainable with an unskilled manual wage.

This protective or amplifying effect was present in General Household Survey data during the relatively full employment of the mid-1970s. The effect became stronger, in the sense that social class difference in the labour market effects of chronic disease became wider, with the economic recession of the 1980s when unemployment levels and rates of economic inactivity rose. In other words, the 'social protection' type of interaction between health and social circumstances becomes more important when the general external environment becomes more hostile. Comparison between the British and Swedish experiences suggests that these effects respond to the social policy context. Among manual workers in Sweden, the labour market consequences of long-term illness are less disadvantageous than in Britain, perhaps due to Sweden's more interventionist labour market policies. Further, if labour market exclusion does result, it may be less damaging to health because Sweden's welfare benefits, compared with Britain's, are closer to normal wage and salary levels (Burstrom and Whitehead 2000).

4.4 Life-course influences on health and mortality at older ages

Much of the best-quality information about life-course influences on health comes from the British birth cohort studies. These studies started in 1946, 1958, 1970, and 2000, so the members of even the oldest of the cohorts have yet to reach the high morbidity and mortality age groups. Consequently, with rare exceptions (Kuh *et al.* 2002), they are, as yet, silent about life-course influences on premature mortality and contain comparatively sparse data on serious morbidity (Hardy *et al.* 2004). For the present, one must look elsewhere in order to investigate life-course influences on the health outcomes relevant to the older age groups.

4.4.1 US National Longitudinal Survey

One of the first life-course studies of mortality at older ages used data from the National Longitudinal Survey of Labour Market Experience of Mature Men (NLS) in the United States of America; a panel survey of some 5000 men aged 45–59 years in 1966. The data set contains retrospective occupational, educational, and family histories, and a range of prospective information, including deaths, during the follow-up period from 1966 to 1983. These deaths, at ages 45–76 years, have been analysed in relation to preceding life-course events (Mare 1990).

The chance of premature death in this data set is graded in the expected direction (namely, the greater the social advantage, the lower the mortality risk) with factors across the life course: father's occupation; length of schooling; first occupation on entering the labour market; occupation in middle age; and family assets in middle age. Controlling for education largely eliminates the association between father's occupation and later mortality risk, which suggests that the influence of childhood socio-economic circumstances is transmitted mainly through later experiences and, particularly, educational attainment. Multivariate analysis further suggests that about half of the mortality differential associated with education results from the occupational and financial advantage enjoyed subsequently by men with more schooling. First occupation retains an independent effect on mortality risk at least 25 years later, especially if the first occupation was professional or managerial. Most of the effect of occupation in middle age on subsequent mortality risk appears to result from the differences in wealth and family assets associated with occupation. In summary, the risk of premature death during late middle age or early old age in the NLS is influenced independently by factors across the life course, most importantly length of schooling, type of first occupation, and, in middle age, family wealth and assets and type of occupation.

4.4.2 **Norwegian linked data**

A second pioneer study of life-course influences on mortality at older ages used Norwegian linked register data from the national censuses of 1960, 1970, and 1980, and vital registration statistics up to 1985. The approximately 180,000 deaths during this period have been examined in relation to lifetime socio-economic variables, expressed as both the type of social circumstances and the temporal sequencing of these circumstances (Salhi et al. 1995; Wunsch et al. 1996).

Mortality risk among men was found to be highest for life courses which combine an education which ended at primary level; employment in manual occupations followed by early retirement from work; and housing conditions which were poor in earlier life and often remain poor through to later life. Unfavourable life courses for women similarly involve low education, starting in poor housing conditions, and economic inactivity. Favourable life courses for women, in contrast, are characterized by initially good housing conditions and, rarely, working in manual occupations. Neither high educational level nor high-level employment appear to be important. The life courses associated with low mortality risk among men combine education to secondary level or higher; initial white-collar employment, followed by promotion to high-level employment or a move to self-employment; and good housing conditions in later life. These results, despite using different methods to analyse different data from a different continent, are broadly similar to those from the US National Longitudinal Survey.

4.4.3 **West of Scotland Collaborative Study**

A third source of comparable information is the West of Scotland Collaborative Study which, in the early 1970s, screened some 5500 male employees, mostly aged 35–64 years, in a representative range of workplaces. Information on cardiovascular health and cardiovascular disease risk factor status was collected, as well as a limited amount of data concerning the earlier stages of life. Twenty-one years of follow-up mortality data were available by the mid-1990s.

In this data set, the conventional risk factors vary in their relationship to the life course (Blane *et al.* 1996). The behavioural risk factors (recreational exercise and cigarette smoking) are related to the subjects' own social class during adulthood, but are not related to their father's social class when they were children. In contrast, most of the physiological risk factors (diastolic blood pressure, serum cholesterol concentration, and forced expiratory volume in one second) are associated with both father's and own social class, but in such a way that the associations are stronger with adulthood than with childhood. One physiological risk factor, body mass index, was related to the father's social class during the subject's childhood, but not to adult class. Broadly similar findings have been described in the Whitehall II Study[5] (Brunner *et al.* 1999). These results can be interpreted as showing that behaviour is determined primarily by current social context (probably the norms of the person's significant others), while physiological status reflects the accumulated influences of both past and present.

The life-course dimension to these analyses was taken a step further by including social class based on first occupation (Davey Smith *et al.* 1997). Each individual now could be assigned to three social class positions: social class during childhood, based on father's occupation; social class at labour market entry, based on own first occupation; and social class during adulthood, based on own occupation at the time of screening. The number of times, between zero and three, that subjects were assigned to manual as opposed to non-manual social classes was related to many aspects of physiological status, with the best health being found among those who had been in non-manual social classes at all three stages of life (Table 4.6). Systolic blood pressure, diastolic blood pressure, serum cholesterol concentration, height, body mass index, forced expiratory volume in one second (FEV_1), and the symptoms of angina and chronic bronchitis were all related in a graded, stepwise fashion to this measure of cumulative lifetime social class. Each move away from thrice non-manual produced worsening health. All-cause mortality during the 21 years of follow-up showed the same relationship with lifetime cumulative class, being more than 50 per cent higher in the group

---

[5] An interesting exception was tobacco smoking among women, where an association with father's social class remained after adjustment for the woman's own socio-economic position; possibly because a woman's social position is more dependent on their class of origin (Marmot *personal communication* 2.9.04).

Table 4.6 Cumulative social class at three stages of life and all-cause mortality among men in the West of Scotland Collaborative Study; relative death rates; (n = 5766)

Cumulative social class	Age adjusted	Age and risk factor adjusted[a]
All three non-manual	1.00	1.00
Two non-manual, one manual	1.29	1.30
Two manual, one non-manual	1.45	1.33
All three manual	1.71	1.57

Source: Davey Smith et al. (1997), adapted from Table 6.

[a] Risk factors: cigarette smoking, diastolic blood pressure, serum cholesterol concentration, body mass index, adjusted FEV_1, angina, bronchitis, and electrocardiogram ischaemia.

assigned to the manual social classes on all three occasions than in those assigned thrice to non-manual classes.

In terms of understanding the causes of the health effects of accumulating disadvantage, it is important to note that adjustment for a range of behavioural and physiological risk factors produces only modest attenuation in the risk of death. This phenomenon—of a gradient in health by the level of social disadvantage accumulated across the life course—may be a general tendency. A similar gradient in long-term illness was found in the ONS Longitudinal Study when disadvantage was measured in terms of both social class and labour market position (Bartley and Plewis 2002). Also, broadly similar results have been described in other countries (Stronks et al. 1996; Pensola 2003; Hallqvist et al. 2004; Naess et al. 2004), although a question remains about the potentially misleading effect of urbanization (Blane 2004).

Further analyses of mortality in the West of Scotland Collaborative Study showed that specific diseases and causes of death may relate to the life course in different ways (Davey Smith et al. 1998). Some causes of death (cancers—apart from stomach and lung, accidents, and violence) are related to adult, but not to childhood, social class. Most of the other prevalent causes of death (coronary heart disease, stroke, lung cancer, stomach cancer, and respiratory disease) are related independently to both childhood and adult social class. Adjustment for adult socio-economic circumstances and adult risk factors: eliminates the association between lung cancer and childhood class; attenuates the relationship of childhood class with death due to coronary heart disease and respiratory disease; but does not alter the relationship between childhood class and stroke and stomach cancer. In other words, stroke and stomach cancer mortality in adulthood appear to be associated to an unusual extent, and independently of any continuity of social disadvantage throughout life, with adverse socio-economic circumstances during childhood.

The fall during the twentieth century in deaths due to stomach cancer and stroke is unexplained, although refrigeration, with the consequent diminution in consumption of salted, smoked, and pickled foods, has long been suspected (Charlton and Murphy 1997).

A different explanation, however, is suggested by the finding that these causes of death during adulthood are related strongly to childhood deprivation. A concern with childhood poverty was a constant theme of twentieth-century social policy and social science (Hall *et al.* 1978). Key developments and events have included:

1   At the turn of the century—Rowntree's surveys of poverty; the 1904 Interdepartmental Committee; and the introduction of school meals.

2   In the 1930s—Eleanor Rathbone's Family Endowment Society and its campaign for family allowances; and the study of child nutrition by the British Medical Association and Boyd Orr at the Rowett Institute.

3   During the Second World War—food rationing policy; and the Beveridge Report.

4   Post-war—the welfare state.

If adult mortality due to stomach cancer and stroke is unusually sensitive to deprivation earlier in childhood, the long fall in mortality from these causes could be an unintended consequence of the series of scientific studies and policy initiatives which have progressively reduced childhood deprivation. Aetiological mechanisms, other than reduced consumption of salted and pickled foods, would be required; height (in the case of stroke) and *Helicobacter pylori* infection (in the case of stomach cancer) have been suggested (Davey Smith *et al.* 1998).

4.4.4 Boyd Orr cohort

The Boyd Orr cohort derives from a survey of diet and health that was conducted in 16 locations in England and Scotland during 1937–39. Socio-economic information and detailed dietary information was collected, and a detailed medical examination was made on the children of each household. Eighty-five per cent (N = 4211) of these children were retraced successfully in the mid-1990s, of whom 696 had died (Gunnell *et al.* 1996). Various aspects of these children's health and nutrition have been shown to influence their adult mortality risk (Gunnell *et al.* 1998a,b; Frankel *et al.* 1998).

In 1996, a random sample, stratified by childhood socio-economic circumstances, was drawn from the full Boyd Orr cohort, for more complete life-course investigation (Blane *et al.* 1999c). Retrospective information about the period 1937–39 to 1997–98 was collected by life-grid interview, and physiological measurements were made. The process of life-course accumulation of social advantage or disadvantage was described in relation to this stratified random sample in section 4.3.1. The effect of social accumulation on the health of these cohort members was investigated in terms of slow physical growth in childhood, exposure to low job control in adulthood, and raised blood pressure in early old age (Montgomery *et al.* 2000). Physical growth during childhood was estimated by including, in the same model, both childhood and adult height, measured in, respectively, 1937–39 and 1997–98. (Only those aged between five and eight were included in the analyses, in order to avoid the pubertal growth spurt.)

Table 4.7 Systolic blood pressure in early old age and childhood and adult heights; those male and female members of a stratified random sample of the Boyd Orr cohort who were aged 5–8 years in 1937–39 (N=149); heights divided into fifths of their distribution

	Model A		Model B	
	Mean difference* (95% confidence interval)	p value	Mean difference* (95% confidence interval)	p value
Childhood height				
Shortest 1	29.0 (14.9, 43.1)	0.000	28.5 (5.6, 51.5)	0.015
2	14.6 (1.1, 28.2)	0.035	13.9 (−5.3, 33.1)	0.16
3	13.8 (−0.7, 28.3)	0.06	12.3 (−7.8, 32.4)	0.23
4	11.8 (−1.4, 25.0)	0.08	10.2 (−7.7, 28.2)	0.26
Tallest 5	0.0		0.0	
Adult height				
Shortest 1	19.3 (5.8, 32.9)	0.006	0.7 (−20.0, 21.5)	0.94
2	15.1 (1.7, 28.4)	0.027	1.2 (−17.6, 20.0)	0.90
3	12.8 (−0.2, 25.8)	0.054	2.8 (−14.4, 20.0)	0.75
4	10.7 (−2.4, 23.7)	0.11	3.8 (−12.0, 19.6)	0.64
Tallest 5	0.0		0.0	

Source: Montgomery *et al.* (2000), adapted from Table 1. * mmHg above reference group (tallest fifth).

Model A: adjusted for age, sex, BMI, hypertensive medication, childhood factors (health, BMI, food expenditure, household crowding, father's social class), adult factors (number of years of tobacco smoking, number of years with low job control, social class), and factors in early old age (welfare benefit status, current tobacco smoking, car ownership); childhood height and adult height modelled separately.

Model B: as model A, but childhood height and adult height included in the same model.

Separately, after adjustment for a wide range of child and adult socio-demographic and socio-economic characteristics, both childhood and adult height were related to systolic blood pressure, with those in the shortest fifth of both height distributions being at particular risk. When both childhood and adult height were included in the same model, only the relationship between the shortest child height and raised systolic blood pressure in early old age remained (Table 4.7). The same results were found when pulse pressure was examined (the results for diastolic blood pressure were in the same direction, but failed to reach conventional levels of statistical significance).

Childhood height had been shown to predict forward among women to the number of years during adulthood spent in occupations with low job control (Holland *et al.* 2000). The small number of subjects who were in both the shortest childhood height group and had accumulated, as an adult, the largest number of years with low job control showed adjusted relative increases of 35.2 mmHg (95% CI 6.0, 64.4; p=0.02) and 25.8 mmHg (95% CI 3.5, 48.2; p=0.02) for systolic blood pressure and pulse pressure respectively (Montgomery *et al.* 2000). Taken together, these results were interpreted as evidence that pre-pubertal growth rate, perhaps as a critical period effect, is associated with the formation of mechanisms involved in the control of blood pressure in later life. As well as this critical period effect, it may be that the material and psychosocial conditions which produce slow child growth also are indicating a particularly disadvantaged life course trajectory that includes increased exposure to low job control; and that slow physical growth during childhood may interact with low job control during adulthood to raise further the systolic blood pressure and pulse pressure in early old age.

Finally, it is worth noting that there may be considerable heterogeneity in the way life-course processes influence the various aspects of health in early old age. Blood pressure in early old age, as we have seen, may be influenced by a childhood factor (physical growth), possibly in interaction with an adult factor (job control). In contrast, in the full Boyd Orr cohort, the consumption, in early old age, of a healthy diet (Maynard *et al.* 2005) appears to be influenced primarily by contemporaneous factors, although some life-course influences can be identified qualitatively (Blane *et al.* 2003) and one childhood factor (level of vegetable consumption during childhood) has an independent association at conventional levels of statistical significance with a healthy diet in early old age (Maynard *et al.* 2004).

The relationship to the life course appears to be attenuated further in the case of quality of life in early old age. Although some influences from adulthood can be identified in the Boyd Orr stratified random sample (Blane *et al.* 2004), quality of life in early old age in this data set appears to be influenced primarily by contemporaneous factors acting in early old age (Wiggins *et al.* 2004). It is possible that life-course influences are strongest where they can be objectified physiologically, in the form of health; of intermediate influence, where they shape preferences and taste; and of smallest direct influence, on psychological reactions to everyday life.

4.4.5 In summary

The US National Longitudinal Survey, the Norwegian record linkage data set, the West of Scotland Collaborative Study, and the UK Boyd Orr cohort provide the first information about the types of life course which are associated with physiological damage and premature death in late middle age and early old age. Many of the characteristics of these life courses might be suspected from cross-sectional studies—poor material and psychosocial circumstances during childhood, for example; the statutory minimum schooling; first employment in the low-skilled or secondary labour market; and occupational and residential deprivation during adulthood.

A life-course perspective adds new insights to the cross-sectional picture. There does not appear to be a phase of life which has special priority for health status and the risk of premature death in the high morbidity/high mortality age groups. Each phase of life appears capable of adding its own protection or disadvantage. Behaviour may be the most malleable form of protection or disadvantage, in the sense that it can respond to the norms of the person's current social context, while physiological status accumulates the results of past events, habits, and hazardous exposures. Second, the elements of the life course appear to be interdependent: educational attainment is a major transmission belt for the long-term effects of childhood circumstances; and family assets are a major component of the effects of adult occupation. Finally, the general advantage or deprivation associated with a social class position would appear to have a sizeable long-term influence on health, over and above the effect of the generally recognized behavioural and physiological risk factors; and the various phases of the life course may have different weights for different diseases and causes of death.

4.5 **Policy implications**

The life-course perspective has important implications for social policy making in relation to health—implications which are additional to the need to deal with immediate threats to health, such as disadvantage of income (Morris *et al.* 2002; Morris and Deeming 2004) and housing (Blane *et al.* 2000; Mitchell *et al.* 2002). Bartley and colleagues have drawn on the biological concept of *critical periods* (when if anything goes wrong, permanent damage can result) to coin the analogous concept of *critical social transitions*, by which they mean a life-course change in social status, the outcome of which can have long-term effects on future life chances (Bartley *et al.* 1997). Such transitions include the move from primary to secondary school, labour market entry, establishing own residence, occupational change, onset of chronic illness, and retirement from paid employment. The life course relates in two ways to these critical social transitions.

First, previous levels of accumulated advantage or disadvantage influence whether or not some types of transition, such as those associated with tertiary education, redundancy, and early chronic disease, will occur. The relationship between parental social class and the chances of admission to a university education (Halsey 1988) and the considerably higher risk of redundancy associated with manual as opposed to non-manual employment (Gershuny and Marsh 1994) are well documented. The 1946 British birth cohort study provides a more detailed understanding of the life- course antecedents of the transition to physical disability during early middle age (Kuh *et al.* 1994). Father's social class during the subject's childhood is the strongest early life predictor of the chances of being physically disabled by age 43 years; and this early disadvantage is transmitted into later life primarily through educational attainment and occupational social class location in early adulthood. The effects, in terms of loss of income and employment, of becoming physically disabled in early middle age are, in turn, considerably greater for those with less advantaged pasts.

Second, previous levels of accumulated advantage or disadvantage also influence whether a critical transition results in a favourable or an unfavourable outcome. As mentioned, previous disadvantage makes labour market exclusion more likely after the early onset of chronic disease (Bartley and Owen 1996). Similarly, the more favourable routes out of redundancy, such as retraining, new skills, and re-employment in a perhaps better-paid occupation, are more likely among those with educational qualifications and a family and social network which can offer encouragement and temporary financial support. Conversely, redundancy following previous disadvantage is more likely to result in either long-term unemployment or casual re-employment in the insecure and hazardous secondary labour market (Walker *et al.* 1985).

In the past, social policy has assumed implicitly that these critical social transitions are distributed randomly and, over the long term, approximately equally among the population; and consequently, that protection against them can be financed by social insurance, in which everyone saves a little during the good times to prevent destitution if and when misfortune strikes. A life- course perspective identifies the flaw in this 'safety net' approach to social welfare. Those at greatest risk of misfortune (say, redundancy and unemployment) are least likely to have previously enjoyed stable employment and hence are least likely to have accumulated sufficient insurance contributions to finance the welfare benefits that they require (Sinfield 1981). As a result, those most in need of a safety net are least able to provide one.

The life-course perspective identifies a further limitation of the traditional 'safety net' approach. Adversity is not randomly distributed; instead it tends to cluster and to accumulate present on top of past disadvantage. Consequently, any single misfortune tends to identify the most vulnerable individuals who have accumulated the greatest number of previous handicaps. What is required is not so much a safety net which allows the individual to re-establish their habitual life, but a 'springboard' which also repairs the damage caused by past disadvantage. A modernized social policy which took account of life-course influences would recognize that:

1 Critical social transitions identify at-risk individuals who, in the absence of effective interventions, are likely to require frequent and, cumulatively over a lifetime, considerable welfare, health, and social support.

2 Effective policy interventions require not only safety nets, to prevent the accumulation of further disadvantage, but also springboards to repair past damage and set people on a more advantaged life trajectory.

Another policy implication of the life-course perspective comes from its complexity, where the relative importance of its different stages depends upon whether one is interested in, for example, physiological status or behaviour or quality of life, or cardiovascular disease or stomach cancer. Given these complex variations, it is sensible to treat each of the phases of the life course as equally important to overall health, and not to prioritize any one stage. Disadvantage is cumulative, so the move to a more advantaged trajectory can be made at any age. Late middle age and early old age are key age groups for social policy because of their impact on health and welfare expenditure. What is important in terms of the least physiological damage and the lowest risk of premature death at these ages, the evidence suggests, is the proportion of the life course spent in advantaged social positions: best is lifelong advantage; worst is lifelong disadvantage; and intermediate is anything which, for some proportion of life, has shifted the life course from the latter to the former trajectory. In this sense, it is never too late, and always good sense, for social policy to offer a 'helping hand'.

Acknowledgements

Dr Blane's research is supported by an Economic and Social Research Council Priority Research Network , Grant Number L326253061.

References

Acheson, D., Barker, D., Chambers, J., Graham, H., Marmot, M., and Whitehead, M. (1998). *Independent inquiry into inequalities in health*. The Stationery Office, London.

Barker, D.J.P. (1994). *Mothers, babies and disease in later life*. BMJ Publishing, London.

Bartley, M. (2004). *Health inequality: an introduction to theories, concepts and methods*. Polity Press, Cambridge.

Bartley, M. and Owen, C. (1996). Relation between socioeconomic status, employment and health during economic change, 1973–93. *BMJ* **313**, 445–9.

Bartley, M. and Plewis, I. (1997). Does health-selective mobility account for socioeconomic differences in health? Evidence from England and Wales, 1971 to 1991. *J. Hlth. Soc. Behav.* **38**, 376–86.

Bartley, M. and Plewis, I. (2002). Accumulated labour market disadvantage and limiting long-term illness: data from the 1971–1991 Office for National Statistics Longitudinal Study. *Int. J. Epidemiol.* **31**, 336–41.

Bartley, M., Blane, D., and Montgomery, S. (1997). Health and the life course: why safety nets matter. *BMJ* **314**, 1194–6.

Bartley, M., Power, C., Blane, D., Davey Smith, G., and Shipley, M. (1994). Birth weight and later socioeconomic disadvantage: evidence from the 1958 British cohort study. *BMJ* **309**, 1475–8.

Belli, R.F. (1998). The structure of autobiographical memory and the event history calendar: potential improvements in the quality of retrospective reports in surveys. *Memory* **6**, 383–406.

Belli, R.F. (2000). Computerised event history calendar methods: facilitating autobiographical recall. *Proceedings of the Section on Survey Research Methods*, American Statistical Association.

Berkman L.F. and Kawachi I. (eds) (2000). *Social epidemiology*. Oxford University Press, Oxford.

Berney, L.R. and Blane, D. (2004). The life grid method of collecting retrospective information from people at older ages. *Research Policy and Planning* **21**, 13–21.

Berney, L., Blane, D., Davey Smith, G., Gunnell, D., Holland, P., and Montgomery, S. (2000). Socioeconomic measures in early old age as indicators of previous lifetime exposure to environmental health hazards. *Sociol. Hlth. Illness* **22**, 415–30.

Blane, D. (2004). Urbanisation and the life course. *Int. J. Epidemiol.* **33**, 1–2.

Blane, D., Abraham, L., Gunnell, D., Maynard, M., and Ness, A. (2003). Background influences on dietary choices in early old age. *J. Royal Soc. Promotion Hlth.* **123**, 204–9.

Blane, D, Bartley, M., and Davey Smith, G. (1997). Disease aetiology and materialist explanations of socioeconomic mortality differentials. *Eur. J. Publ. Hlth* **7**, 385–91.

Blane, D., Bartley, M., and Mitchell, R. (2000). The 'Inverse Housing Law' and respiratory health. *J. Epidemiol. Commun. Hlth.* **54**, 745–9.

Blane, D., Berney, L., Davey Smith, G., Gunnell, D., and Holland, P. (1999c). Reconstructing the life course: a 60 year follow-up study based on the Boyd Orr cohort. *Public Health* **113**, 117–24.

Blane, D., Davey Smith, G., and Hart, C. (1999a). Some social and physical correlates of intergenerational social mobility: evidence from the West of Scotland Collaborative Study. *Sociology* **33**, 169–83.

Blane, D., Harding, S., and Rosato, M. (1999b). Does social mobility affect the size of the socioeconomic mortality differential? Evidence from the Office for National Statistics Longitudinal Study. *J. Roy. Stat. Soc.* **162**, 59–70.

Blane, D., Hart, C.L., Davey Smith, G., Gillis, C., Hole, D.J., and Hawthorne, V.M. (1996). Association of cardiovascular disease risk factors with socioeconomic position during childhood and during adulthood. *BMJ* **313**, 1434–8.

Blane, D., Higgs, P., Hyde, M., and Wiggins, R. (2004). Life course influences on quality of life in early old age. *Soc. Sci. Med.* **58**, 2171–9.

Brunner, E., Shipley M.J., Blane D., Smith G.D., and Marmet M.G. (1999). When does cardiovascular risk start? Past and present socioeconomic circumstances and risk factors in adulthood. *J. Epidemiol. Commun. Hlth.* **53**, 757–64.

Burstrom, B. and Whitehead, M. (2000). Inequality in the social consequences of illness: how do people with long-term illness fare in the British and Swedish labour markets? *Int. J. Hlth. Services* **30**, 435–51.

Cambois, E. (2004). Careers and mortality in France: evidence on how far occupational mobility predicts differentiated risks. *Soc. Sci. Med.* **58**, 2545–58.

Caselli, G., Duchene, J., Egidi, V., Santini, A., and Wunch, G. (1991). A matter of life and death: methodologies for studying the life history analysis of adult mortality. In: *Socioeconomic differential mortality in industrialised countries*, Vol. 7, pp. 242–77. Comité International de Cooperation dans les Recherches Nationales en Demographie (CICRED), Paris.

Chandola, T., Bartley, M., Sacker, A., Jenkinson, C., and Marmot, M. (2003). Health selection in the Whitehall II Study. *Soc. Sci. Med.* **56**, 2059–72.

Charlton, J. and Murphy, M. (ed.) (1997). *The health of adult Britain*. HMSO, London.

Dannefer, D. (2003). Cumulative advantage/disadvantage and the life course: cross-fertilizing age and social science theory. *J. Gerontology* **58B**, S327–S337.

Davey Smith, G., Hart, C.L., Blane, D., Gillis, C., and Hawthorne, V.M. (1997). Lifetime socioeconomic position and mortality: prospective observational study. *BMJ* **314**, 547–52.

Davey Smith, G., Hart, C., Blane, D., and Hole, D. (1998). Adverse socioeconomic conditions in childhood and cause specific adult mortality: prospective observational study. *BMJ* **316**, 1631–5.

Drever, F. and Whitehead, M. (1997). *Health inequalities*. The Stationery Office, London.

Elstad, J.I. (2001). Health-related mobility, health inequalities and gradient constraint: discussion and results from a Norwegian study. *Eur. J. Public Hlth.* **11**, 135–40.

Elstad, J.I. (2003). Social causation, health-selective mobility and the reproduction of socioeconomic health inequalities over time: panel study of adult men. *Soc. Sci. Med.* **57**, 1475–89.

Frankel, S.J., Gunnell, D.G., Peters, T.J., Maynard, M., and Davey Smith, G. (1998). Childhood energy intake and adult mortality from cancer: the Boyd Orr cohort study. *BMJ* **316**, 499–504.

Gershuny, J. and Marsh, C. (1994). Unemployment in work histories. In: *Social change and the experience of unemployment* (ed. D. Gallie, C. Marsh, and C. Vogler), pp. 66–114. Oxford University Press, Oxford.

Giele, J.Z. and Elder, G.H. (ed.) (1998). *Methods of life course research: qualitative and quantitative approaches*. Sage, London.

Gliksman, M.D., Kawachi, I., Hunter, D., Colditz, G.A., Manson J.A.E., and Stampfer, M.J. (1995). Childhood socioeconomic status and risk of cardiovascular disease in middle aged US women: a prospective study. *J. Epidemiol. Commun. Hlth.* **49**, 10–15.

Gunnell, D.J., Davey Smith, G., Frankel, S.J., Nanchahal, K., Braddon, F.E.M., Pemberton, J., *et al.* (1998b). Childhood leg length and adult mortality: follow-up of the Carnegie (Boyd Orr) Survey of Diet and Health in pre-war Britain. *J. Epidemiol. Commun. Hlth.* **52**, 142–52.

Gunnell, D.J., Frankel, S., Nanchahal, K., Braddon, F.E.M., and Davey Smith, G. (1996). Lifecourse exposure and later disease: a follow-up study based on a survey of family diet and health in pre-war Britain (1937–39). *Public Health* **110**, 85–94.

Gunnell, D.J., Frankel, S.J., Nanchahal, K., Peters, T.J., and Davey Smith, G. (1998a). Childhood obesity and adult cardiovascular mortality: a 57 year follow-up study based on the Boyd Orr cohort. *Am. J. Clin. Nutr.* **67**, 1111–18.

Hall, P., Land, H., Parker, R., and Webb, A. (1978). The introduction of family allowances. In: *Change choice and conflict in social policy* (ed. P. Hall, H. Land, R. Parker, and A. Webb), pp. 157–230. Heinemann, London.

Hallqvist, J., Lynch, J., Bartley, M., Lange, T., and Blane, D. (2004). Can we disentangle life course processes of accumulation, critical period and social mobility? An analysis of disadvantaged socio-economic positions and myocardial infarction in the Stockholm Heart Epidemiology Program. *Soc. Sci. Med.* **58**, 1555–62.

Halsey, A.H. (1988). *British social trends since 1900*. Macmillan, Basingstoke.

Hardy, R., Wadsworth, M.E.J., Langenberg, C., and Kuh, D. (2004). Birthweight, childhood growth and blood pressure at 43 years in a British birth cohort. *Int. J. Epidemiol.* **33**, 121–9.

Hart, C., Smith, G.D., and Blane, D. (1998). Social mobility and 21 year mortality in a cohort of Scottish men. *Soc. Sci. Med.* **47**, 1121–30.

Heady, J.A., Morris, J.N., Kegan, A., and Raffle, P.A.B. (1961). Coronary heart disease in London busmen. *Br. J. Prevent. Soc. Med.* **15**, 143–53.

Holland, P., Berney, L., Blane, D., Davey Smith, G., Gunnell, D., and Montgomery, S. (2000). Life course accumulation of disadvantage. *Soc. Sci. Med.* **50**, 1285–95.

Karvonen, S., Rimpela, A.H., and Rimpela, M.K. (1999). Social mobility and health related behaviours in young people. *J. Epidemiol. Commun. Hlth.* **53**, 211–17.

Kuh, D.L.J. and Ben Shlomo, Y. (ed.) (2004). *A life course approach to chronic disease epidemiology* (2nd edn). Oxford University Press, Oxford.

Kuh, D.J.L., Hardy R., Langenberg C., Richards, M., and Wadsworth, M.E.J. (2002). Mortality in adults aged 26–54 years related to socioeconomic conditions in childhood and adulthood: post-war birth cohort study. *BMJ* **325**, 1076–80.

Kuh, D.L.J., Wadsworth, M.E.J., and Yusuf, E.J. (1994). Burden of disability in a post war birth cohort in the UK. *J. Epidemiol. Commun. Hlth.* **48**, 262–9.

Langenberg C., Hardy R., Kuh D.L.J., Brunner E., and Wadsworth, M.E.J. (2003). Central and total obesity in middle aged men and women in relation to lifetime socioeconomic status: evidence from a national birth cohort. *J. Epidemiol. Commun. Hlth.* **57**, 816–22.

Lawlor D.A., Ebrahim S., Davey Smith, G. (2002). Socioeconomic position in childhood and adulthood and insulin resistance. *BMJ* **325**, 805–10.

Mare, R.D. (1990). Socioeconomic careers and differential mortality among older men in the United States. In: *Measurement and analysis of mortality: new approaches* (ed. J. Vallin, S. D'Souza, and A. Palloni), pp. 362–87. Clarendon Press: Oxford.

Marmot, M.G. and Wadsworth, M.E.J. (ed.) (1997). Fetal and early childhood environment: long-term health implications. *Br. Med. Bull.* **53**, (Issue 1).

Maynard, M., Gunnell, D., Abraham, L., Blane, D., Bates, C., and Ness, A. (2005). Selecting a healthy diet score: lessons from a study of diet and health in early old age (the Boyd Orr cohort). *Public Health Nutrition* **8**, 321–6.

Maynard, M., Gunnell, D., Abraham, L., Ness, A., Bates, C., and Blane, D. (2004). What influences diet in early old age? Prospective and cross-sectional analyses of the Boyd Orr cohort. *Eur. J. Public Hlth.* (forthcoming).

Mitchell, R., Blane, D., and Bartley, M. (2002). Elevated risk of high blood pressure: climate and the inverse housing law. *Int. J. Epidemiol.* **31**, 831–8.

Montgomery, S.M., Bartley, M.J., Cook, D.G., and Wadsworth, M.E.J. (1996). Health and social precursors of unemployment in young men in Great Britain. *J. Epidemiol. Commun. Hlth.* **50**, 415–22.

Montgomery, S., Bartley, M., and Wilkinson, R. (1997). Family conflict and slow growth. *Arch. Dis. Child.* **77**, 326–30.

Montgomery, S., Berney, L., and Blane, D. (2000). Pre-pubertal growth and blood pressure in early old age. *Arch. Dis. Child.* **82**, 358–63.

Morris, J.N. and Deeming, C. (2004). Minimum incomes for healthy living (MIHL): next thrust for UK social policy? *Policy and Politics* **32**, 441–54.

Morris, J.N., Donkin, A.J.M., Wonderling, D., Wilkinson, P., and Dowler, E.A. (2002). A minimum income for healthy living. *J. Epidemiol. Commun. Hlth.* **54**, 885–9.

MRC Vitamin Study Research Group (1991). Prevention of neural tube defects: results of the Medical Research Council Vitamin Study. *Lancet* **338**, 131–7.

Naess, O., Claussen, B., Thelle, D., and Davey Smith, G. (2004). Cumulative deprivation and cause-specific mortality: a census based study of life course influences over three decades. *J. Epidemiol. Commun. Hlth.* **58**, 599–603.

Notkola, V., Punsar, S., Karvonen, M.J., and Haapakoski, J. (1985). Socioeconomic conditions in childhood and mortality and morbidity caused by coronary heart disease in adulthood in rural Finland. *Soc. Sci. Med.* **21**, 517–23.

Pensola, T. (2003). *From past to present: effect of lifecourse on mortality and social class. Differences in mortality in middle adulthood.* The Population Research Institute, Helsinki.

Power, C., Bartley, M., Davey Smith, G., and Blane, D. (1996). Transmission of social and biological risk across the life course. In: *Health and social organisation* (ed. D. Blane, E. Brunner, and R. Wilkinson), pp. 188–203. Routledge, London.

Power, C., Manor, O., and Leah, L. (2002b). Are inequalities in height underestimated by adult social position? *BMJ* **325**, 131–4.

Power C., Manor O., and Matthews S. (2003). Child to adult socioeconomic conditions and obesity in a national cohort. *Int. J. Obes. Relat. Metab. Disord.* **27**, 1081–6.

Power C., Stansfeld S., Matthews S., Manor O., and Hope S. (2002a). Childhood and adulthood risk factors for socioeconomic differentials in psychological distress: evidence from the 1958 British birth cohort study. *Soc. Sci. Med.* **55**, 1989–2004.

Salhi, M., Caselli, G., Duchene, J., *et al.* (1995). Assessing mortality differentials using life histories: a method and applications. In: *Adult mortality in developed countries: from description to explanation* (ed. A.D. Lopez, G. Caselli, and T. Valkonen), pp. 57–79. Clarendon Press, Oxford.

Sinfield, R.A. (1981). *What unemployment means.* Martin Robertson, Oxford.

Smithells, R.W., Sheppard, S. and Schorah, C.J. (1976). Vitamin deficiencies and neural tube defects. *Arch. Dis. Child.* **51**, 944–50.

Stronks, K., van de Mheen, H. and Looman, C.W.N. (1996). Behavioural and structural factors in the explanation of socioeconomic inequalities in health: an empirical analysis. *Sociol. Hth. Illness* **18**, 653–74.

van de Mheen, H., Stronks, K., and Mackenbach, J. (1998). A life course perspective on socioeconomic inequalities in health. In: *The sociology of health inequalities* (ed. M. Bartley, D. Blane, and G. Davey Smith), pp. 193–216. Blackwell, Oxford.

Wadsworth, M.E.J. (1997). Health inequalities in the life course perspective. *Soc. Sci. Med.* **44**, 859–70.

Walker, A., Noble, I., and Westergaard, J. (1985). From secure employment to labour market insecurity. In: *New approaches to economic life* (ed. B. Roberts, R. Finnegan, and D. Gallie), pp. 1947. Manchester University Press, Manchester.

Wamala, S., Lynch, J., and Kaplan, G.A. (2001). Women's exposure to early and later socioeconomic disadvantage and coronary heart disease risk: the Stockholm Female Coronary Risk Study. *Int. J. Epidemiol.* **30**, 275–84.

Wiggins, R., Higgs, P., Hyde, M., and Blane, D. (2004). Quality of life in the third age: key predictors of the CASP-19 measure. *Aging and Society* (forthcoming).

Wilkinson, R.G. (1996). *Unhealthy societies: the afflictions of inequality*. Routledge, London.

Wunch, G., Duchene, J., Thiltges, E., and Salhi, M. (1996). Socioeconomic differences in mortality: a life course approach. *Eur. J. Popn.* **12**, 167–85.

Chapter 5

Health and labour market disadvantage: unemployment, non-employment, and job insecurity

Mel Bartley, Jane Ferrie, and Scott M. Montgomery

5.1 **Introduction**

This chapter assembles evidence on the implications for population health of early 21st-century labour market conditions in industrialized nations. It takes an approach informed by the most recent research done on the basis of longitudinal data and, where possible, from studies which include objective measures of both physical and psychological health at more than one point in time. The availability of such data helps to overcome some of the major problems in deciding whether changes in labour market conditions have a health impact sufficient to justify policy debate and response.

What do we mean by 'early 21st-century labour market conditions'? It is generally agreed that although the numbers of people who report themselves as 'unemployed and actively looking for work' has fallen in nations such as the USA and the UK since peaks in the late 1980s, conditions are very different from those of the 1970s. The labour market has to some extent 'polarized' . On the one hand, there are more jobs that require high levels of education and skill in new high-technology industries and, even more, in services such as banking, law, and health care. On the other hand, the jobs available to those without advanced education and training have increasingly become what are known as 'Mac-jobs' (after the Mcdonalds catering empire) (Ritzer 1993). The paradigmatic Mac-job is in the fast food industry and consists of the relatively unskilled work involved in preparing and serving such meals.

In many mainland European nations, however, large-scale replacement of unemployment by low-paid work has not yet taken place. Unemployment rates in Germany and France, for example, are still very high. To some extent it could be said that mainland Europe and Scandinavia 'lag behind' the USA and UK, in that the economic crisis of the 1980s in the latter nations hit mainland Europe and Scandinavia about ten years later. Policy responses to this crisis are, therefore, still to be worked out. It is still an open question as to whether citizens of these nations will experience the rise of low-wage, insecure employment in the place of the old heavy industrial jobs, or whether some innovative economic and social policies will lead to a different course of events. Because there is now this dichotomy between national responses to economic change, this chapter will first review the evidence on the relationship of unemployment to mental and physical health, and then discuss what is known about the health effects of the 'flexible labour market' policies that have been adopted in the USA and UK.

5.2 **Health effects of unemployment**

Research has repeatedly shown a higher prevalence of ill health (Cook 1982; Bartley 1987, 1991, 1994; Korpi 2001) and excess mortality (Iversen *et al.* 1987; Moser *et al.* 1987, 1990; Morris *et al.* 1994; Harding *et al.* 1998; Mesrine 2000) in men and women who are unemployed. Figs. 5.1 and 5.2 show rates of poor self-rated health by employment status in men and women in England in 1998. Men who are unemployed, and women who are either unemployed or keeping house full time, are more likely to describe their health as generally fair or poor.

Damage to psychological health is also found by the vast majority of studies, an effect which appears to be independent of pre-existing health and to be reversed on re-employment in many cases (Banks and Jackson 1982; Warr 1984; Weich and Lewis 1998; Claussen 1999; Montgomery *et al.* 1999; Jenkins *et al.* 1997). However, it is not a simple step from this observation to a causal relationship between unemployment

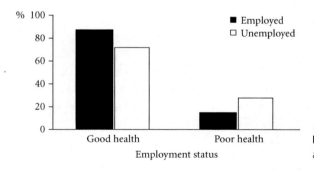

Fig. 5.1 Employment status and health: men.

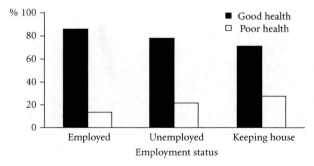

Fig. 5.2 Employment status and health: women.

and health. Those who are ill may be more likely to lose their jobs and find it harder to regain employment (Korpi 2001; Earle 2002). Or there may be indirect effects whereby men and women with other characteristics, such as lower levels of education, which are known to be related to health risks, are also less likely to be employed. When considering the policy implications of the relationship of unemployment to health, it is obviously essential to assess the possibility that this is a consequence of selection (Martikainen and Valkonen 1996).

5.2.1 Selection

Although there is a cross-sectional association of unemployment with illness, physical health does not necessarily decline during a spell of unemployment; a number of studies failed to find an increase in morbidity amongst those who were continuously unemployed for up to 18 months (Bartley 1987, 1991). Those who are ill may be more likely to lose their jobs and find it harder to regain employment, because of their illness. This is known as selection (Valkonen and Martikainen 1995; Mathers and Schofield 1998; Breslin 2003).

The 'direct health selection' hypothesis asserts that poorer health itself increases the risk of unemployment (Bartley 1991; Valkonen and Martikainen 1995; Martikainen & Valkonen 1996, 1998). Ill health has been clearly shown to be a risk for both initial job loss and for subsequent chances of re-employment (Claussen et al. 1993). However, studies where a whole workplace closes down, so that there is no possibility for job loss to be affected by health, have also shown increases in illness in those made redundant (Cobb and Kasl 1977; Beale 1985, 1992; Kivimaki et al. 2000; Ferrie et al. 2001b, 2002).

Another test of the 'direct selection' hypothesis can be made by using longitudinal data on unemployment and mortality (Moser et al. 1990). The number of longitudinal studies of unemployment and mortality is growing slowly, as such data sets require a great deal of effort and cost to collect and maintain. In those which do exist, people who are unemployed at the beginning of any follow-up period are always found to have higher mortality than those who are employed. The question is: could this be because the unemployed are already more likely to have life-threatening illnesses which precede their unemployment? One way of deciding whether this is the case is to examine the trend in mortality over a long period of time. If high mortality in the unemployed was found only because life-threatening diseases were more prevalent in the unemployed than the employed, longitudinal data would show high mortality in the unemployed in the early periods of follow-up, with a sharp decline in mortality rate with increasing length of time. This is because those amongst the unemployed who were ill would eventually all die: if they were the sole reason for the excess risk of death, then the excess mortality in the cohort should disappear at this point.

Research using linked census-based data from England and Wales (the OPCS Longitudinal Study) (Moser et al. 1990; Bethune 1997) and from the Nordic countries (Iversen et al.1987; Martikainen 1990) have not identified this pattern of mortality. On the contrary, the unemployed display a higher risk of mortality no matter how long the cohorts are followed. This finding makes it rather unlikely that direct selection into unemployment of those with life-threatening disease can account for the relationship between unemployment and excess mortality .

There may still be some tendency for those who remain unemployed to be 'different' to those who do not, even if this difference does not take the form of a life-threatening disease (Caspi 1998). Perhaps people at high risk of unemployment may also have certain personality characteristics, for example (this could be the 'factor X' in Fig. 5.3). However, this is a more complex hypothesis, and not necessarily the same as 'selection'. These ideas have to be considered alongside other evidence on the life-course accumulation of social and health disadvantage. Whether or not we consider that there may be differences in the previous life histories of those at higher and lower risk of unemployment, we need to consider the mechanisms through which a relationship to health may occur. The indirect selection hypothesis states that characteristics such as personality traits are 'confounders'. In this case, the mechanism would be that both unemployment and health are related to a certain personality trait. This makes it appear that unemployment is related to health, whereas in fact, the true causal relationship is that by which the personality trait affects both health and unemployment separately. If this is the mechanism, we would find that those with the personality trait were equally likely to develop poor health whether or not they became unemployed, and there should be no greater illness in people who do not possess the relevant trait whether they are employed or unemployed.

One study which has been able to test this hypothesis in relation to mental health is the 1958 British birth cohort study (Montgomery *et al.* 1999). The study contains extensive data on psychological development throughout the school years and young adult life, as well as complete employment histories from leaving school to age 33. It can, therefore, address the possibility that the high level of psychological morbidity found in unemployed men and women is due to a pre-existing vulnerability to poor mental health. The researchers were able to date the onset of symptoms of depression and anxiety which required medical care in cohort members, and relate this to both

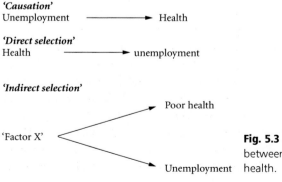

Fig. 5.3 Possible relationships between unemployment and health.

recent unemployment and a measure of the total amount of unemployment which an individual had accumulated since first entering the labour market.

Even after taking into account pre-existing mental health, recent unemployment was clearly related to the onset of symptoms, although in the cohort as a whole, the amount of accumulated past unemployment was not. However, when those with a prior tendency to depression were excluded from the analysis, this had the effect of strengthening the relationship between longer-term accumulation of unemployment and the onset of episodes of depression and anxiety. This showed that it is not only men with pre-existing poor mental health who are vulnerable to the psychologically damaging consequences of job loss. It provides strong evidence that longer-term unemployment causes deterioration in mental health in those who were previously healthy. It was recent, rather than the total amount of unemployment a person experienced, which put him at risk for subsequent deterioration in mental health. This indicates that interventions need initially to be targeted at those who have recently lost their jobs, when the decline in mental health may be steepest. What might be the reasons for this effect of unemployment? Several have been put forward, and here we will consider three of these: poverty; the fact that unemployment is a stressful life event; and changes in health-related behaviours at the time of unemployment.

5.2.2 Poverty

Some research into the relationship between unemployment and ill health has argued for putting poverty back into the centre of the inquiry (Fryer 1992). Low living standards are not an inevitable consequence of unemployment; this is a result of the levels at which benefits are set. During the 1980s, levels of income replacement for the unemployed were lowered. It was argued that under conditions of increasing automation of unskilled and semi-skilled work, levels of benefit available to the unemployed exceeded the market worth of their labour (Gaffikin and Morrisey 1992)—that is, the wage rate which employers were willing to pay. If the level of pay at which an unemployed person will accept new work—the 'reservation wage'—is too high, employers will not take them on. If benefit levels are too high, the state is raising the reservation wage and, therefore, may be contributing to the problem of high unemployment. In the UK, benefits were cut in a number of ways from the early 1980s, and this was indeed followed by a decrease in the real value of the lowest wages and a general redistribution of income away from the poorest sections of society, so that between 1979 and 1991, while the average household experienced an increase in real income of 36%, that of the poorest 10% fell by 14% after housing costs (Sinfield 1993). In 1981, the households in the lowest 10% of the income distribution shared out 4.1% of total income (including benefits and net of direct taxation) in the population between them (this had fallen to 2.9% by 1993), while the richest 10% shared out 21.3% in 1981 and 26.2% in 1993 (Goodman et al. 1997).

Job insecurity, in addition, has the desired effect (according to this model) of aiding the imposition of the 'right to manage'. As well as exerting downward pressure on wages, a shortage of jobs may reduce the propensity of employees to question health and safety provisions, or otherwise assert employment rights.

Many studies link the health effects of unemployment directly to financial problems. Jackson and Warr report that the proportional change in family income between employment and unemployment predicted subjects' scores on the General Health Questionnaire (GHQ), a widely used measure of psychological health (Jackson and Warr 1984). In studies by White and colleagues, long-term unemployed people who had to borrow money in the past year had a risk of depression as measured by GHQ score (4.5) which was more than double that of those who did not have to borrow (2.0). These researchers also found that those obliged to borrow were also more likely to report deterioration in physical health (White 1991). Others have documented the ways in which increasing financial pressures, as savings are used up and worn-out items need to be replaced, are responsible for the growing inactivity and social isolation of many unemployed people (Bradshaw *et al.* 1983). In the OPCS/DSS survey of living standards in unemployment, GHQ scores were related to debt (Heady and Smyth 1989). In the MRC's 1946 cohort study, after financial hardship was controlled for, the relationships between unemployment and psychological symptoms in both men and women were weakened or disappeared (Rodgers 1991). Figs. 5.4 and 5.5 show that among unemployed men, and among both unemployed women and those keeping house only, rates of car and home ownership were lower, and fewer households had central heating in the English health survey in 1993.

These British findings are echoed in other countries. Kessler *et al.* found that financial strain was the strongest mediating factor between unemployment and reported ill health in their American study, being far more important than reduced social integration or an increased number of life events (Kessler *et al.* 1987). A Dutch study found, similarly, that present or anticipated financial problems, as well as loneliness, were the major mediating factors between unemployed status and reported health problems in both men and women (Kleinhesselink and Spruit 1992; Leeflang *et al.* 1992).

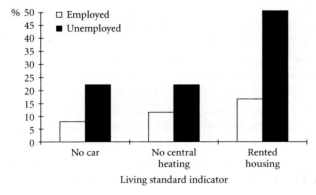

Fig. 5.4 Employment status and living standards: men.

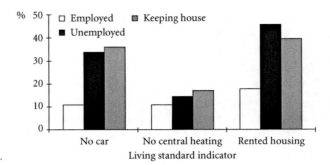

Fig. 5.5 Employment status and living standards: women.

Eventually, it seems, many of the unemployed adapt to straitened financial and social circumstances. Several studies agree that there appears to be no further deterioration in psychological well-being after a period of between one year and 18 months (Warr and Jackson 1985; Hamilton *et al.* 1993). This adds weight to the argument for providing early assistance to those who become unemployed. Other evidence suggests that adaptation to unemployment was accompanied by lowered expectations of oneself, and perhaps a degree of alienation and cynicism. In Warr and Jackson's study, GHQ scores did not deteriorate between 18 and 27 months of continuous unemployment, although they remained at a level far above those of comparable employed samples (Warr and Jackson 1987). The authors compare the adaptive process to that found in institutionalized inmates of prisons or hospitals.

5.2.3 Unemployment as a stressful life event

Research shows job loss to be a highly stressful life event, which has been characterized as a form of bereavement (Fagin and Little 1984). In modern welfare states, starvation and physical privation are no longer thought to accompany the loss of paid work (Gravelle 1985). Many researchers have suggested that work has a number of non-financial benefits to the individual, termed by Jahoda 'latent consequences', and it is the loss of these which results in the threatening character of unemployment (Ezzy 1993). Jahoda's latent consequences of employment included giving a time structure to the day, self esteem, and the respect of others (Jahoda 1979; Fryer 1987). Warr has developed a somewhat similar 'vitamin theory' of the benefits of work for mental health, which include physical and mental activity, use of skills, decision latitude, interpersonal contact, social status, and 'traction' (a reason to go on through the day and from one day to the next) (Warr 1987).

Figure 5.6, based on the English national health survey for 1993, shows low levels of psychological well being, as measured by the GHQ, in both men and women who were unemployed. In the Scandinavian countries, where benefits are relatively generous, and financial effects might not be expected to be as great, similar effects are seen. A study in Stockholm of men with irregular work histories and a variety of problems which

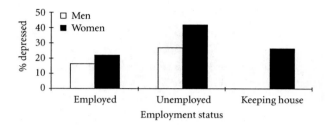

Fig. 5.6 Employment status by depression on GHQ: men and women.

required frequent social service assistance, found that those who were employed, even in low-paid casual jobs, were all more active and integrated (and psychologically healthier) than the unemployed (Isaksson 1989). Amongst unemployed industrial workers in Finland, those who regained work experienced a considerable improvement in psychological health, regardless of their financial circumstances either before or after re-employment (Lahelma 1992). Italian workers laid off from their jobs experienced raised amounts of both psychological and physical illness despite receiving the whole of their normal wage (Rudas *et al.* 1991). These studies provide evidence of the non-financial benefits of work for psychological health. 'Stress' may affect physical health as well as psychological health, as a result perhaps of chronically increased levels of anxiety.

5.2.4 **Health-related behaviour**

There is evidence that unemployment is associated with some forms of health-damaging behaviour, although previous research has yielded inconsistent findings on the link (Cook 1982; Lee *et al.* 1990, 1991; Power and Estaugh 1990; Montgomery *et al.* 1998; Morris *et al.* 1992). Associations between unemployment and health behaviours need to be seen in the context of the longer-term development of health behaviours (Wadsworth *et al.* 1999).

Self-destructive behaviour amongst unemployed men has been widely investigated (Platt 1986; Wilson and Walker 1993; Crawford and Prince 1999; Blakely 2003). In the OPCS Longitudinal Study, men unemployed at the 1971 Census had an SMR[1] for suicide of 236: this excess risk was greatest in those aged 35 to 44 (Moser *et al.* 1990). However, male suicide continued to rise as unemployment fell in the late 1980s (Charlton *et al.* 1993). Parasuicide ('attempted suicide') has also been found to be higher in unemployed men (Platt and Kreitman 1985; Platt 1986). There seems to be agreement that it is not unemployment per se which precipitates suicidal behaviour. Rather, as Kessler *et al.* have also found in their American studies, unemployment increases the likelihood of other adverse life events and lessens the psychological and social resources needed to cope with these (Kessler *et al.* 1988). Longitudinal research in England and Wales also shows that spells of unemployment have longer-term effects, such as loss of home and marriage breakdown (Fox and Shewry 1988).

---

[1] SMR = Standardized Mortality Ratio.

5.2.5 **Health and labour market 'flexibility'**

The nature and prevalence of unemployment changed dramatically in the UK and USA during the 1990s and early part of the 21st century; officially recorded unemployment decreased. However, this trend was not accompanied by a recovery in the numbers of relatively secure industrial jobs that had disappeared in the recessions of the 1980s. In the USA, unemployment fell as tightening rules for benefit receipt resulted in the take-up of low-paid jobs, many of which are relatively insecure. An increasing number of US citizens must now do more than one job in order to meet the basic costs of life. In the UK, in January 2005, while the numbers claiming unemployment benefits had fallen to under 850,000 (the lowest since 1975), there were around 3 million men of working age who were neither employed nor unemployed in the sense of 'actively seeking work' (National Statistics 2004, 2005). Rather, these people form a new group of 'non-employed'.

The proportion of all men aged 16–64 who were employed in 1971 in the UK was nearly 81%, before the onset of the economic recession of the late 1970s and 1980s. This fell to 68.5% by 1991 (Lindsay and Doyle 2003). The largest group of those without jobs in the early 2000s were not unemployed, but rather economically inactive (that is, not even looking actively for work). The majority of non-employed persons described themselves as unable to work due to ill health. Men without formal qualifications were at far greater risk of long-term work disability of this kind. In 1979, just over 3% of those aged 25–54, without qualification, were inactive due to illness; by 2002, the proportion had risen by almost six times, to over 17% (Nickell and Quintini 2002). Around 50% suffered from disabling conditions of a psychiatric nature (Nickell 2004).

The question therefore arises of the hidden costs of labour market flexibility. In theory, the right of owners and managers of firms to hire and fire without regulation by trade union rights or employment laws could make it more likely that firms will expand their workforces and that more jobs will therefore be provided. Workers with lower levels of job security are thought to be more likely to work hard, so that a 'flexible' labour market may increase national levels of productivity and, thereby, national wealth. However, there are now thought to be other possible effects of these policies on the health and economic activity of the population (Burchell 1999; Bohle *et al.* 2001).

Studies of factory closures in the 1970s, 80s, and 90s consistently found health begins to be affected at the time when people anticipate unemployment but are still at work (Cobb and Kasl 1977; Beale 1985, 1992; Kivimaki *et al.* 2000; Ferrie *et al.* 2001*b*, 2002). Job insecurity and threat of job loss have been found to result in increased psychological disturbance and physiological changes as well as increased need for medical care (Beale 1986; Ferrie *et al.* 2001*a*). In a study in Malmo, Sweden, the relationship between threatened redundancy and psychological and physiological health measures appeared to vary according to the degree of future financial uncertainty. Male shipyard workers aged over 58, threatened with redundancy, who knew that they would be offered relatively generous early retirement settlements, experienced no deterioration in psychological or physical health (Mattiasson *et al.* 1990).

Some studies suggest that low-quality jobs do not necessarily protect physical or mental health: in some cases unsatisfactory jobs can be as depressing as unemployment (Winefield *et al.* 1991; Graetz 1993). In the British Social Change and Economic Life Initiative, those with insecure work who had been obliged to take lower-status jobs in the recent past had a score on the GHQ not significantly different from the unemployed (Burchell 1996).

Job insecurity may also constitute a psychosocial hazard in itself. A recent investigation of the effects of privatization in the British Civil Service took advantage of the availability of detailed physical and psychological screening over a ten-year period during which some departmental functions were sold to the private sector and others were converted into agencies in preparation for privatization. In the department which was entirely sold off to the private sector, a deterioration in health status was seen during the 'period of anticipation' before the finalization of the change (Ferrie *et al.* 1995). Immediately before the sale, significant increases were also seen in cardiovascular risk factors (Ferrie *et al.* 1998*b*). After the sale of this department to the private sector, a follow-up survey found that 40% of respondents were out of employment, and 50% of those in employment were in insecure jobs (Ferrie 1997) (Fig. 5.7). Amongst the other departments in the study which were not completely privatized, the workers most threatened by job insecurity were found to have experienced increases in reported symptoms, long-term illness, and adverse sleep patterns. Those whose civil service departments had been transferred to agency status were also found to have relatively higher blood pressure compared to those untouched by the changes (Ferrie *et al.* 1998*a*).

As evidence gathers on the health effects of job insecurity, there has been relatively little research on what happens to those who are excluded from paid employment due to their state of health. An obvious response to this is that we know these people are ill already, so there is no point in such research. However, a great paradox remains, at least in the UK labour market, that as the health of the working age population improved between 1975 and 2000, in terms of mortality at working ages, the numbers of people unable to work where illness is cited as the reason, tripled. In 1972, over 80% of men with a professional or management occupation, and 70% of semi- or unskilled workers, who reported long-term illnesses, were nevertheless employed. By 1992, around

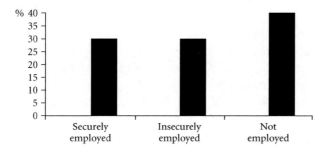

Fig. 5.7 Employment status after PSA privatization.

75% of 'ill' managers and professionals were in paid work but under 50% of 'ill' semi- or unskilled workers (Bartley and Owen 1996). At any given time, the employed labour force includes all sorts of people with varying types of health problem.

What seems to have happened as labour markets became more 'flexible' in the UK was that employers became more demanding of good health in their employees. It is also possible that the new types of employment in service industries were more demanding in terms of psychological adjustment. The 'Mac-job' is more likely to involve close supervision and contact with the public for example, than work on build-ing sites and in mining or shipbuilding. In addition, the old heavy industries had been strongly unionized. Unions and management in many workplaces agreed to move industrially injured workers to less hazardous jobs (for example, miners who began to experience chest pain and breathing difficulties took work above the ground) (Bartley 1991). As the highly-unionized heavy industries disappeared, so did those jobs and working practices.

Perhaps the best way to approach the study of the relationship between health and labour market status is that unemployment and work insecurity are part of a process through which health disadvantage is accumulated over the life course. Research taking this perspective turns away from any simple opposition between 'selection' and 'causa-tion', and shows that unemployment occurs as part of a much longer-term sequence of events in the life of the individual. It is now becoming possible to look at these processes using cohort studies that follow individuals from childhood to middle age. We can see, for example, that those most likely to experience unemployment may also be more vulnerable to excess mortality and morbidity because of earlier experience of hardship and disadvantage. Their experience of unemployment itself, therefore, con-tributes to a process of accumulation of health risks (Montgomery *et al.* 1996; Power and Matthews 1997; Holland *et al.* 2000; Bartley and Plewis 2002).

5.3 Effect of unemployment and job insecurity on population health

A growing body of international comparative research suggests that societies with higher levels of unemployment and job insecurity may actually produce different sorts of life histories in individual members than those that provide larger numbers of secure jobs. It has been all too easy to take for granted some of the effects of quasi-full employment on the wider society, one of the most important of which was that employers carried many of the social overhead costs of labour power. In order to recruit and retain skilful workers in a tight labour market where there are plenty of jobs, most large firms undertook extensive training, recruiting school leavers at an early age into apprenticeships. Schools, therefore, had far fewer restless and unmoti-vated youths to deal with than would otherwise have been the case—benefiting all children in the school. 'Internal labour markets' (the availability of promotion within a firm based on experience rather than on qualifications) offered people the chance to advance in their jobs even in the absence of school qualifications, from a later starting point. Increasing numbers of firms offered occupational pensions, thus raising the living standards of the retired population at little cost to the state (Sinfield 1981).

As part of the 'McDonaldization' of the labour market, the costs of training and of supporting those who are no longer able to work are now increasingly being borne by the individual (the disappearance of apprenticeships and the appearance of student loans, critical illness policies, and private pensions are examples). As we have seen, there has also been an increase in the numbers of persons who have become economically inactive, which in many countries far exceeds the increase in the numbers officially unemployed and seeking work (Nickell 2003). In combination, the increase of insecure, low-paid 'Mac-jobs' and of the numbers of people dependent on long-term sickness benefit also may have had the effect of sharpening overall inequality of income.

The relationship between job insecurity and levels of economic inactivity is seldom considered. It has been assumed that men of working age are inactive because they are ill, and women are keeping house, so that the state of the labour market is not responsible (as it is for unemployment). However, we know that in times of low unemployment, the great majority of men with long-term illness are in fact employed, and thus deriving most of their income from paid work. As unemployment rises, men with some degree of illness are increasingly forced into economic inactivity, and thus into dependency on benefits (Bartley and Owen 1996). The effect of home responsibilities on women's labour force participation is also known to vary widely according to the demand for labour and the supply of child care. As the proportion of working-age men with jobs has declined in the UK, the proportion of women in paid work has risen sharply (Lindsay and Doyle 2003). However, the majority of these jobs are part-time and do not pay a wage sufficient to maintain the living standard of a single individual (let alone a person with dependents). A single adult or sole breadwinner could not afford to accept many of these jobs, as the resultant income would be lower than the level of welfare benefit, given that benefits cover the cost of housing. As wages for lower-paid forms of work drop relative to housing costs, it becomes more dangerous to relinquish benefits in order to accept a job. This is of course especially true if the post is insecure, where a few weeks without pay could result in eviction and homelessness. The city of London has, at the same time, one of the largest number of unfilled vacancies for unskilled work and one of the highest unemployment rates in the UK. The reason for this is that housing costs are so high relative to even the average wage, let alone a low wage, in London, that many workers cannot actually afford to accept the lower-paid jobs that they are offered.

5.4 Policy implications

A full audit of the health impact of rising job insecurity needs to locate paid employment in the life trajectory of individual men and women. The idea of a 'healthy worker', or of a worker with no other demands on their physical and mental resources than employment, is a myth. There is no clear dividing line between good and bad health, even at a single time point. When jobs are scarce, trivial physical or psychological factors may become sources of discrimination (as was found in the 1930s for the wearing of spectacles) (Bartley 1987).

When looking more realistically at human beings passing through the life course, the distinction between 'healthy workers' and 'unhealthy non-workers' seems even more artificial. Biological endowment and material and emotional experiences during childhood confer varying amounts of 'health resources' or 'health potential' to the young person (Dahl and Kjaersgaard 1993). Physical strength must be replaced on a regular basis, hence the importance of reasonable working hours, breaks, and holidays during which energies are renewed. However, leisure time is of less benefit in the renewal of physical health if it is experienced in poor conditions and at the expense of low resources and social stigmatization, as is the case during unemployment.

In the real world, the occupations with more adverse working conditions and lower rates of pay also tend to have higher rates of job insecurity. It is of no surprise, therefore, that the ageing process itself is known to take place at differential rates according to the employment history of the individual: more arduous work being associated with faster ageing (House *et al.* 1994). Unlike physical resources, psychological and social resources are more likely to increase than depreciate with the experiences involved in employment. Deterioration in psychological health during unemployment is therefore more immediate, and improvement on re-employment happens quickly. Stable employment contributes to building up skills, work experience, and social networks, although some forms of work will also have a psychological cost. In youth, important considerations of establishing an independent identity arise, and work is part of this. Entry into stable work is now often preceded by long periods of job insecurity. The process of identity formation is, therefore, far more at risk, with accompanying rises in rates of relationship breakdown, poor mental health, addiction, and accidental and self-inflicted harm.

Work is known to aid the development of secure identity and self-esteem, and to facilitate the formation of stable relationships (Wadsworth 1991). Persons living outside of partnerships are at increased health risk, and unemployment is a major risk factor for relationship breakdown (Jensen 1990; Kinnunen and Pulkkinen 1998). Little research has been done to directly relate the high risk of partnership breakdown in households affected by unemployment to health outcomes, although what there is points clearly to increases in risk for both men and women. Likewise, we know very little about the effects of unemployment in the household on the health of children and their chances of educational and occupational attainment, though once again what we do know is disquieting.

During the 1990s, new cohort data added a considerable amount to our understanding of why unemployment is associated with poor health. We began to see that unemployment takes place as part of a process of accumulation of disadvantage which may begin in childhood, and that a spell of unemployment often occurs as part of a more general pattern of hazardous and insecure work. The old assumptions behind the notion of a social insurance or welfare state 'safety net' are seen to be too simple. To use a metaphor, the people most likely to fall into the net bear a heavier weight of disadvantage than those who are less likely to need its support (Bartley *et al.* 1997).

In the UK, health needs' indices used in the planning of health services have traditionally used unemployment as one factor predictive of high need. However, if policies are designed using average needs' indices which take no account of the impact of chronic job insecurity, this may now be insufficient. Income support levels are determined, as discussed above, with the intention of meeting only the most basic material needs. This takes no account whatever of the fact that those who experience greater amounts of unemployment are likely to carry with them additional burdens produced by earlier disadvantage and hardship. There is a need for 'springboards' rather than mere 'safety nets': positive help in the shape of social, emotional, and improved financial support, as well as the opportunity for education and training. The benefits of such policies would extend beyond individuals themselves during a single spell of unemployment. Policies designed as 'springboards' would automatically work counter to the tendency of unemployment to lower the value of the human resources an individual brings with them to the labour market (Bartley *et al.* 1997).

However, research has not fully kept up with more recent labour market change. Too little is known about other forms of labour market disadvantage such as economic inactivity and prolonged employment in very low-waged work. It is now necessary to take a more global view. Developed industrial nations have reacted in very different ways to the challenges of economic and technological change. Japan, for example, has experienced over a decade of recession with a relatively small increase in unemploy-ment (although to levels unprecedented in that nation's post-war history) and little increase in job insecurity. France and Germany have also resisted the trend towards increasing insecurity at the cost of very high rates of unemployment. Nordic nations have maintained relatively high levels of both employment and job security by main-taining what are regarded as very high levels of taxation. Economic growth appears to be highest in the UK and USA, which have adopted similar policies of labour market deregulation.

This is seen as posing a dilemma for policy makers. How are the possible economic disadvantages of a labour market containing relatively large numbers of secure and well-paid jobs to be weighed against the social advantages? In such a labour market, as the demand for traditional skills reduces, if skilled workers are not willing to settle for lower-paid, less secure 'Mac-jobs', this will result in a high level of unemployment, as we see in Germany. Of course, the idea that traditional skills such as carpentry, plumbing, and welding are no longer in demand is by no means an uncontroversial generalization, but this is how the argument goes. The alternative, at present, is seen as the 'American jobs miracle', where traditional forms of working-class employment have been replaced by lower-paid work in the service economy, such as catering and personal service.

There is a large agenda here for social epidemiology to begin to trace out the implications of these different labour market policies for other factors known to be among the important 'social determinants' of health, such as education, housing, and family formation and stability. In this way, we can assess any possible health costs to be counted against the presumed economic benefits of each different type of solution to the challenges of rapid change.

Acknowledgement

Mel Bartley's work for this chapter was partly supported by ESRC Grant no. RES 000 23 0588.

References

Banks, M.H. and Jackson, P.R. (1982). Unemployment and the risk of minor psychiatric disorder in young people: cross-sectional and longitudinal evidence. *Psychol Med* **12**:189–98.

Bartley, M. (1987). Unemployment and health: causation or selection—a false antithesis? *Sociol Health Illn* **10**:41–67.

Bartley, M. (1991). Health and labour force participation: stress, selection, and the reproduction costs of labour power. *J Soc Policy* **20**:327–64.

Bartley, M. (1994). Unemployment and ill health: understanding the relationship. *J Epidemiol Community Health* **48**(4):333–7.

Bartley, M., Blane, D., and Montgomery, S. (1997). Health and the life course: why safety nets matter. *BMJ* **314**: 1194–9.

Bartley, M. and Owen, C. (1996). Relation between socioeconomic status, employment and health during a time of economic change 1973–1993. *BMJ* **313**:445–8.

Bartley, M. and Plewis, I. (2002). Accumulated labour market disadvantage and limiting long-term illness: data from the 1971–1991 Office for National Statistics' Longitudinal Study. *Int J Epidemiol* **31**:336–41.

Beale, N. (1985). Job loss and family morbidity: a study of a factory closure. *J R Coll Gen Pract* **35**(280):510–4.

Beale, N. (1986). Job loss and family morbidity. *J R Coll Gen Pract* **36**(285):176–7.

Beale, N. (1992). A critical review of the effect of factory closures on health. *Br J Ind Med* **49**(1):70.

Bethune, A. (1997). Unemployment and mortality. In: *Health Inequalities* (ed. M. Drever and M. Whitehead), pp. 156–67. HMSO, London.

Blakely, T.A. (2003). Unemployment and suicide. Evidence for a causal association? *J Epidemiol Community Health* **57**(8):594–600.

Bohle, P., Quinlan, M., and Mayhew, C. (2001). The health and safety effects of job insecurity: an evaluation of the evidence. *Economic and Labour Relations Review* **12**(1):32–60.

Bradshaw, J., Cooke, J., and Godfrey, C. (1983). The impact of unemployment on the living standards of families. *J Soc Policy* **12**:433–52.

Breslin, F.C. (2003). Factors influencing the impact of unemployment on mental health among young and older adults in a longitudinal, population-based survey. *Scand J Work Environ Health* **29**(1):5–14.

Burchell, B. (1996). Who is affected by unemployment? In: *Unemployment and social change* (ed. D. Gallie, C. Marsh, and C. Vogler). Oxford University Press, Oxford.

Burchell, B.J. (1999). The unequal distribution of job insecurity, 1966–86. *International Review of Applied Economics* **13**(3):437–58.

Caspi, A., Wright, B.R.E., Moffitt, T.E., and Silva, P.A. (1998). Early failure in the labor market: childhood and adolescent predictors of unemployment in the transition to adulthood. *Am Sociol Rev* **63**(3):424–51.

Charlton, J., Kelly, S., Dunnell, K., Evans, B., and Jenkins, R. (1993). Suicide deaths in England and Wales: trends in factors associated with suicide deaths. *Popul Trends* **71**:34–42.

Claussen, B. (1999). Health and re-employment in a five-year follow-up of long-term unemployed. *Scand J Public Health* **27**(2):94–100.

Claussen, B., Bjorndal, A., and Hort, P.F. (1993). Health and re-employment in a 2-year follow-up of long-term unemployed. *J Epidemiol Community Health* **47**:14–18.

Cobb, S. and Kasl, S.C. (1977). *Termination: the consequences of job loss.* DHEW-NIOSH Publication no 77–224. US National Institutes for Occupational Safety and Health, Cincinnati.

Cook, D.G., Cummins, R.O., Bartley, M.J., and Shaper, A.G. (1982). Health of unemployed middle-aged men in Great Britain. *Lancet* **1**(8284):1290–4.

Crawford, M.J. and Prince, M. (1999). Increasing rates of suicide in young men in England during the 1980s: the importance of social context. *Soc Sci Med* **49**(10):1419–23.

Dahl, E. and Kjaersgaard, P. (1993). Trends in socioeconomic mortality differentials in post-war Norway—evidence and interpretations. *Sociol Health Illn* **15**(5):587–611.

Earle, A. (2002). What causes job loss among former welfare recipients: the role of family health problems. *J Am Med Womens Assoc* **57**(1):5–10.

Ezzy, D. (1993). Unemployment and mental health: a critical review. *Soc Sci Med* **37**(1):41–52.

Fagin, L. and Little, M. (1984). *The forsaken families.* Penguin Books, Harmondsworth.

Ferrie, J. (1997). Labour market status, insecurity and health. *Journal of Health Psychology* **2**:373–97.

Ferrie, J.E., Martikainen, P., Shipley, M.J., Marmot, M.G., Stansfeld, S.A., and Smith, G.D. (2001*a*). Employment status and health after privatisation in white collar civil servants: prospective cohort study. *BMJ* **25**(1):647–51.

Ferrie, J.E., Shipley, M.J., Marmot, M.G., Martikainen, P., Stansfeld, S., and Davey Smith, G. (2001*b*). Job insecurity in white collar workers: towards an explanation of associations with health. *J Occup Health Psychol* **6**(1):26–42.

Ferrie, J.E., Shipley, M.J., Marmot, M.G., Stansfeld, S., and Davey Smith, G. (1998*a*). The health effects of major organisational change and job insecurity. *Soc Sci Med* **46**(2):243–54.

Ferrie, J.E., Shipley, M.J., Marmot, M.G., Stansfeld, S., and Smith, G.D. (1995). Health effects of anticipation of job change and non-employment: longitudinal data from the Whitehall II study. *BMJ* **311**(7015):1264–9.

Ferrie, J.E., Shipley, M.J., Marmot, M.G., Stansfeld, S.A., and Smith, G.D. (1998*b*). An uncertain future: the health effects of threats to employment security in white-collar men and women. *Am J Public Health* **88**(7):1030–6.

Ferrie, J.E., Shipley, M.J., Stansfeld, S.A., and Marmot, M.G. (2002). Effects of chronic job insecurity and change in job security on self reported health, minor psychiatric morbidity, physiological measures, and health related behaviours in British civil servants: the Whitehall II study. *J Epidemiol Community Health* **54**(5):450–4.

Fox, A.J. and Shewry, M. (1988). New longitudinal insights into relationships between unemployment and mortality. *Stress Med* **4**(1):11–19.

Fryer, D. (1987). Monmouthshire and Marienthal: sociographies of two unemployed communities. In: *Unemployed people* (ed. D. Fryer and P. Ullah). Open University Press, Milton Keynes.

Fryer, D. (1992). A plea for a greater emphasis on the role of poverty in psychological research on unemployment and mental health in the social context. In: *On the mysteries of unemployment* (ed. C.H.A. Verhaar and J.G. Janussen). Kluwer, Amsterdam.

Gaffikin, F. and Morrisey, M. (1992). *The new unemployed: joblessness and poverty in the market economy*. Zed Books, New Jersey.

Goodman, A., Johnson, P., and Webb, S. (1997). *Inequality in the UK*. Oxford University Press, Oxford.

Graetz, B. (1993). Health consequences of employment and unemployment: longitudinal evidence for young men and women. *Soc Sci Med* **36**(6):715–24.

Gravelle, H. (1985). *Does unemployment kill?* Nuffield Trust, York.

Hamilton, V.L., Hoffman, W.S., Broman, C.L., and Rauma, D. (1993). Unemployment, distress and coping: a panel study of autoworkers. *J Pers Soc Psychol* **65**:234–47.

Harding, S., Bethune, A., Maxwell, R., and Brown, J. (1998). Mortality trends using the Longitudinal Study. In: *Health inequality* (ed. F. Drever and M. Whitehead), pp. 143–55. HMSO, London.

Heady, P. and Smyth, M. (1989). *Living standards during unemployment*. HMSO, London.

Holland, P., Berney, L., Blane, D., Smith, G.D., Gunnell, D.J., and Montgomery, S.M. (2000). Life course accumulation of disadvantage: childhood health and hazard exposure during adulthood. *Soc Sci Med* **50**(9):1285–95.

House, J.S., Lepkowski, J.M., Kinney, A.M., Mero, R.P., Kessler, R.C., and Herzog, A.R. (1994). The social stratification of aging and health. *J Health Soc Behav* **35**(3):213–34.

Isaksson, K. (1989). Unemployment, mental health and the psychological functions of work in male welfare clients in Stockholm. *Scand J Soc Med* **17**(2):165–9.

Iversen, L., Andersen, O., Andersen, P.K., Christoffersen, K., and Keiding, N. (1987). Unemployment and mortality in Denmark. *BMJ* **295**:879–84.

Jackson, P.R. and Warr, P.B. (1984). Unemployment and psychological ill-health: the moderating role of duration and age. *Psychol Med* **14**(3):605–14.

Jahoda, M. (1979). The impact of unemployment in the 1930s and the 1970s. *Bull Br Psychol Soc* **32**:309–14.

Jenkins, R., Lewis, G., Bebbington, P., Brugha, T., Farrell, M., Gill, B., *et al.* (1997). The national psychiatric morbidity surveys of Great Britain—initial findings from the household survey. *Psychol Med* **27**(4):775–89.

Jensen, P. (1990). Unemployment and marital dissolution. *J Popul Econ* **3**(3):215–29.

Kessler, R.C., Turner, J.B., and House, J.S. (1987). Intervening processes in the relationship between unemployment and health. *Psychol Med* **17**(4):949–61.

Kessler, R.C., Turner, J.B., and House, J.S. (1988). Effects of unemployment on health in a community survey: main, modifying and mediating effects. *J Soc Issues* **44**:69–85.

Kinnunen, U. and Pulkkinen, L. (1998). Linking economic stress to marital quality among Finnish marital couples—mediator effects. *J Family Issues* **19**(6):705–24.

Kivimaki, M., Vahtera, J., Pentti, J., and Ferrie, J.E. (2000). Factors underlying the effect of organisational downsizing on health of employees: longitudinal cohort study. *BMJ* **320**(7240):971–5.

Kleinhesselink, D.J. and Spruit, I.P. (1992). The contribution of unemployment to socioeconomic health differences. *Int J Epidemiol* **21**(2):329–37.

Korpi, W. (2001). Accumulating disadvantage: longitudinal analyses of unemployment and physical health in representative samples of the Swedish population. *Eur Sociological Rev* **17**(3):255–74.

Lahelma, E. (1992). Unemployment and mental well-being: elaboration of the relationship. *Int J Health Serv* **22**(2):261–74.

Lee, A.J., Crombie, I.K., Smith, W.C., and Tunstall–Pedoe, H.D. (1990). Alcohol consumption and unemployment among men. *Br J Addict* **85**:1156–70.

Lee, A.J., Crombie, I.K., Smith, W.C., Tunstall–Pedoe, H.D. (1991). Cigarette smoking and employment status. *Soc Sci Med* **32**:1309–12.

Leeflang, R.L.I., Klein–Hesselink, D.J., and Spruit, I.P. (1992). Health effects of unemployment II: men and women. *Soc Sci Med* **34**:351–62.

Lindsay, C. and Doyle, P. (2003). Experimental consistent time series of historical Labour Force Survey data. *Labour Market Trends* September 2003:467–75.

Martikainen, P. (1990). Unemployment and mortality among Finnish men. *BMJ* **301**:407–11.

Martikainen, P.T. and Valkonen, T. (1996). Excess mortality of unemployed men and women during a period of rapidly increasing unemployment. *Lancet* **348**(9032):909–12.

Martikainen, P.T. and Valkonen, T. (1998). The effects of differential unemployment rate increases of occupation groups on changes in mortality. *Am J Public Health* **88**(12):1859–61.

Mathers, C.D. and Schofield, D.J. (1998). The health consequences of unemployment: the evidence. *Med J Aust* **168**(4):178–82.

Mattiasson, I., Lindgarde, F., Nilsson, J.A., and Theorell, T. (1990). Threats of unemployment and cardiovascular risk factors: longitudinal study of quality of sleep and serum cholesterol concentrations in men threatened with redundancy. *BMJ* **301**:461–6.

Mesrine, A. (2000). The high death rate among job seekers: a catalyst effect of unemployment? (La surmortalite des chomeurs: un effet catalyseur du chomage?) *Economie et statistique* **33**(4):33–48.

Montgomery, S.M., Bartley, M.J., Cook, D.G., and Wadsworth, M.E.J. (1996). Health and social precursors of unemployment in young men in Great Britain. *J Epidemiol Community Health* **50**(4):415–22.

Montgomery, S.M., Cook, D.G., Bartley, M.J., and Wadsworth, M.E.J. (1998). Unemployment, cigarette smoking, alcohol consumption and body weight in young British men. *Eur J Public Health* **8**(1):21–7.

Montgomery, S.M., Cook, D.G., Bartley, M.J., and Wadsworth, M.E. (1999). Unemployment predates symptoms of depression and anxiety resulting in medical consultation in young men. *Int J Epidemiol* **28**(1):95–100.

Morris, J.K., Cook, D.G., and Shaper, A.G. (1992). Non-employment and changes in smoking, drinking, and body weight. *BMJ* **304**(6826):536–41.

Morris, J.K., Cook, D.G., Shaper, A.G. (1994). Loss of employment and mortality. *BMJ* **308**(6937):1135–9.

Moser, K.A., Goldblatt, P.O., Fox, A.J., and Jones, D.R. (1987). Unemployment and mortality—comparison of the 1971 and 1981 longitudinal study census samples. *BMJ* **294**(6564):86–90.

Moser, K.A., Goldblatt, P.O., Fox, A.J., and Jones, D. (1990). Unemployment and mortality. In: *Longitudinal Study: mortality and social organisation*. HMSO, London.

National Statistics (2005). *Labour market at a glance* (press release), 10 Jan 2005.

National Statistics (2004). *Labour market trends* (Table S9), December 2004.

Nickell, S. (2003). *Poverty and worklessness in Britain*. Royal Economic Society Presidential Address at the RES Conference at Warwick University, Coventry, 8th April 2003.

Nickell, S. (2004). Poverty and worklessness in Britain. *The Economic Journal* **114**:C1–C25.

Nickell, S. and Quintini, G. (2002). The recent performance of the UK labour market. *Oxford Review of Economic Policy* **18**(2):202–20.

Platt, S. (1986). Parasuicide and unemployment. *Br J Psychiatry* **149**:401–5.

Platt, S. and Kreitman, N. (1985). Parasuicide and unemployment among men in Edinburgh 1968–82. *Psychol Med* **15**(1):113–23.

Power, C. and Estaugh, V. (1990). Employment and drinking in early adulthood. *Br J Addict* **85**:487–94.

Power, C. and Matthews, S. (1997). Origins of health inequalities in a national population sample. *Lancet* **350**(9091):1584–9.

Ritzer, G. (1993). *The McDonaldization of society*. Pine Forge Press.

Rodgers, B. (1991). Socio-economic status, employment and neurosis. *Soc Psychiatry Psychiatr Epidemiol* **26**:111–222.

Rudas, N., Tondo, L., Musio, A., and Mosia, M. (1991). Unemployment and depression: results of a psychometric evaluation. *Minerva Psichiatr* **32**:205–9.

Sinfield, A. (1981). *What unemployment means*. Martin Robertson, Oxford.

Sinfield, A. (1993). *Poverty, inequality and justice*. New Waverly Papers No. 6, Edinburgh.

Valkonen, T. and Martikainen, P.T. (1995). The association between unemployment and mortality: causation or selection? In: *Adult mortality in developed countries: from description to explanation* (ed. A. Lopez, G. Caselli, and T. Valkonen), pp. 210–22. Clarendon, Oxford.

Wadsworth, M.E.J. (1991). *The imprint of time*. Oxford University Press, Oxford.

Wadsworth, M.E., Montgomery, S.M., and Bartley, M.J. (1999). The persisting effect of unemployment on health and social well-being in men early in working life. *Soc Sci Med* **48**(10):1491–9.

Warr, P.B. (1984). Reported behaviour changes after job loss. *Br J Soc Psychol* **23**(3):271–5.

Warr, P. (1987). *Work, unemployment and mental health*. Oxford University Press, London.

Warr, P. and Jackson, P. (1985). Factors influencing the psychological impact of prolonged unemployment and of re-employment. *Psychol Med* **15**:795–807.

Warr. P. and Jackson, P. (1987). Adapting to the unemployed role: a longitudinal investigation. *Soc Sci Med* **25**(11):1219–24.

Weich, S. and Lewis, G. (1998). Material standard of living, social class, and the prevalence of the common mental disorders in Great Britain. *J Epidemiol Comm Hlth* **52**(1):8–14.

White, M. (1991). *Against unemployment*. PSI, London.

Wilson, S.H. and Walker, G.M. (1993). Unemployment and health—a review. *Public Health* **107**(3):153–62.

Winefield, A.H., Tiggeman, M., and Goldney, R.D. (1991). The psychological impact of unemployment and unsatisfactory employment in young men and women. *Br J Psychol* **82**:473–80.

Chapter 6

Health and the psychosocial environment at work

Michael Marmot, Johannes Siegrist, and Tores Theorell

6.1 Introduction

There has been a slow recognition that the importance of work for health goes beyond traditional occupational diseases (Schilling 1989). Indeed, it is likely that work makes a greater contribution to diseases and ill health not thought of as 'occupational'. Early research concentrated on the possible role of physical activity in the workplace (Morris *et al.* 1953). Other work, more in the spirit of traditional occupational health, has specified a number of physical and chemical exposures (e.g. lead, carbon disulphide, carbon monoxide, nitroglycerin, nitroglycol) (Schnall *et al.* 2000). More recently, the workplace has been seen as an appropriate setting for health promotion activities, providing the opportunity to influence lifestyles such as smoking, diet, and physical activity, and to conduct screening for disease risk (Breucker and Schroer 1996).

There is now evidence that psychosocial factors at work influence risk of physical and mental illness and may play an important role in contributing to the social gradient in ill health. There have been different approaches to measurement of work stress. Recent research has focused on a few explicit theoretical concepts. Among these, the models of job demand–control (Karasek 1979; Karasek and Theorell 1990) and effort–reward imbalance (Siegrist *et al.* 1986; Siegrist 1996) have received special attention.

A number of different diseases have been related to psychosocial conditions in the workplace, most notably coronary heart disease (CHD), musculoskeletal disorders, and mental illness. This chapter touches on two types of question: the relation between conditions at work and disease; and the contribution this relationship may make to the explanation of variations in disease in society. Because variations in coronary heart disease have been studied extensively, we put special emphasis on that disease, but as the chapter will endeavour to show, other disease end-points are important.

6.2 Changes in the distribution of coronary heart disease

It is worth reviewing the changing distribution of CHD internationally to put into context the possible contribution of work stress to the development of ill health and disease. There have been two major changes in the epidemiology of CHD over recent years:

1 A changing social class distribution of the disease (Marmot 1992);
2 A rise and fall in CHD in different countries (Uemura and Pisa 1988).

In many European countries, as in the USA, as CHD became a mass disease, it rose first in higher socio-economic groups and, subsequently, in lower, to the extent that the social distribution changed to the now familiar pattern of an inverse social gradient: higher rates as the social hierarchy is descended. More recently, the decline in CHD mortality both in the UK and the USA has been enjoyed, to a greater extent, by higher socio-economic groups, leading to a widening of the social gap (White *et al.* 2003; Armstrong *et al.* 2004; Cooper *et al.* 2000). Concerns that the predominance of CHD in higher socio-economic groups may relate to the stress of their occupations go back at least to Osler (1910) who wrote that work and worry were major causes of the disease. The fact that CHD is now more common in lower socio-economic groups does not, by itself, refute the potential importance of work 'stress' (Marmot 2004). Research has moved on from the simplistic notion that high responsibility or dealing with multiple tasks represents work stress.

Cardiovascular mortality has been declining in North America, Australia, and many countries of 'western' Europe, whilst it has been on the rise in the countries of central and eastern Europe and in the newly independent states of the former Soviet Union. Of the six-year life expectancy gap between the countries of 'east' and 'west' in Europe, more than half is due to cardiovascular disease, and especially to CHD. This gap in life expectancy grew from around the late 1960s to the present (Marmot and Bobak 2005), corresponding to the time when cardiovascular disease was on the rise in the east and declining in the west. The concepts and data reviewed in this chapter may provide some explanation for the inverse social gradient in cardiovascular disease in the 'west' and increased mortality in the 'east'.

6.3 Explanations of the social distribution of coronary heart disease

There is now a widely validated body of knowledge on risk factors for CHD that relate to development of atherosclerosis, and a somewhat less secure body of knowledge relating to predisposition to thrombosis. The major risk factors are high levels of blood pressure and plasma total cholesterol and smoking. Although smoking, in particular, shows a strong social gradient (Marmot *et al.* 1991), these risk factors account for no more than one third of the social gradient in cardiovascular disease (Marmot *et al.* 1978, 1984). Similarly, smoking is high in many countries of central and eastern Europe and may relate to the high rates of cardiovascular disease (Marmot and Bobak 2005), but data from the international MONICA studies (Kuulasmaa *et al.* 2000) show that international variations in smoking, high blood pressure, and raised plasma cholesterol account for less than half of the international variation in CHD mortality rates.

We are left then with two types of question. First, what accounts for the social and international variation in unhealthy behaviours such as atherogenic diet, smoking, and sedentary life style? Second, given that these factors appear to be inadequate explanations of social and international variations in cardiovascular mortality, what else could account for the observed differences? We have argued elsewhere that one must look for explanations in the nature of social and economic organization of societies (Marmot 2004). One particular feature is the nature of working life, both because what happens in the workplace may be important for health and because work and the operation of the labour market play a central role in the organization of social and economic life, which in turn are important in the social determinants of health. The evidence that supports the importance of work for cardiovascular and other diseases is presented below.

6.3.1 The changing nature of work

In advanced societies, work continues to play an important role for health and well being in adult life. Having a job is often a prerequisite for a continuous income and, more so than any other social circumstance, employment characteristics determine adult socio-economic status. Beyond economic livelihood, a person's occupation is important for socialization. It provides opportunities for personal growth and development, including the favourable experience of self in a core social role, and allows participation in social networks beyond primary groups.

The nature of work has undergone profound changes during recent decades. Today, fewer jobs are defined by physical demands and more by mental and emotional demands. While jobs in mass production are decreasing, employment in the service sector continues to rise. Computer-based information processing is becoming a part of a growing number of job profiles. In a large survey of European workers (Paoli and Merllié 2001), 60 per cent work at very high speeds, 40 per cent are confined to monotonous work, 49 per cent indicate permanent and direct contact with clients, and 25 per cent are working on shift rotation.

These changes in the nature of work have coincided with changes in the labour market. Women and older people comprise a growing proportion of the work force. Part-time working and flexible work arrangements have also increased. Perhaps most importantly for health, job instability, forced mobility, and unemployment are becoming more prevalent, resulting in an increase in job career discontinuity, forced early retirement, and job loss. Surveys report that 30 per cent of workers are currently in insecure jobs (Ferrie et al. 1999), and a significant proportion of middle-aged men and women are no longer participating in the labour market due to early, often involuntary retirement (Brugiavini 2001).

6.3.2 Social inequalities in the quality of work and health

Social inequalities in the quality of work and in access to the labour market have been reported in numerous studies, such that it can be concluded that the benefits and costs of working life are unequally distributed across society. This conclusion also holds true for the health burden of working life. A social gradient of health according to occupational standing has been documented for all-cause mortality, coronary heart disease morbidity and mortality, psychiatric disorders (especially depression), and chronic bronchitis (Siegrist and Marmot 2004). These social inequalities in health deserve particular attention considering that after the first years of childhood, midlife is the time when social differences in mortality are most pronounced. Therefore, elucidating the role of work in explaining health inequalities in midlife is a major research task.

This research faces two challenges: first, the identification of health-adverse (or 'toxic') and health-promoting (or 'salutogenic') components within complex working conditions in advanced societies, where a focus is put on the increasingly important psychosocial dimension of the work environment; and, second, the demonstration of the usefulness of theoretical models of the psychosocial work environment with relevance to health in explaining social inequalities in health. In the next section, these two challenges are dealt with.

6.4 Theoretical models of psychosocial work environment with relevance to health

6.4.1 General theoretical background

Research on psychosocial work-related stress differs from traditional biomedical occupational health research by the fact that stressors cannot be identified by direct physical or chemical measurements. Rather, theoretical concepts are needed to delineate particular stressful job characteristics such that they can be identified at a level of generalization that allows for their identification in a wide range of different occupations. These concepts are then translated into measures with the help of selected psychological and sociological research methods (questionnaires, observation techniques, etc.). While several concepts of psychosocial work-related stress have been developed (Cooper 1998; Dunham 2001; Perrewé and Ganster 2002), two models have received special attention recently: the demand–control model and the effort–reward imbalance model. Before describing them in more detail, their common theoretical background is explained.

A psychosocial work environment with relevance to health is defined by the interaction between a person's cognitions, emotions, and behaviours, and the material and social work context. A combination of sociological and psychological approaches is therefore needed to account for this interaction. While the primary interest of sociology remains at the level of collective (social) phenomena, it nevertheless needs to direct its analysis at the individual level of behaviour as well, and, in particular, at those general patterns of motivations that determine the broad range of diverse overt behaviours (Coleman 1990).

With this theoretical focus in mind, we underline two general (and perhaps universal) patterns of human motivations in their relation to the social environment: first, the need for physical and mental well being as a prerequisite for the organism's reproduction and the individual's productivity; and, secondly, the need of experiencing a positive self. Positive experience of self, while closely linked to well being, is contingent on a social environment that provides opportunities of belonging, acting, or contributing and of receiving favourable feedback. Conversely, a social structure that excludes individuals from belonging, acting, or contributing, and that prevents them from receiving favourable feedback, diminishes or even destroys positive experience of self.

The term 'psychosocial environment' has been defined as the socio-structural range of opportunities that is available to an individual person to meet his or her needs of well being, productivity, and positive self experience (Siegrist and Marmot 2004). Two aspects of positive self experience are of particular importance for well being and health: self efficacy and self esteem. Self efficacy has been defined as the belief a person has in his or her ability to accomplish tasks (Bandura 1986). This belief is based on a favourable evaluation of one's competence and of expected outcomes. A psychosocial environment conducive to self efficacy enables the person to practise his or her skills, to experience control in terms of successful agency. At the psychological level, self efficacy induces feelings of mastery. It is therefore assumed that a psychosocial environment that offers options of experiencing self efficacy produces favourable effects on health and well being, whereas opposite effects are expected in individuals who are confined to a restrictive, control-limiting psychosocial environment (as defined in the demand–control model, see below).

A similar relationship is assumed with respect to self esteem (i.e. the continued positive experience of a person's self worth). A psychosocial environment conducive to self esteem enables the person to connect him or herself with significant others and to receive appropriate feedback for well-accomplished tasks. Self esteem strengthens feelings of belonging, approval, and success. If a psychosocial environment prevents the person from experiences of belonging and approval, recurrent feelings of disappointment and frustration emerge. Reward deficiency is particularly stressful if invested efforts are not reciprocated (as is the case in the effort–reward imbalance model, see below).

In summary, we maintain that the psychosocial environment serves as a concept that bridges the social opportunity structure with the individual's strong need of favourable self efficacy and self esteem. Furthermore, we maintain that health and well being are to a considerable extent influenced by the quality and intensity of these processes. In adult life, employment and the quality of work define one of the most important psychosocial environments. Therefore, theoretical models with relevance to work and health are introduced (6.4), and their empirical significance (6.5) and policy implications (6.6) are discussed.

6.4.2 **The demand–control model**

In the sixties, research on job conditions and CHD had explored working demands and working hours (e.g. Hinkle *et al.* 1968). In the 1970s, several research traditions found evidence for a favourable effect on mental health produced by skill development (Hackman and Lawler 1971) and autonomy at work (Kohn and Schooler 1973; Gardell 1971). It was Karasek's original contribution to formulate a two-dimensional concept of work stress, the demand–control model, where a high level of psychological demands combined with a low level of decision latitude (low level of decision authority and low level of skill utilization) was predicted to increase the risk of stressful experience and subsequent physical illness (in particular CHD) (Karasek 1979). This combination may, in the long run, influence the worker's coping patterns. If a situation is uncontrollable, it is likely to induce negative expectancy in the process of coping with the demands (Eriksen and Ursin 2004). In 1981, Karasek et al. first found evidence of a predictive role of high demand and low control conditions in CHD, using data on a representative Swedish sample (Karasek et al. 1981). Since then, a large number of prospective and cross-sectional studies on associations of stressful work as defined by high demand and low control (job strain) with cardiovascular risk and disease and other disorders have been conducted (see below).

The original hypothesis that excessive psychological demands interact with lack of decision latitude in generating increased risk of stress-related disease was supplemented by a second hypothesis which concerns the learning of new patterns of behaviour and skills on the basis of psychosocial job experience. According to this, learning for adults accrues over a lifetime of work experience. It may contribute to the worker's possibility to exert control over his or her working situation and, thus, have an impact on broader conditions of adult life. According to this hypothesis, the active situation is associated with the development of strong feelings of self efficacy or mastery which is assumed to produce 'salutogenic' effects. Another way of expressing this in 'coping' terms is to say that the active work situation may increase positive expectancy (Eriksen and Ursin 2004). Moreover, experiencing self efficacy in active job situations increases the likelihood of spending an active life outside work, enriched by social, cultural, or political initiatives. This positive 'work–life balance' further reinforces well being and health, whereas confinement to job strain and associated lack of self efficacy limits a person's potential of experiencing a positive 'work–life balance' (see Karasek and Theorell 1990).

It is obvious that some of the 'classic' high-strain jobs are found in mass industry, especially under conditions of piece work and machine-paced assembly line work. Nevertheless, a number of strain jobs were also identified in the service sector. The concept therefore proves to be relevant in different employment sectors, and will remain important in the foreseeable future due to changing patterns of employment. For example, the rate of temporary employment is increasing in western Europe, particularly for those with low education. It is in these kinds of employment that lack of control will be a major problem. Even in those with a high education, the increasing demands for flexibility will create new decision latitude problems. The ever-increasing demands for effectiveness from the workforce are raising the levels of psychological demands for all workers. This is particularly reflected in Swedish national welfare statistics which show that the 1990s were characterized by increasing work demands in the whole workforce and, the late 1990s, by decreasing decision authority (Westerlund *et al.* 2004).

The original demand–control concept was modified to include social support at work as a third dimension (Johnson and Hall 1988) and to assess work control in a life-course perspective—'total job control exposure' (Johnson *et al.* 1990). Another important innovation has been the exploration of health effects produced by intervention studies that are based on the theoretical concept, and several promising intervention studies have been reported recently (see 6.6.2 below).

In summary, job profiles defined by high quantitative demands in combination with low control over task performance limit the experience of self efficacy among workers and elicit stressful experience with adverse long-term consequences on health. These effects are enhanced if social support in the workplace is lacking. Moreover, stress-related disease risks are augmented with increasing exposure time.

6.4.3 The effort–reward imbalance model

A complementary theoretical model—the effort–reward imbalance model—builds on the notion of social reciprocity, a fundamental principle of interpersonal behaviour and an 'evolutionary old' grammar of social exchange. Social reciprocity is characterized by mutual co-operative investments based on the norm of return expectancy, where efforts are assumed to be equalized by respective rewards. Failed reciprocity, resulting from a violation of this norm, elicits strong negative emotions and sustained stress responses because it operates against this fundamental principle.

This principle of social reciprocity lies at the core of the employment contract which defines distinct obligations or tasks to be performed in exchange for equitable rewards. The model of effort–reward imbalance is based on the assumption that efforts spent at work are not reciprocated by equitable rewards under specific conditions. These rewards include money, esteem, and career opportunities, including job security. The model of effort–reward imbalance claims that lack of reciprocity between the costs and gains (i.e. high cost/low gain conditions) elicits negative emotions with propensity to sustained autonomic and neuroendocrine activation.

In structural terms, this imbalance results from the fact that the social exchange between employee and employer is based on an incomplete contract which does not specify the full range of detailed obligations and benefits. In incomplete contracts, assumptions of trust in mutual commitment are made. However, under the following conditions, incomplete contracts are likely to result in high cost/low gain conditions. First, the risk of non-reciprocity in exchange is particularly high if employees have no alternative choice in the labour market. This is the case, for instance, if their skills are poor or if they subscribe to short-term contracts. Less frequently, non-reciprocity at work is experienced by workers as a negative life event, such as contract violation or failed contract.

Second, employees themselves may contribute to effort–reward imbalance at work either intentionally or unintentionally. For instance, they may, for a certain period, accept job arrangements that are considered unfair for strategic reasons, as they tend to improve their chances of career promotion and related rewards at a later stage. This pattern is often observed in the early stages of professional careers, among others. Failed success after long-lasting investment is particularly harmful to a person's well being and health.

Third, there are psychological reasons for a continued mismatch between efforts and rewards at work. People characterized by a motivational pattern of excessive work-related overcommitment and a high need for approval may suffer from inappropriate perceptions of demands and their own coping resources more often than their less involved colleagues (Siegrist 1996, 2002). Perceptual distortion prevents them from accurately assessing cost/gain relations. As a consequence, they underestimate the demands and overestimate their own coping resources, while not being aware of their own contribution to non-reciprocal exchange.

In summary, the proposed theoretical model is based on the sociological hypothesis that structured social exchange, as mediated through core social roles (the work role), is rooted in contracts of reciprocity of cost and gain. Conditions of failed social reciprocity are, in part, structural (or extrinsic) and, in part, personal (or intrinsic). Structural conditions of recurrent experience of high effort and low reward at work include lack of alternative choice in the labour market, lack of mobility, low level of skills, and confinement to a short-term contract. Personal conditions include strategic choices of the workers (although these often may be induced by social pressure) and characteristics of individual coping with the demands and rewards at work (overcommitment).

Three hypotheses are tested:

1 People characterized by an imbalance between (high) effort and (low) reward (failed reciprocity) are at elevated risk of stress-related diseases (over and above the risk associated with each one of the components).

2 People scoring high on 'overcommitment' are at elevated risk of stress-related diseases.

3 Relatively highest risk of stress-related diseases is expected in people who are characterized by the co-manifestation of conditions 1 and 2.

In section 6.5.2, a test of these hypotheses is presented, although most of the evidence relates to the first hypothesis. Details on the measurement of effort–reward imbalance at work can be found elsewhere (Siegrist *et al.* 2004). However, it should be mentioned that 'effort' and 'reward' are measured by two unidimensional scales containing six and 11 Likert-scaled items, respectively. Imbalance is assessed by applying a standardized algorithm (ratio effort/reward). 'Overcommitment' is also measured by a Likert scale containing six items in its short version. Reliability, factorial structure, and different types of validity (convergent, discriminant, criterion validity) of these scales were analysed, including comparison of self-report data with contextual information (where available) (Siegrist *et al.* 2004).

6.5 Empirical evidence

6.5.1 The demand–control model

The importance of work-related psychosocial factors to the development of ill health and disease can be illustrated from the Whitehall studies of British civil servants. The finding of dramatic differences in mortality by grade of employment in the first Whitehall study, which could not be explained by conventional risk factors alone (Marmot *et al.* 1984), led to the initiation of a second longitudinal study of civil servants—the Whitehall II study of 10,308 male and female civil servants. A major aim of this second study has been to investigate occupational and other social influences on health and disease in a white-collar office-based population. In pursuing the work environment as providing possible explanations, we have examined characteristics of the demand–control model. One hypothesis is that the lower the grade of employment in the civil service, the lower the level of control over the job, the lower the use of skills, and the higher the level of monotony. Such characteristics may be related to the higher rate of cardiovascular and other diseases in lower employment grades. Our initial analyses of the psychosocial work environment confirmed the above, with men and women in lower employment grades reporting lower levels of control, less varied work and use of skills, and a slower pace of work. Overall, fewer of the lower grades expressed themselves as satisfied with their work situation (Marmot *et al.* 1991).

The social distribution of psychosocial working conditions raises a problem of confounding. An association between working conditions and ill health could arise because of a direct causal connection or because people with low control over their working lives are of low status. It could be that other characteristics associated with low status, not the work, are important. Adjusting, statistically, for social position is one way of dealing with the problem, but it runs the risk of over adjustment. If it is indeed job strain that accounts for the link between low social position and disease, adjusting for social position controls for the variance of interest. It is preferable, if possible, to adjust for the potential confounders, not for social position itself.

Coronary heart disease and other risks and diseases

The relationship between the demand–control model and risk of CHD has been studied extensively in a number of countries, and several reviews have been published more recently (Belkic *et al.* 2004; Hemingway and Marmot 1998; Schnall *et al.* 2000; Kuper *et al.* 2002). The overall conclusion has been that there is solid evidence for a relationship, although negative findings were also reported in a minority of studies (see below).

The design of the Whitehall II study is longitudinal and this has enabled us to assess the psychosocial work environment over a period of time and examine its relationship to the development of new CHD. In addition to self-reported measures, we have used independent measures of the psychosocial work environment to address the question of whether job stress is influenced by subjective perceptions or by more objective appraisals of the work, or by both. Our results showed that both men and women with low control, either self-reported or independently assessed, had a higher risk of newly reported CHD during a mean follow-up period of five years. This association could not be explained by employment grade, negative affectivity, or classical coronary risk factors. In this initial follow-up, the importance of the full job strain model was not supported since job demands and social supports and the interactions between work characteristics were not related to the risk of new CHD (Bosma *et al.* 1997). A later follow-up of the same cohort, however, showed that job strain was associated with greater CHD risk than the other combinations in the model (active, passive, and relaxed) (Kuper and Marmot 2003).

In addition to Whitehall II, other studies have looked at the association of characteristics of the work environment to heart disease. The Swedish case control study of over 2000 men and women in Stockholm (SHEEP) has investigated the role of psychosocial work-related factors in the development of acute myocardial infarction (AMI). Men who reported high demands and low control in their job were at greater risk of developing AMI. This relationship was more pronounced for manual workers (Hallqvist *et al.* 1998). Similarly, in a prospective study of blue-collar workers in Finland, high demand and low control predicted cardiovascular mortality over a 25-year period (Kivimaki *et al.* 2002) after adjustment for main biological risk factors. A currently unpublished European study (JACE) comprised a five-year mean follow-up of large cohorts of employed men. Again, job strain was significantly and independently associated with an elevated AMI risk (M. Kornitzer personal communication 2004).

An investigation of the psychosocial work environment in the ten years preceding the onset of AMI showed that a recent decrease in the amount of control at work was associated with an elevated risk of disease. Again, this effect was greater in manual workers and in men under 55 years of age (Theorell *et al.* 1998). These data regarding loss of control and its effect on CHD illustrate that illness susceptibility after reported loss of control increases gradually over time. This knowledge offers new approaches towards preventing clinically overt CHD (see 6.6).

Investigations with negative findings need to be considered as well. One reason may be the specific populations under study. For example, the studies by Reed *et al.* (1989) and Suadicani *et al.* (1993) included men who were relatively old, particularly at the end of the follow-up period when a large proportion had retired. The same is probably the case with a recently published study by Eaker *et al.* (2004) which was based upon a ten-year follow-up of the Framingham offspring cohort. The sample in the study of Hlatky *et al.* (1995) was not representative as selection factors may have operated in determining who underwent coronary angiography. In the bus drivers studied by

Netterstrom and Suadicani (1993), psychosocial stress at work may have been denied to some extent. This interpretation is in line with findings from a different investigation of bus drivers, using observational techniques instead of self reports (Greiner *et al.* 1997; see also Belkic *et al.* 2004).

These results will influence the subsequent use and development of this theoretical model in future research studies. Thus, improved measurement of the psychosocial work environment will be needed, and additional techniques of data analysis will be required (Hallqvist *et al.* 1998). Table 6.1 summarizes studies of psychosocial work characteristics in terms of the demand–control model and coronary heart disease.

Musculoskeletal diseases are one of the most important work-related health problems. There are several cross-sectional studies (for instance, Joksimovic *et al.* 2002; Vingård *et al.* 2000) that have shown relationships between either the demand–control model or the effort–reward imbalance model and musculoskeletal disorder. There are few prospective studies, however. In a prospective study of 902 metal workers in Finland, Kaila–Kangas *et al.* (2004) showed that low self-reported job control was associated with increased risk of developing severe back pain resulting in hospitalization. On the other hand, a large prospective Dutch study (Hoogendoorn *et al.* 2002) showed essentially negative predictive results for the demand–control model in relation to low back pain. With regard to musculoskeletal disorders, the findings have been more difficult to interpret than those for cardiovascular disease. Part of this is due to the fact that psychosocial conditions at work are often correlated with physical conditions. When physical working conditions are controlled for, the effect of the psychosocial conditions are often attenuated. In rehabilitation, however, psychosocial conditions seem to be particularly important.

Another health indicator, functional gastrointestinal disorder, has been analysed in relation to the demand–control model. In one such study, lack of social support at work was found to worsen the prognosis of this illness (Westerberg and Theorell 1997). There is also a substantial literature exploring possible physiological and behavioural pathways which may link job strain to the development of poor health. Early longitudinal studies (Karasek and Theorell 1990) including physiological concomitants of spontaneous job strain variations in employed subjects who were followed on repeated occasions, with three-month intervals, showed decreasing plasma testosterone (in men) as well as increasing sleep disturbance (in men and women) with increasing job strain. Lowered testosterone in men and sleep disturbance are associated with decreasing regeneration. The significance of this lies in the fact that a high level of regeneration protects the body against adverse effects of long-lasting mobilization of energy. At the same time, increasing mean levels of systolic blood pressure were observed with increasing job strain, mirroring elevated levels of mobilization of energy (see also Schnall *et al.* 2000). In a recent Canadian large-scale study, a high level of long-lasting exposure to job strain predicted rising systolic and diastolic blood pressure in both men and women (Brisson *et al.* 2004).

Table 6.1 Studies of psychosocial work characteristics and coronary heart disease

Author, year, country, study	Total sample (% women)	Age at entry	Exposure	Follow-up (years)	Type of events (no.)	Adjustments	Relative risk
Theorell and Floderus–Myred 1977, Sweden, building construction workers	5187 (0%)	41–64	Workload index	2	Fatal CHD and NF MI (31)	Age	1.98
La Croix and Haynes 1984, USA, Framingham Heart Study	876 (37%)	45–64	Job control and demands (individual and ecological)	10	Fatal CHD, NF MI, coronary insufficiency and angina (not stated)	Age, smoking, blood pressure, cholesterol	Women: 2.9 Men: no association Ecological exposure was associated with risk in men and women
Alfredsson et al. 1985, Sweden, five Swedish counties	958,096 (51%)	20–64	Hectic work, few chances to learn new things, and monotonous work (ecological)	1	NF MI hospitalizations (1201)	Age, smoking, 10 socio-demographic factors, heavy lifting	*Men* Hectic work + non-learning: SMR = 128 (109–148) Hectic monotonous work: SMR = 118 (102–135) *Women* Hectic monotonous work: SMR = 164 (112–233)
Haan 1988, Finland, study of metal workers	902 (33%)	17–65	Job strain— physical strain, variety, and control (individual)	10	Fatal CHD and NF CHD (60)	Age, sex, smoking, blood pressure, cholesterol, relative weight, alcohol	Strain (low control, low variety, high physical strain) 4.95 (p = 0.03)
Reed et al. 1989, USA, Honolulu Heart Program	4737 (0%)	45–65	Strain—decision latitude and psychological demands (ecological)	18	Fatal CHD and NF MI (359)	Age, smoking, blood pressure, cholesterol, exercise, glucose	Job strain inversely associated with CHD incidence (p = 0.07) No significant effect of either job control or demand

Study	N (% women)	Age	Exposure	Follow-up (years)	Outcome	Adjustments	Results
Netterstrom and Suadicani 1993, Denmark, urban bus drivers	2045 (0%)	21–64	Job variety and satisfaction (individual)	10	Fatal CHD (59)	Age	Choose same job: 2.2 (1.2–4.0) Not looking for new job: 6.5 (1.6–27.0) Job is special: 1.9 (1.1–3.1) Cannot use skills: 1.5 (0.9–2.5) High work pace: 0.9 (0.5–1.6) Passengers complain: 0.6 (0.4–1.2) Job varied: 1.6 (0.9–1.9) Job very varied: 2.5 (1.4–4.5)
Suadicani et al. 1993, Denmark, Copenhagen Male Study	1638 (0%)	59.7 (mean age)	Job influence, monotony, pace, satisfaction, ability to relax (individual)	4	Fatal CHD and NF MI (46)	Age, smoking, blood pressure, cholesterol, HDL, triglycerides, BMI, alcohol, exercise, hypertension, selenium, social class	Only inability to relax after work associated with CHD: 2.9 (1.3–6.1)
Alterman et al. 1994, USA, Western Electric Study	1683 (0%)	38–56	Job strain — decision latitude and psychological demands (ecological)	25 (fatal) 10 (NF)	Fatal CHD (283) and NF CHD (115)	Age, smoking, blood pressure, cholesterol, alcohol, family history of CVD, education	Per tertile increase in exposure — *Fatal CHD* Job control: 0.76 (0.59–1.00) Job demands: 0.78 (0.48–1.26) Job strain: 1.40 (0.92–2.14) *NF CHD* Job control: 0.87 (0.57–1.31) Job demands: 1.07 (0.54–2.12) Job strain: 1.54 (0.85–2.80)

Table 6.1 (Continued)

Author, year, country, study	Total sample (% women)	Age at entry	Exposure	Follow-up (years)	Type of events (no.)	Adjustments	Relative risk
Bosma et al. 1997, UK, Whitehall II Study	10,308 (33%)	35–55	Job control, job demands, social support at work (individual and ecological)	5.3 (mean)	Diagnosed CHD (166), angina (328)	Age, sex, smoking, blood pressure, cholesterol, BMI, drugs for hypertension	Low job control— CHD: 1.26 (0.67–2.39) Angina: 2.02 (1.22–3.34) Job demands and social support at work not related Ecological and individual measures similar
Lynch et al. 1997, Finland, Kuopio Ischemic Heart Disease Risk Factor Study	1727 (0%)	42, 48, 54, or 60	Job demands, resources, income (individual)	10.8	Fatal CHD and NF MI (89)	Age, behavioural, biological, and psychosocial covariates	Demands/resources/income (compared to low/high/high) High/low/low: 1.57 (0.78–3.18)
Steenland et al. 1997, USA, NHANES1	3575 (0%)	25–74	Job strain—job control and job demand (ecological)	16	Fatal CHD and NF MI (519)	Age, smoking, blood pressure, cholesterol, BMI, diabetes, education	High control: 0.71 (0.54–0.93) High demands: 0.81 (0.61–1.09) Job strain: 1.08 (0.81–1.49)
Bosma et al. 1998, UK, Whitehall II Study	10,308 (33%)	35–55	Job control (also ecological), job demands, social support at work, effort-reward imbalance (individual)	5.3 (mean)	Angina pectoris and doctor-diagnosed ischaemia (413)	Age, sex, smoking, cholesterol, BMI, hypertension, employment grade, negative affectivity	Effort reward imbalance: 2.15 (1.15–4.01) Low control (individual): 2.38 (1.32–4.29) Low job control (ecological): 1.56 (1.08–2.27) Job demands and social support at work unrelated
Moore et al. 1999, Canada, Quebec	869 (0%)	42–60	Occupational stress (individual)	10	Fatal CHD, NF MI, angina (79)	None	Dissatisfied with: Work environment: 1.16 (0.62–1.15) Work schedule: 1.30

Study	N (%)	Age	Exposure	Follow-up	Outcome (N)	Adjustments	Results
Sacker et al. 2001, Health Survey for England	4235 (0%)	20–64	Job strain		Self-reported heart disease, angina, possible MI, doctor-diagnosed heart disease, any heart disease	Age, socio-economic status, diet, smoking, leisure time, cholesterol, BMI, diabetes, blood pressure	(0.73–2.29) Job context: 1.01 (0.52–1.97) Work responsibility: 0.89 (0.44–1.80) Support at work: 1.06 (0.61–1.86) Frequent stress at work: 1.19 (0.70–2.02) High strain: Angina: 2.46 (1.23–4.92) Possible MI: 1.46 (1.01–2.12) Doctor-diagnosed heart disease: 1.50 (1.02–2.20) Any heart disease: 1.60 (1.20–2.13)
Lee et al. 2002, USA, Nurses' Health Study	35,038 (100%)	46–71	Job strain	4	Fatal CHD (38), NF MI (108)	Age, smoking, alcohol intake, BMI, history of hypertension, diabetes mellitus, and other covariates	High-strain jobs: 0.71 (0.42–1.19) Passive jobs: 1.08 (0.69–1.69) Active jobs: 0.91 (0.54–1.53)
Kivimaki et al. 2002, Finland	812 (33%)	18–27, 28–47, over 48	Job strain, effort–reward imbalance	25.6	Fatal CHD (73)	Smoking, physical activity, systolic blood pressure, cholesterol, BMI	High job strain: 2.22(1.04–4.73) High effort–reward imbalance: 2.42 (1.02–5.73)
Kuper and Marmot 2003, UK, Whitehall II Study	10,308 (33%)	35–55	Job strain, job demands, decision latitude	11	Fatal CHD, NF MI (men:239, women: 59) all CHD (men: 591, women:325)	Age, sex, grade, coronary risk factors	All CHD: High demand and low control: 1.38 (1.1–1.75)

Table 6.1 (*Continued*)

Author, year, country, study	Total sample (% women)	Age at entry	Exposure	Follow-up (years)	Type of events (no.)	Adjustments	Relative risk
Eaker et al. 2004, Framingham offspring study	3039 (44%)	18–77	Job strain	10	Fatal CHD (men:160, women: 54) NF CHD (men: 118, women:31)	Age, systolic blood pressure, cholesterol, BMI, smoking, diabetes	Fatal CHD *Men* Job strain: 1.1(0.66–2.00) High strain: referent Low strain: 0.85(0.48–1.5) Passive: 0.99(0.59–1.68) *Women* Job strain: 1.00(0.37–2.75) High strain: referent Low strain: 0.76(0.24–2.42) Passive: 1.37(0.63–2.97)
Hlatky et al. 1995, USA, Duke Medical Center, employed patients undergoing coronary angiography	1489 (24%)	41–59	Job strain, decision latitude and psychological demands (individual)	4 (mean)	Fatal CHD (42) and NF MI (70)	Ejection fraction, extent of coronary atherosclerosis, myocardial ischaemia	Job strain Fatal CHD: 1.01 (0.51–2.01) Total CHD: 0.96 (0.62–1.46)
Hoffmann et al. 1995, Switzerland	222 (0%)	30–60	Job work load	1	Poor medical outcome (death,	Age, severity of MI, exercise, overprotection by	High workload was positively associated with outcome (p = 0.01)

Study	N (%)	Age	Exposure	Follow-up	Outcomes	Adjustments	Results
patients 7 weeks (mean) after first MI					reinfarction, New York Heart Association Class ≥III, exercise capacity <100W) (19)	friends, external locus of control	
Orth-Gomer et al. 2000, Sweden, Stockholm Female Coronary Risk Study, women post acute coronary event	292 (100%)	30–65	Job strain (job demands, job control) (Karasek)	4.8 (mean)	Fatal CHD, NF MI, revascularization procedure (81)	Age, smoking, blood pressure, HDL, triglycerides, oestrogen status, diabetes, diagnosis at index event, symptoms of heart failure, education	Severe work stress: 1.67 (0.64–4.32) Age adjusted only: Low control: 1.62 (0.84–3.01) High demands: 1.21 (0.63–2.32)
Welin et al. 2000, Sweden, Gothenburg, patients 3–6 days post first MI	275 (16%)	<65	Extra work, mental strain at work	10	All-cause mortality (67), fatal CHD (41), NF MI (55)	None	No association between fatal CHD and extra work (p = 0.26), mental stress at work (p = 0.99) No association with total mortality or NF MI

Adapted from Kuper et al. 2002 with permission from Thieme Medical Publishers, Inc.

Abbreviations: CHD: coronary heart disease; NF: non-fatal; MI: myocardial infarction

Additional cardiovascular risk factors, such as blood lipids, plasma fibrinogen, and markers of inflammation that are relevant to atherosclerosis, were explored with respect to job strain. The evidence is growing that psychosocial factors may contribute to elevated plasma fibrinogen, an indicator of inflammatory activity and increased coagulation (Brunner *et al.* 1996; Siegrist and Peter 1997). A recent review showed that several studies have been published on plasma fibrinogen. Among those studies which had more than a thousand participants, there were significant relationships between job strain and/or low decision latitude on one hand and elevated plasma fibrinogen on the other hand (Theorell 2002). Enhanced coagulation and increased inflammatory activity could both be regarded as phenomena that accompany energy mobilization. Studies of immunological reactions have also been published. Some of them have been on immunoglobulins and some on cytokines. For instance, in a longitudinal study of spontaneous variations in job strain, increasing immunoglobulin G was observed with rising job strain, particularly in subjects who had poor social support in their general life situation (Theorell *et al.* 1990). In an epidemiological study, the serum interleukin-6 concentration was shown to be higher in men with low decision latitude than in other male participants (Theorell and Hasselhorn 2002).

Although results are not consistent, these newly explored risk factors are important in understanding the pathophysiological processes underlying the statistically documented associations with AMI.

In summary, extensive research in several countries has shown that job strain is a risk factor for coronary heart disease as well as for other disease outcomes. The associations seem to hold even after adjustment for other established risk factors.

Sickness absence

In the original Whitehall study, grade of employment was associated with mortality from a range of specific causes (Marmot *et al.* 1984). This suggested the possibility that, in addition to searching out the determinants of specific medical diagnoses, it was appropriate to search for determinants of general susceptibility to illness. Second, we take the view that ill health is important not only because it may hasten the time of death but because it interferes with social, psychological, and physical functioning during life. One way of looking at sickness absence is that it is a measure that integrates decrements in social, psychological, and physical functioning. Short spells of absence are more likely to represent decrements in psychological and social functioning; long spells are more likely to represent decrements in physical functioning or 'real illness'. Third, sickness absence is a measure of great economic importance to employers. Studies of the determinants of sickness absence may, therefore, be of interest not only to those whose primary interest is in the aetiology of illness, but to those interested in the health of the economy and of individual firms (Marmot and Feeney 1996).

There was a clear association between grade of employment and sickness absence. Men in the lowest grade had six times the absence rate of men in the highest grade for both short (<7 days) and long (> = 7 days) spells of absence. Women showed a similar, although slightly reduced, gradient. As might be expected, the worse people rated their own health, the higher the sickness absence rates; sickness absence was also related to individual characteristics such as smoking and to problems outside work including financial problems and inadequate support (North *et al.* 1993).

Characteristics of the psychosocial work environment were also related to sickness absence. Men and women who rated their jobs as low on control, low on variety and use of skills, reported low support at work, and a slow pace of work had higher rates of short and long spells of sickness absence compared with those who rated their jobs high on these characteristics (North *et al.* 1993). Psychosocial work characteristics were also associated with sickness absence for psychiatric disorder and back pain. Low variety and use of skills and low support from colleagues and supervisors were associated with higher rates of short spells for psychiatric reasons in men and women (Stansfeld *et al.* 1997), and low control showed the most consistent effect, predicting both short and long spells of sickness absence for back pain in men and women (Hemingway *et al.* 1997).

One question we asked was how much of a contribution did work and other characteristics make to generating the social gradient in ill health as measured by sickness absence? Respective analyses suggest that about 25% of the social gradient in men and about 35% of the gradient in women is accounted for by these psychosocial work-related characteristics (North *et al.* 1993). When the analysis was stratified by employment grade, it was found that within the lower grades, there was support for the demand–control model, with jobs characterized by high work demands and low control predicting sickness absence (North *et al.* 1996). In white-collar workers, the findings were not significant.

Taken together, the health burden of an adverse psychosocial work environment in terms of the demand–control support model is considerable. Equally, the economic consequences of reduced health and increased sickness absence are substantial, calling for increased efforts of prevention.

6.5.2 Effort–reward imbalance model

Prospective epidemiological studies

As was shown, several sources of information on associations between psychosocial stress at work and health are available, such as data from cross-sectional and case-control studies, from prospective epidemiological observational investigations, from studies using ambulatory monitoring techniques or experimental designs, and from intervention trials. The prospective epidemiological observational study is considered a gold standard approach in this field because of its temporal sequence (exposure assessment precedes disease onset), the quantification of subsequent disease risk following exposure (relative risk of exposed vs. non-exposed subjects), and, ideally, large sample size (based on statistical power calculation and allowing for adjustment for confounding variables in multivariate analysis). For these methodological reasons, the selective presentation of associations between effort–reward imbalance at work (exposure) and different types of disease is mainly based on prospective studies (for recent reviews of available evidence including other study designs see van Vegchel *et al.* 2005; Tsutsumi and Kawakami, 2004). To further explore the validity of reported findings, some ambulatory monitoring data are included. The absence of evidence from intervention studies reflects the lack of such research.

Table 6.2 summarizes the results of several independent epidemiological reports on associations of effort–reward imbalance at work and disease onset that are available to date. Relative risks of health outcomes are calculated by estimating odds ratios (OR) or hazard ratios (HR), based on multivariate logistic regression analysis. The confidence intervals of these risks are not reported here, but all except two ratios are statistically significant in the expected direction—the higher the ratio, the more powerful the risk factor.

Significantly elevated odds ratios or hazard ratios vary between 1.3 (lowest) and 4.5 (highest), with an overall mean of about 2.0. This means that people who experience failed reciprocity at work (high effort and low reward) are twice as likely to suffer from one or more of the health risks under study in the near future, compared to people who are free from this type of chronic psychosocial stress. Elevated risks cannot be attributed to the influence of relevant confounding factors.

The observation period in these studies varies widely from one year to about 25 years (mean eight years) and, in most studies, the measurement of exposure (effort–reward imbalance) is restricted to baseline assessment. We now know that cumulative or chronic effort–reward imbalance over a longer period of time is associated with higher risk, compared to single (baseline) assessment (Chandola *et al.* 2005; Godin *et al.* 2005). It is therefore possible that the relative risks indicated in Table 6.2 represent conservative estimates. However, it must be noted that, in some studies, proxy measures of effort–reward imbalance were used as the original scales were not available at the time of study onset.

As can be seen from Table 6.2, available evidence is generally stronger for men than for women, and it is stronger for coronary heart disease than for other health outcomes. Yet, evidence is of similar strength independent of whether self-reported 'soft' end-points or clinically defined 'hard' end-points are used. Seven out of 12 studies rely on data from the UK Whitehall II study of British civil servants (Marmot *et al.* 1991). Two studies come from Finland (different samples) and the remaining investigations are from Belgium, France, and Germany.

More recently, a large Swedish cohort study based on a group of some 20,000 working men and women showed that a proxy measure of effort–reward imbalance at work predicted the risk of a long spell of sick leave over a one-year observation period (Jeding *et al.* 2005).

Table 6.2 Effort–reward imbalance at work and health outcomes: review of prospective epidemiological studies

First author, year	Total sample (% women)	Country	Observation period (years)	Health outcome	Relative risk (odds ratio: OR, hazard ratio: HR)
Siegrist 1990	416 (0%)	Germany	6.5	Incident fatal or NF CHD	OR 4.5
Lynch 1997	2297 (0)	Finland	8.1	Incident CHD (myocardial infarction)	HR 2.3
Bosma 1998	10,308 (33)	UK	5.3	Incident CHD, including angina	OR 2.2
Kuper 2002	10,308 (33)	UK	11.0	Incident CHD	HR 1.3 (1.8*)
Kivimäki 2002	812 (32)	Finland	25.6	Cardiovascular disease mortality	HR 2.3
Kumari 2004b	8067 (30)	UK	10.5	Incident type II diabetes	Men: OR 1.6; women: OR 0.9#
Stansfeld 1999	10,308 (33)	UK	5.3	Mild to moderate psychiatric psychiatric disorder (mostly depression)	Men: OR 2.6; women: OR 1.6
Godin 2005	1986 (64)	Belgium	1.0	Depression Anxiety Somatization	Men: OR 2.8; women: OR 4.6 Men: OR 2.3; women: OR 4.5 Men: OR 2.0; women: OR 3.6
Kuper 2002	6918 (33)	UK	11.0	Poor self-rated functioning (SF36)	Physical: OR 1.4 Mental: OR 2.3
Stansfeld 1998	10,308 (33)	UK	5.3	Poor self-rated functioning (SF 36)	Physical: Men: OR 1.4; women: OR 2.0 Mental: Men: OR 1.8; women: OR 2.3 1.8 men
Niedhammer 2004	6286 (30)	France	1.0	Poor self-rated health	Men: OR 1.8; women: OR 2.2
Head 2004	8280 (31)	UK	5.3	Alcohol dependence	Men: OR 1.9; women: OR 1.2#

* Effort–reward imbalance in combination with low social support at work.
# Statistically non-significant.
Abbreviations: CHD: coronary heart disease; SF 36: short form 36 health survey.

In summary, there is solid evidence indicating that failed reciprocity in a core social role, the work role, represents an independent risk factor of a variety of highly prevalent diseases, especially so among middle-aged men.

Naturalistic and experimental studies

Findings from epidemiological studies are supplemented by the results of naturalistic and experimental studies where physiological function is measured in relation to behaviour and psychological states. Ambulatory monitoring of physiological parameters such as heart rate (HR) and blood pressure (BP) allow a direct assessment of everyday work-related psychosocial influences on physiological functioning. In contrast, experimental studies in the laboratory provide a strict standardization of relevant conditions under study, at the expense of ecological validity of findings. Both approaches are useful and have been applied to the effort–reward imbalance model.

In one ambulatory monitoring study, BP, HR, and heart rate variability were monitored on three days in 109 male, white-collar employees of a Dutch computer company. The group classified as having high imbalance between effort and reward had significantly higher work and home systolic BP than men with low or no imbalance, higher HR during work, and lower heart rate variability during all periods of monitoring (Vrijkotte et al. 2000). In this study, overcommitment was not associated with the three indicators of cardiovascular reactivity, but was found to be highly correlated with indicators of a disturbed metabolic system (Vrijkotte et al. 1999).

In an investigation on biological correlates of effort–reward imbalance and overcommitment to work conducted in a subgroup of the Whitehall II cohort, significantly elevated cortisol responses to waking and elevated systolic BP over the day were found in the group of highly committed men, compared to those with low overcommitment (Steptoe et al. 2004). In particular, as documented in the Fig. 6.1, a significant interaction between overcommitment, socio-economic position, and time of day was observed with highest BP in overcommitted men belonging to the lowest occupational position. No association between the effort:rewards ratio and biological variables was found in this study, and findings were restricted to men.

A different approach was chosen in an experimental study on middle managers who underwent a mental stress test. In the chronically stressed high effort/low reward group, significantly lower responsiveness to challenge was observed in heart rate, adrenaline, and cortisol, compared to the low stress group (Siegrist et al. 1997). Attenuated autonomic and neurochemical stress reactions may mirror functional adaptation to excessive simulation due to a chronically adverse psychosocial work environment.

In a recent experiment, regional brain activity was analysed, using functional magnetic resonance imaging, in subjects exposed to monetary gain and loss. The group defined by highest scores on the scales measuring effort, reward, and overcommitment showed significantly altered activation in several pre-defined areas of the brain reward system, compared to the group with lowest scores (Siegrist et al. 2005).

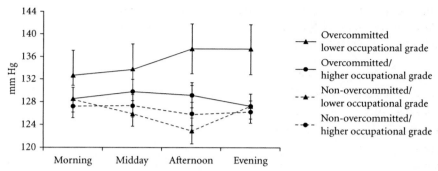

Fig. 6.1 Mean systolic blood pressure, in men, averaged over morning, midday, afternoon, and evening periods. (From Steptoe *et al.* 2004, with permission)

Taken together, these findings are important in understanding the mechanisms through which psychosocial influences at work may operate in triggering the development of somatic diseases, such as coronary heart diseases.

6.5.3 Links between psychosocial work environment and inequalities in health

How useful are these models in explaining part of the social gradient of disease in mid life? In particular, are the models mediating the association of socio-economic status with health or do they operate as effect modifiers in this association? Both arguments, mediation and effect modification, can be applied to the psychosocial variables under study. For instance, low control at work and, to a lesser extent, low reward at work, were shown to be more prevalent among lower status groups (Bosma *et al.* 1998; Niedhammeret *al.* 2000; Siegrist *et al.* 2004). Low control was also shown to predict CHD incidence in British civil servants, after adjustment for relevant confounders (Marmot *et al.* 1997). As CHD was more prevalent among lower employment grade civil servants, it was hypothesized that low control at work mediates the inverse association of socio-economic status with CHD. In multivariate analysis, low control in the workplace accounted for about half the social gradient of CHD (i.e. reduced the odds ratio of CHD in the low employment grade group from about 1.4 to about 1.2) after respective adjusting. Importantly, the relation between low control and CHD was not removed by adjusting for SES (Marmot *et al.* 1997). Similar findings were obtained in a Czech case-control study of CHD patients (Bobak *et al.* 1998).

As low control at work reduces self efficacy and positive outcome expectancy, these psychological conditions are hypothesized to be more frequent in lower status groups. Moreover, they might mediate part of the association between low socio-economic status and CHD.

The effect modification hypothesis posits that susceptibility to an exposure is higher among lower-status compared to higher-status people and, therefore, that among people with lower socio-economic status, the effect size produced by the exposure, is higher. This hypothesis was tested in several prospective and case-control studies that documented a stronger effect of high demand and low control at work, or of high effort and low reward at work, on the risk of CHD incidence in lower-status groups (Johnson and Hall 1988; Hallqvist *et al.* 1998; Kuper *et al.* 2002*b*). For instance, Kuper *et al.* (2002*b*) analysed the relation of effort–reward imbalance to CHD incidence (quartiles of the effort–reward ratio) in a 11-year follow-up period in the Whitehall II study. While they found an increased risk of CHD in the upper quartile of scores of the effort–reward ratio within the total study population, this effect was relatively strongest in the lowest employment group (clericals). In the clerical as compared to the administrative group, the odds ratio of effort–reward imbalance was 1.56 versus 1.19 for all CHD, and was 1.71 versus 1.27 for fatal CHD/non-fatal acute myocardial infarction.

6.6 Further developments and policy implications

6.6.1 Conceptual and methodological developments

It was mentioned before that a variety of work stress models were proposed and tested in addition to those described above in detail. We do not claim that the demand–control model and the effort–reward imbalance model cover the whole range of an adverse psychosocial work environment. Rather, they are distinct from others in that they have been widely tested and in that they have the potential of being applied to a variety of different occupations and even to other types of recurrent activities beyond employment (Chandola *et al.* 2004; Knesebeck and Siegrist 2003). Several further developments are needed and, in fact, have been initiated more recently. One such extension includes the combination of the two models into a single-study design (Peter *et al.* 2002; Ostry *et al.* 2003) and their comparison with complementary models, such as the model of organizational justice (Kivimäki *et al.* 2004), among others.

A different line of extension concerns the behavioural consequences of work-related stress (safety, injury risk, vigilance and fatigue, quality of performance, addictive behaviour). Less research so far has been conducted on these important topics. Similarly, the work–home interface needs to be explored in more detail, with particular emphasis on spillover from work to home and vice versa, and on the compensatory effects that may occur between the two spheres (Westman 2002).

As was shown, several studies indicate that an adverse psychosocial work environment, as measured by the two models, is more important for men's health than for women's health. Whether this finding is attributable to different gender roles, different exposure conditions, or the effect of unmeasured protective factors, or whether effects vary according to the occupational groups and health indicators under study needs to be clarified in future research. As the nature of work changes at an unprecedented pace, new types of work organization evolve, such as home work, flexible work (e.g. freelancers), precarious work, or multiple work arrangements. While adverse health effects of long-term unemployment are well documented, the health effects of these newly evolving patterns of work and employment are still poorly understood.

Further developments are needed at the measurement level as well. It was already pointed out that self-report measures may have limited validity due to reporting bias and that additional contextually validated measurements are required. Moreover, multiple measurements over time are preferable to a single (baseline) measurement of work stress because they add to the robustness of findings. Although 'reporting bias' and 'residual confounding' provide continuous challenges to this field of research, the overall evidence of links between work stress and health is nevertheless solid.

6.6.2 Policy implications

What are the policy implications of this evidence? In this chapter, we have argued that two theoretical models hold particular promise in explaining at least part of the social variation in disease, and especially CHD, a variation that may be attributed, in part, to work stress as defined by the demand–control and effort–reward imbalance models. High demand/low control conditions and high cost/low gain conditions at work are unequally distributed both between and within societies and may potentially provide a framework in which to understand the contribution of psychosocial factors at work to the development of disease.

The conceptual differences between the models have direct implications for the design of intervention measures to improve health; whereas the emphasis of the demand–control model is on change of the task structure (such as job enlargement, job enrichment, and increasing the amount of support within the job). The reduction of high cost/low gain conditions includes action at three levels: the individual level (e.g. reduction of excessive need for control); the interpersonal level (e.g. improvement of esteem reward); and the structural level (e.g. adequate compensation for stressful work conditions by improved pay and related incentives, opportunities for job training, learning new skills, and increased job security). Both models can be used concomitantly in preventive efforts, as documented below.

Practical experiments in Scandinavia have shown that it is possible to increase the interest among employers in improving decision latitude and other aspects of the working conditions for employees and that this may improve employee health (Theorell et al. 2001; Theorell 2004). A necessary condition for success is that work is done both on the individual and the organizational level and that top-down approaches are avoided.

One intervention study illustrating this approach was conducted in a one-year low-intensity educational programme of managers of an insurance company. Accordingly, the aim was to stimulate managers to improve their employees' participation in decisions, to monitor demand levels to keep them at optimal levels, to stimulate support (from work mates and from supervisors), to stimulate development of competence, and to provide rewards for efforts. The educational sessions took place for two hours (half an hour of lecture followed by group discussion) every second week for a working year. Half the organization served as control group in the evaluation. Assessments were made before the programme started, after six months, and, finally, after one year.

The most interesting results were those obtained from the employees (excluding the managers themselves). At baseline and after six months, there were no differences between the groups. After one year, however, there were several significant differences between the groups: the serum cortisol levels (measured in the morning) had decreased in the experimental group but not in the control group employees. In addition, self-reported decision authority had developed more favourably in the experimental group's employees than in the other employees (Theorell *et al.* 2001).

This study was conducted during a period of structural changes in Swedish working life and one interpretation of this is that the managerial programme had managed to decrease uncertainty in the employees and that this may have had psychological as well as physiological effects.

A further example is a British study which comprised six office work sites. They were randomly allocated to experimental and control group with three work sites in each one. In the experimental group, a one-year programme for increased employee participation was implemented. Assessments, compared to the baseline, revealed significantly improved self ratings of performance and mental health, as well as objectively recorded decrease in sick leave after one year in the experimental group (Bond and Bunce 2001).

Other researchers have also shown improved health parameters after interventions aiming at improved psychosocial working conditions (for a review, see Wahlstedt 2001). It is, however, often difficult to make evaluations of such interventions, and there are several reasons for this including:

1 Ongoing structural changes in the labour market may interrupt well-planned evaluations due to mergers, downsizing, and outsourcing.

2 Randomization of individuals participating in the programmes is not meaningful, whereas randomization of whole work sites may be a good alternative. The result of this is that very large samples are required.

3 Big efforts are required from the work sites. This means that many employers may hesitate to participate in evaluations.

4 The intervention procedures have to be negotiated often during a relatively short period. This means compromising and, frequently, a small, insufficiently intensive intervention is the result.

5 Interventions that are subjected to evaluation should be scientifically founded and also practically sound. Many evaluations of interventions do not fulfil this criterion.

The result of all these difficulties is that the literature on evaluations of effects of this kind of psychosocial work environment work is small and, accordingly, there is no scientific consensus on their health effects. However, the knowledge regarding health effects of the psychosocial work environment can also be used for interpretations of societal changes and their effects on public health.

There are three major incentives for investing in an improved quality of work organization, including fair employment contracts. The first one is responsibility. When asbestos was shown to cause certain types of cancer, preventive steps were taken by occupational health agencies to minimize the risk. A similar case can be made for injury prevention at work. Similarly, should we not consider reducing work-related stress to the extent supported by scientific evidence? Responsibility may not be a convincing argument for some parts of the world's current economy. Yet, the European Commission has recently proposed an agenda for corporate social responsibility, and a number of other initiatives support this approach at the global level, such as the ILO's Tripartite Declaration on Multinational Enterprises and Social Policy and the OECD Guidelines for Multinational Enterprises. In all these initiatives, the protection and promotion of the health of employees is considered an important task of employment policy.

Costs of inactivity define a second incentive. While interest in short-term profit may run against this argument, it is nevertheless evident that the costs of an unhealthy work organization create a financial burden to companies and organizations as well as to society at large. A conservative estimate of annual costs of work-related stress in the 15 European Union nations is 20 billion Euro (Dunham 2001). This estimate considers the total sum of direct and indirect health costs of that fraction of the highly prevalent diseases mentioned above that is attributable to work-related stress. This is no more than about 10 per cent of the total variance of these diseases.

Return on investment is a third incentive for improving quality of work organization, including fair employment contracts. Up to now, few studies only have been available demonstrating substantial medium-term cost savings of such investments. Yet, particularly impressive in this regard is a US study by Jeffery Pfeffer who explored common organizational features of those US companies that were most successful in terms of shareholder value over a number of years (Pfeffer 1998). He came up with the following list of common characteristics:

1 employment security;

2 selective hiring of new personnel;

3 self-managed teams and decentralized decision making as the basic principles of organizational design;

4 comparatively high compensation, contingent on organizational performance;

5 extensive training;

6 reduced status distinctions and barriers across levels;

7 extensive sharing of financial and performance information throughout the organization.

It is almost certain that Pfeffer was not aware of the models of work stress discussed here (in particular, the effort–reward imbalance model and the demand–control model) as his interest was exclusively an economic one. However, it is evident that several of the features of economically successful organizations are similar to those which result from recommendations based on the scientific results presented in this chapter.

Therefore, in conclusion, a substantial part of policy implications derived from research on psychosocial stress at work and health concur with these economically driven improvements of work organization, including employment contract. Joint efforts are needed from stakeholders, professionals, and national/international organizations to further improve the quality of working life and, thus, to reduce social inequalities in health.

References

Alfredsson, L., Spetz, C.–L., and Theorell, T. (1985). Type of occupation and near-future hospitalization for myocardial infarction and some other diagnoses. *Int. J. Epidemiol.* **14**:378–88.

Alterman, T., Shekelle, R.B., Vernon, S.W., and Burau, K.D. (1994). Decision latitude, psychologic demand, job strain, and coronary heart disease in the Western Electric study. *Am. J. Epidemiol.* **139**:620–7.

Armstrong, D.L., Strogatz, D., and Wang, R. (2004). United States coronary mortality trends and community services associated with occupational structure, among blacks and whites, 1984–1998. *Soc. Sci. Med.* **58(11)**:2349–61.

Bandura, A. (1986). *Social Foundations of Thought and Action* (Vol. 1). Englewood Cliffs, NJ: Prentice–Hall.

Belkic, K.L., Landsbergis, P.A., Schnall, P.L., and Baker, D. (2004). Is job strain a major source of cardiovascular disease risk? *Scand. J. Work Environ. Health* **30(2)**:85–128.

Bobak, M., Hertzman, C., Skodova, Z., and Marmot, M. (1998). Association between psychosocial factors at work and non-fatal myocardial infarction in a population based case-control study in Czech men. *Epidemiology* **9**:43–7.

Bond, F.W. and Bunce, D. (2001). Job control mediates change in a work reorganization intervention for stress reduction. *J. Occup. Health Psychol.* **6**:290–302.

Bosma, H., Marmot, M.G., Hemingway, H., Nicholson, A., Brunner, E.J., and Stansfeld, S. (1997). Low job control and risk of coronary heart disease in the Whitehall II (prospective cohort) study. *BMJ* **314**:558–65.

Bosma, H., Peter, R., Siegrist, J., and Marmot, M.G. (1998). Two alternative job stress models and the risk of coronary heart disease. *Am. J. Publ. Health* **88**:68–74.

Breucker, G. and Schroer, A. (ed.) (1996). *International experiences in workplace health promotion.* European Health Promotion, Series 6. Copenhagen: World Health Organization.

Brisson, C., Guimont, C., Vezina, M., Moisan, J., Dagenais, G.R., Milot, A. *et al.* (2004). *Psychosocial work environment and evolution of blood pressure: the contribution of job control and physical work demands.* Abstract at the International Congress of Behavioural Medicine, Mainz, 2004.

Brugiavini, A. (2001). Early retirement in Europe. *European Review* **9**: 501–15.

Brunner, E.J., Davey Smith, G., Marmot, M.G., Canner, R., Beksinska, M., and O'Brien, J. (1996). Childhood social circumstances and psychosocial and behavioural factors as determinants of plasma fibrinogen. *Lancet* **347**:1008–13.

Chandola, T., Kuper, H., Singh–Manoux, A., Bartley, M., and Marmot, M. (2004). The effect of control at home on CHD events in the Whitehall II study: gender differences in psychosocial domestic pathways to social inequalities in CHD. *Soc. Sci. Med.* **58**:1501–9.

Chandola, T., Siegrist, J., and Marmot, M. (2005). Do changes in effort–reward imbalance at work contribute to an explanation of the social gradient in angina? *Occupational & Environmental Medicine* **62**: 223–30.

Coleman, J.S. (1990). *Foundations of Social Theory.* Cambridge: Belknap Press.

Cooper, C.L. (ed.) (1998). *Theories of Organizational Stress.* Oxford: Oxford University Press.

Cooper, R., Cutler, J., Desvigne–Nickens, P., Fortmann, S.P., Freidman, L., Havlik, R. *et al.* (2000). Trends and disparities in coronary heart disease, stroke, and other cardiovascular disease in the United States. *Circulation* **102**:3137–47.

Dunham, J. (2001). *Stress in the Workplace. Past, Present and Future.* London: Whurr.

Eaker, E.D., Sullivan, L.M., Kelly–Hayes, M., D'Agostino, Sr., R.B., and Benjamin, E.J. (2004). Does job strain increase the risk for coronary heart disease or death in men and women? The Framingham Offspring Study. *Am. J. Epidemiol.* **159(10)**:950–8.

Eriksen, H.R. and Ursin, H. (2004). Subjective health complaints, sensitization, and sustained cognitive activation (stress). *J. Psychosom. Res.* **56(4)**:445–8.

Ferrie, J.E., Griffiths, J., Marmot, M.G., and Ziglio, E. (1999). *Labour market changes and job insecurity: a challenge for social welfare and health promotion.* Copenhagen: WHO Regional Publications.

Gardell, B. (1971). Alienation and mental health in the modern industrial environment. In: *Society, stress and disease. The psychosocial environment and psychomatic diseases* (ed. L. Levi). London: Oxford University Press.

Godin, I., Kittel, F., Coppieters, Y., and Siegrist, J. (2005). A prospective study of cumulative job stress in relation to mental health. *BMC Public Health* **5**:67–76.

Greiner, B.A., Ragland, D.R., Krause, N., Syme, S.L., and Fisher, J.M. (1997). Objective measurement of occupational stress factors—an example with San Francisco urban transit operators. *J. Occup. Health Psychol.* **4**:325–42.

Haan, M.N. (1988). Job strain and ischaemic heart disease: an epidemiologic study of metal workers. *Annals of Clinical Research* **20**:143–5.

Hackman, J.R. and Lawler, E.E. (1971). Employee reactions to job characteristics. *J. Appl. Psychol.* **55**:259–86.

Hallqvist, J., Diderichsen, F., Theorell, T., Reuterwall, C., Ahlbom, A., and SHEEP study group. (1998). Is the effect of job strain on myocardial infarction due to interaction between high psychological demands and low decision latitude. Results from the Stockholm Heart Epidemiology Program (SHEEP). *Soc. Sci. Med.* **46(11)**:1405–15.

Head, J., Stansfeld, S.A., and Siegrist, J. (2004). The psychosocial work environment and alcohol dependence: a prospective study. *Occupational and Environmental Medicine* **61**: 219–24.

Hemingway, H. and Marmot, M. (1998). Psychosocial factors in the primary and secondary prevention of coronary heart disease: a systematic review. In: *Evidence based cardiology* (ed. S. Yusuf, J. Cairns, J. Camm, E. Fallen, and B. Gersch). London: BMJ Publishing Group.

Hemingway, H., Shipley, M., Stansfeld, S., and Marmot, M. (1997). Sickness absence from back pain, psychosocial work characteristics and employment grade among office workers. Whitehall II Study. *Scandinavian Journal of Work, Environment and Health* **23**:121–9.

Hinkle, L.E., Whitney, L.H., Lehman, E.W., Dunn, J., Benjamin, B., King, R., *et al.* (1968). Occupation, education and coronary heart disease. *Science* **161**:238–46.

Hlatky, M.A., Lam, L.C., Lee, K.L., Clapp–Channing, N.E., Williams, R.B., Pryor, D.B., *et al.* (1995). Job strain and the prevalence and outcome of coronary artery disease. *Circulation* **92**:327–33.

Hoffmann, A., Pfiffner, D., Hornung, R., and Niederhauser, H. (1995). Psychosocial factors predict medical outcome following a first myocardial infarction. Working Group on Cardiac Rehabilitation of the Swiss Society of Cardiology. *Coronary Artery Disease* **6**:147–52.

Hoogendoorn, W.E., Bongers, P.M., de Vet, H.C., Ariens,G.A., van Mechelen,W., and Bouter, L.M. (2002). High physical work load and low job satisfaction increase the risk of sickness absence due to low back pain: results of a prospective cohort study. *Occupational and Environmental Medicine* **59**:323–8.

Jeding, K., Oxenstierna, G., Ferrie, J., Westerlund, H., Siegrist, J., and Theorell, T. (2005). Effort–reward imbalance is associated with increased rates of long-term sickness absence (submitted).

Johnson, J.V. and Hall, E.M. (1988). Job strain, work place social support, and cardiovascular disease: a cross-sectional study of a random sample of the Swedish working population. *Am. J. Public Health* **78**:1336–42.

Johnson, J.V., Stewart, W., Fredlund, P., *et al.* (1990). *Psychosocial Job Exposure Matrix: An Occupationally Aggregated Attribution System for Work Environment Exposure Characteristics* (221 edn). Stockholm: National Institute for Psychosocial Factors and Health.

Joksimovic, L., Starke, D., Knesebeck, O., and Siegrist, J. (2002). Perceived work stress, overcommittment and self-reported musculoskeletal pain: a cross sectional investigation. *International Journal of Behavioural Medicine* **9**:122–38.

Kaila–Kangas, L., Kivimaki, M., Riihimaki, H., Luukkonen, R., Kirjonen, J., and Leino–Arjas, P. (2004). Psychosocial factors at work as predictors of hospitalization for back disorders: a 28-year follow-up of industrial employees. *Spine* **29(16)**:1823–30.

Karasek, R.A. (1979). Job demands, job decision latitude and mental strain: implications for job design. *Admin. Sci. Quart.* **24**:285–308.

Karasek, R. and Theorell, T. (1990). *Healthy work: stress, productivity, and the reconstruction of working life.* New York: Basic Books.

Karasek, R., Baker, D., Marxer, F., Ahlbom, A., and Theorell, T. (1981). Job decision latitude, job demands and cardiovascular disease: a prospective study of Swedish men. *Am. J. Public Health* **71**:694–705.

Kivimaki, M., Ferrie, J.E. Head, J., Shipley, M., Vahtera, J., and Marmot, M.G. (2004). Change in organisational justice: effects on employee health in the Whitehall II study. *J. Epidemiol. Comun. Health* **58**:931–7.

Kivimaki, M., Leino–Arjas, P., Luukkonen, R., Riihimaki, H., Vahtera, J., and Kirjonen, J. (2002). Work stress and risk of cardiovascular mortality: prospective cohort study of industrial employees. *BMJ* **325**:857–60.

Knesebeck, O.V.D. and Siegrist, J. (2003). Reported non-reciprocity of social exchange and depressive symptoms: extending the model of effort-reward imbalance beyond work. *J. Psychosomatic Research* **55**:209–14.

Kohn, M. and Schooler, C. (1973). Occupational experience and psychological functioning: an assessment of reciprocal effects. *American Sociological Review* **38**:97–118.

Kumari, M., Head, J., and Marmot, M. (2004*a*). Prospective study of social and other risk factors for incidence of type II diabetes in Whitehall 2 study. *Annals of Internal Medicine* **164**:1873–80.

Kumari, M., Seeman, T.E., and Marmot, M. (2004*b*). Biological predictors of change in functioning in the Whitehall II study. *Annals of Epidemiology* **14(4)**:250–7.

Kuper, H. and Marmot, M. (2003). Job strain, job demands, decision latitude, and the risk of coronary heart disease within the Whitehall II study. *J. Epidemiol. Commun. Health* **57(2)**:147–53.

Kuper, H., Marmot, M., and Hemingway, H. (2002*a*). Systematic review of prospective cohort studies of psychosocial factors in the etiology and prognosis of coronary heart disease. *Seminars in Vascular Medicine* **2**(3):267–314.

Kuper, H., Singh–Manoux, A., Siegrist, J., and Marmot, M. (2002*b*). When reciprocity fails: effort–reward imbalance in relation to coronary heart disease and health functioning within the Whitehall II Study. *Occupational and Environmental Medicine* **59**(11):777–84.

Kuulasmaa, K., Tunstall–Pedoe, H., Dobson, A., Fortmann, S.P., Sans, S., Tolonen, H., *et al.* (2000). Estimation of contribution of changes in classic risk factors to trends in coronary-event rates across the WHO MONICA Project populations. *Lancet* **355**:675–87.

Lacroix, A. and Haynes, S. (1984). Occupational exposure to high demand/low control work and coronary heart disease incidence in the Framingham cohort. *Am. J. Epidemiol.* **120**:481.

Lee, S., Colditz, G., Berkman, L., and Kawachi, I. (2002). A prospective study of job strain and coronary heart disease in US women. *Int. J. Epidemiol.* **31**(6):1147–53.

Lynch, J., Krause, N., Kaplan, G.A., Tuomilehto, J., and Salonen, J.T. (1997). Workplace conditions, socioeconomic status, and the risk of mortality and acute myocardial infarction: the Kuopio Ischaemic Heart Disease Risk Factor Study. *Am. J. Public Health* **87**:617–22.

Marmot, M.G. (1992). Coronary heart disease: rise and fall of a modern epidemic. In: *Coronary Heart Disease Epidemiology* (ed. M.G. Marmot and P. Elliott). Oxford: Oxford University Press.

Marmot, M. (2004). *Status Syndrome*. London: Bloomsbury.

Marmot, M. and Bobak, M. (2005). Social and economic changes and health in Europe East and West. *European Review* **13**: 15–32.

Marmot, M. and Feeney, A. (1996). Work and health: implications for individuals and society. In: *Health and Social Organisation* (ed. D. Blane, E. Brunner, and R. Wilkinson). London/New York: Routledge.

Marmot, M.G., Adelstein, A.M., Robinson, N., and Rose, G. (1978). The changing social class distribution of heart disease. *BMJ* **2**:1109–12.

Marmot, M.G., Bosma, H., Hemingway, H., Brunner, E., and Stansfeld, S. (1997). Contribution of job control and other risk factors to social variations in coronary heart disease. *Lancet* **350**:235–40.

Marmot, M.G., Davey Smith, G., Stansfeld, S.A., Patel, C., North, F., Head, J., *et al.* (1991). Health inequalities among British Civil Servants: the Whitehall II study. *Lancet* **337**:1387–93.

Marmot, M.G., Shipley, M.J., and Rose, G. (1984). Inequalities in death—specific explanations of a general pattern. *Lancet* **323**:1003–6.

Moore, L., Meyer, F., Perusse, M., Cantin, B., Dagenais, G.R., Bairati, I., *et al.* (1999). Psychological stress and incidence of ischaemic heart disease. *Int. J. Epidemiol.* **28**(4):652–8.

Morris, J.N., Heady, J.A., Raffle, P.A.B., Roberts, C.G., and Parks, J.W. (1953). Coronary heart disease and physical activity of work. *Lancet* **II**:1053–7.

Netterstrom, B. and Suadicani, P. (1993). Self-assessed job satisfaction and ischaemic heart disease mortality: a 10-year follow up of urban bus drivers. *Int. J. Epidemiol.* **22**:51–6.

Niedhammer, I., Siegrist, J., Landré, M.F., Goldberg, M., and Leclerc, A. (2000). Étude des qualités psychométriques de la version française du modèle du déséquilibre efforts/récompenses. *Revue D'Épidémiologie et Santé Publique* **48**: 419–37.

Niedhammer, I., Teck, M.L., Starke, D., and Siegrist, J. (2004). Effort—reward imbalance model and self reported health: cross-sectional and prospective results from the GAZEL cohort. *Soc. Sci. Med.* **58**:1531–41.

North, F.M., Syme, S.L., Feeney, A., Head, J., Shipley, M.J., and Marmot, M.G. (1993). Explaining socioeconomic differences in sickness absence: the Whitehall II study. *BMJ* **306**:361–6.

North, F.M., Syme, S.L., Feeney, A., Shipley, M.J., and Marmot, M.G. (1996). Psychosocial work environment and sickness absence among British civil servants: the Whitehall II Study. *Am. J. Publ. Health* **86**:332–40.

Orth–Gomer, K, Wamala, S.P., Horsten, M., Schenck–Gustafsson, K., Schneiderman, N., and Mittelman, M.A. (2000). Marital stress worsens prognosis in women with coronary heart disease: the Stockholm female coronary risk study. *JAMA* **284**:3008–14.

Osler, W. (1910). The Lumleian Lectures on angina pectoris. *Lancet* 175:839–44.

Ostry,A.S., Kelly, S., Demers, P.A., Mustard, C., and Hertzman,C. (2003). A comparison between the effort–reward imbalance and demand–control models. *BMC Public Health* 3: 10–19.

Paoli, P. and Merllié, D. (2001). *Third European survey of working conditions*. Dublin: European Foundation for the Improvement of Living and Working Conditions.

Perrewé, P.L. and Ganster, D.C. (eds.) (2002). *Historical and current perspectives on stress and health*. Amsterdam: JAI Elsevier.

Peter, R., Siegrist, J., Hallqvist, J., Reuterwall, C., Theorell, T., and the SHEEP Study Group (2002). Psychosocial environment and myocardial infarction: improving risk estimation by combining two alternative job stress models in the SHEEP Study Group. *J. Epidemiol. Commun. Health* **56**: 294–300.

Pfeffer, J. (1998). *Human equation. Building profit by putting people first*. Boston: Harvard Business School Press.

Reed, D.M., Lacroix, A.Z., Karasek, R.A., Miller, D., and MacLean, C.A. (1989). Occupational strain and the incidence of coronary heart disease. *Am. J. Epidemiol.* **129**:495–502.

Sacker, A., Bartley, M., Firth, D., and Fitzpatrick, R. (2001). Dimensions of social inequality in the health of women in England: occupational, material and behavioural pathways. *Soc. Sci. Med.* **52**:763–81.

Schilling, R.S.F. (1989). Health protection and promotion at work. *Br. J. Ind. Med.* **46**:683–8.

Schnall, P., Belkic, K., and Pickering, T.G. (2000). Assessment of the cardiovascular system at the workplace. *Occup. Med.* **15(1)**:189–212.

Siegrist, J. (1996). Adverse health effects of high-effort/low-reward conditions. *J. Occup. Health. Psychol* **1**:27–41.

Siegrist, J. (2002). Effort–reward imbalance at work and health. In: *Historical and Current Perspectives on stress and health* (ed. P.L. Perrewe and D.C. Ganster), pp. 261–91. Amsterdam: JAI Elsevier.

Siegrist, J. and Marmot, M. (2004). Health inequalities and the psychosocial environment—two scientific challenges. *Soc. Sci. Med.* **58**:1463–73.

Siegrist, J. and Peter, R. (1997). Chronic work stress is associated with atherogenic lipids and elevated fibrinogen in middle-aged men. *J. Int. Med.* **242(2)**:149–56.

Siegrist, J., Klein, D., Grunewald, R., and Matschinger, H. (1986). Pressure response and heart rate reaction to a mental stress test in a blue-collar population at cardiovascular risk. *J. Hypertension* 4:S260–2.

Siegrist, J., Klein, D., and Voigt, K.H. (1997). Linking sociological with physiological data: the model of effort–reward imbalance at work. *Acta Physiologica Scandinavia* 161, Suppl. 640: 112–16.

Siegrist, J., Menrath, I., Stücker, T., Klein, M., Kellermann, T., Shah, N.J., *et al.* (2005). Effort–reward imbalance at work moderates brain activity during monetary loss experience (submitted).

Siegrist, J., Peter, R., Junge, A., Cremer, P., and Seidel, D. (1990). Low status control, high effort at work and ischemic heart disease: prospective evidence from blue-collar men. *Soc. Sci. Med.* **31**:1127–34.

Siegrist, J., Starke, D., Chandola, T., *et al.* (2004). The measurement of effort–reward imbalance at work: European comparisons. *Soc. Sci. Med.* **58**:1483–99.

Stansfeld, S., Bosma, H., Hemingway, H., and Marmot, M. (1998). Psychosocial work characteristics and social support as predictors of SF-36 functioning: the Whitehall II study. *Psychosomatic Medicine* **60**:247–55.

Stansfeld, S.A., Fuhrer, R., Shipley, M.J., and Marmot, M.G. (1999). Work characteristics predict psychiatric disorder: prospective results from the Whitehall II Study. *Occupational and Environmental Medicine* **56(5)**:302–7.

Stansfeld, S.A., Rael, E.G.S., Head, J., Shipley, M., and Marmot, M. (1997). Social support and psychiatric sickness absence: a prospective study of British civil servants. *Psychological Medicine* **27**:35–48.

Steenland, K., Johnson, J., and Nowlin, S. (1997). A follow up study of job strain and heart disease among males in the NHANES1 population. *Am. J. Ind. Med* **31**:256–60.

Steptoe, A., Siegrist, J., Kirschbaum, C., and Marmot, M. (2004). Effort–reward imbalance, overcommitment, and measures of cortisol and blood pressure over the working day. *Psychosomatic Medicine* **66**:323–9.

Suadicani, P., Hein, H.O., and Gynetelberg, F. (1993). Are social inequalities as associated with the risk ischaemic heart disease a result of psychosocial working conditions? *Atherosclerosis* **101**:165–75.

Theorell, T. (2002). Job stress and fibrinogen. *Eur. Heart J.* **23(23)**:1799–801.

Theorell, T. (2004). Democracy at work and its relationship with health. In: *Emotional and physiological processes and positive intervention strategies* (ed. P.L. Perrewé and D.C. Ganster). Amsterdam: Elsevier.

Theorell, T. and Floderus–Myrhed, B. (1977). 'Workload' and risk of myocardal infarction—a prospective psychosocial analysis. *Int. J. Epidemiol.* **6**:17–21.

Theorell, T., Emdad, R., Arnetz, B., and Weingarten, A.M. (2001). Employee effects of an educational program for managers at an insurance company. *Psychosomatic Medicine* **63**: 724–33.

Theorell, T., Hasselhorn, H.M., and the MUSIC Norrtalje Study Group (2002). Endocrinological and immunological variables sensitive to psychosocial factors of possible relevance to work-related musculoskeletal disorders. *Work and Stress* **16(2)**:154–65.

Theorell, T., Orth–Gomer, K., and Eneroth, P. (1990). Slow-reacting immunoglobulin in relation to social support and changes in job strain: a preliminary note. *Psychosomatic Medicine* **52**:511–16.

Theorell, T., Tsutumi, A., Hallqvist, J., Reuterwall, C., Fredlund, P., Emlund, N., *et al.* (1998). Decision latitude, job strain, and myocardial infarction: a study of working men in Stockholm. *Am. J. Public Health* **88(3)**:382–88.

Tsutsumi, A. and Kawakami, N. (2004). A review of empirical studies on the model of effort–reward imbalance at work: reducing occupational stress by implementing a new theory. *Soc. Sci. Med.* **59**: 2335–59.

Uemura, K. and Pisa, Z. (1988). Trends in cardiovascular disease mortality in industrialised countries since 1950. *World Health Statistics Quarterly* **41**:155–78.

van Vegchel, N., de Jonge, J., Bosma, H., and Schaufeli, W. (2005). Reviewing the effort–reward imbalance model: drawing up the balance of 45 empirical studies. *Soc. Sci. Med.* **60**:1117–31.

Vingard, E., Alfredsson, L., Hagberg, M., Kilbom, A., Theorell, T., Waldenstrom, M., *et al.* (2000). To what extent do current and past physical and psychosocial occupational factors explain care-seeking for low back pain in a working population? Results from the Musculoskeletal Intervention Center–Norrtalje Study. *Spine* **25(4)**:493–500.

Vrijkotte, D.G.M., Doornen, L.J.P.v., and Geus, E.J.C.d. (1999). Work stress and metabolic and hemostatic risk factors. *Psychosomatic Medicine* **61**:796–805.

Vrijkotte, D.G.M., Doornen, L.J.P.v., and Geus, E.J.C.d. (2000). Effect of work stress on ambulatory blood pressure, heart rate, and heart rate variability. *Hypertension***35**: 880–6.

Wahlstedt, K. (2001). *Postal work—work organizational changes as tools to improve health*. Uppsala: Acta Universitatis Uppsaliensis.

Welin, C., Lappas, G., and Wilhelmsen, L. (2000). Independent importance of psychosocial factors for prognosis after myocardial infarction. *J. Intern. Med.* **247(6)**:629–39.

Westerberg, L. and Theorell, T. (1997). Working conditions and family situation in relation to functional gastrointestinal disorders. The Swedish Dyspepsia Project. *Scand. J. Prim. Health Care* **15(2)**:76–81.

Westerlund, H., Ferrie, J., Hagberg, J., Jeding, K., Oxenstierna, G., and Theorell, T. (2004). Workplace expansion, long-term sickness absence, and hospital admission. *Lancet* **363**: 1193–7.

Westman, M. (2002). Crossover of stress and strain in the family and work place. In: *Historical and Current Perspectives on Stress and Health* (ed. P.L. Perrewé and D.C. Ganster), pp. 143–81. Amsterdam: JAI Elsevier.

White, C., Van Galen, F., and Chow, Y.H. (2003). Trends in social class differences in mortality by cause, 1986 to 2000. *Health Statistics Quarterly* **20**:25–37.

Chapter 7

Transport and health

Mark McCarthy

7.1 **Background**

Epidemiology, the study of health and disease in populations, is quite a new science. Much of the early work on infectious diseases, the leading cause of death and disease until recent times, led to effective control through public policies of sanitation, quarantine, and immunization. Chronic disease epidemiology developed in the mid-twentieth century, and the new paradigm of 'risk factors' emphasized individual responsibility and the opportunities for health promotion through changing behaviour. More recently, however, the importance of public policy in sustaining or damaging health has been re-established. It is the intention of this chapter to show that transport is a crucial contributor to health and disease in contemporary European countries, and that major changes are needed in public policy to reverse existing trends.

The new paradigm in thinking about transport and health has been to shift the debate from 'safety' to health benefits (Davis 1993). 'Safety' has been used by public authorities to create transport systems that are sometimes harmful to health. For example, a law introduced in Victoria, Australia, requiring cyclists to wear helmets led to fewer people cycling—and, therefore, not getting the health benefit that cycling provides (Robinson 2003). Another example of the difference between 'safety' and health has been the use of the financial 'costs' attributed to loss of life in accidents as a justification for further road building. Such calculations are flawed, however, since new roads generate more cars and more journeys by a means of transport that is more dangerous than its alternatives (buses and trains).

Many older epidemiologists learned their basic statistics from textbooks that described the Poisson distribution (of infrequent random events) using Bortkiewicz's example of the number of people kicked to death by horses—infrequent in distribution over time, although when added together (e.g. for a whole year), remarkably consistent. If we substitute the modern people transporter, the car, for the horse in Bortkiewicz's example, we have very similar results—deaths are infrequent and scattered over time according to a Poisson distribution. The unexpectedness of the event, and its possible avoidance, led to the term 'accident'. Epidemiologists though, noting the recurrent nature of these 'accidents', have found associations (environmental, for example opportunities for speeding, or individual, for example drunk driving) which increase the likelihood of an accident happening. (In the literature, there is often argument whether the term used should, instead, be 'injury', emphasizing the actual rather than chance nature of the event. However, the term 'accident' will be retained here, as it has a commonplace meaning and there may be confusion for 'injury' between the event itself and the physical effects.)

7.2 Sustainable development—a global perspective

Essential to debate on transport and health is the concept of 'sustainable development'. The United Nations 'Earth Summit' in Rio de Janiero in 1992 focused world opinion on protecting the Earth's resources, biosystems, and societies for present and future generations. The Earth Summit report mentioned 'health' many times and the World Health Organization and other agencies have reaffirmed the relationship between sustainable development and health.

Sustainable development acknowledges that economic development will continue in all parts of the world and, along with population increase, there will be pressure on scarce resources. One particular focus is the use of energy. The 1997 Kyoto United Nations Conference set international agreements for controlling carbon dioxide, produced from fossil fuels, which is a greenhouse gas with the potential to create global warming. Although oil is needed for much industrial production in developing countries, advanced economies do not rely so much on industrial products as on services; and, in both business and leisure, the use of transport—especially the car—has been growing. Predictions that transfer the existing patterns of car use of Western countries to all the people in developing countries show that the car is quite unsustainable, from the energy perspective, as a means of global transport. (The same will apply to oil-fuelled air travel if current trends persist.) Western economies are using cars at a far greater level of CO_2 production per capita than is acceptable globally, and will have to cut down their car use. Sustainable development provides a critical perspective on transport patterns.

Oil is a dominant economic presence in the world economy. The Gulf wars against Iraq in 1991 and 2003 were launched, in part, to protect Western sources of oil. Development of Russia and the central Asian republics is giving pre-eminence to oil extraction and their transport to developing economic markets. Much oil is used for motor vehicles, and the market is continually growing. World Health Day in 2004, organized by the World Health Organization and launched in Paris by President Chirac, was for the first time focused on road safety. The *World Report on Road Traffic Injury Prevention*, published jointly by the World Health Organization and the World Bank (Peden *et al.* 2004), shows that 1.2 million people die from road accidents worldwide each year, and between 20 and 50 millions are injured, some with permanent disabilities. Mortality rates are highest in Africa and Middle Eastern countries. It is predicted that road crashes will be the third greatest cause of death and disability, worldwide, by the year 2020, just behind clinical depression and heart disease, and ahead of respiratory infections, tuberculosis, and HIV. The impact will be greatest in the rapidly motorising countries.

7.3 **Patterns of travel**

Travel can be by different modes of transport, depending on the distances to be travelled, and including walking, cycling, buses, cars, trains, boats, and aircraft. International comparative data are available only for vehicle travel, not walking (a significant public health limitation). In recent decades, in western Europe, the number of journeys by bus and rail have remained stable or diminished, whereas travel by car and air have increased. By contrast, in countries of central and eastern Europe, and the newly independent states, bus and rail travel remain important means of travel, while car use is expanding from a low base.

The National Travel Survey for Great Britain (GB) shows that 30 per cent of journeys are for work and 20 per cent visiting friends (Department of Transport 2004*a*). Two thirds of trips are by car, either as a driver or motor vehicle passenger (Fig. 7.1). The length of journey is closely related to mode of transport: for journeys over 12 km, cars are, by far, the most used means of transport.

Travel patterns are related to income. While the total *number* of trips between social groups is relatively similar, about 1000 a year (Fig. 7.2), people in low-income families travel further *distance*, by walking and by bus, than people in high-income families, while high-income families travel much further by car (Fig. 7.3).

7.4 **Trends**

The dominant trend of travel in past decades in western societies has been the rise in motor vehicle transport, static use of public transport, and falling journeys and distance for cycling and walking. Even in the last decade, for example, the distance travelled by car has increased, and walking has fallen by the same proportion (Fig. 7.4).

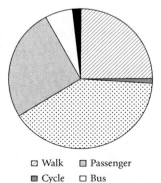

⊘ Walk	▢ Passenger
▨ Cycle	▢ Bus
▨ Driver	■ Rail

Fig. 7.1 Trips per person, by mode, GB, 2003. (*Source:* Department of Transport 2004*a*).

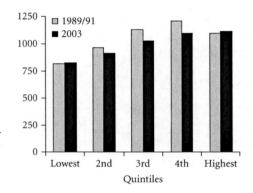

Fig. 7.2 Trips per person, per year, by social group, GB. (*Source*: Department of Transport 2004*a*).

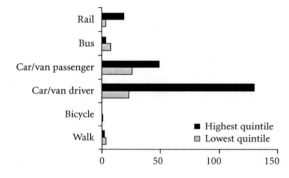

Fig. 7.3 Miles travelled per year, by mode, for highest and lowest quintile income groups, GB, 2003. (*Source*: Department of Transport 2004*a*).

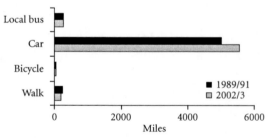

Fig. 7.4 Annual average miles travelled per person, per year, by mode, GB. (*Source*: Department of Transport 2004*a*).

Total journeys increased by only 10 per cent over the same period, and since 2000 have been falling. For freight, there has been an increase in both volume (measured as weight) and distance. Road transport volume doubled in the period 1952–94, but the distance covered increased four-fold. In the same period, rail volume diminished. In the last decade, the distance of freight transported by rail has doubled (Table 7.1). (It is of note that more than a quarter of moving road freight vehicles are empty.)

7.5 **Health impacts of transport**

Transport impacts on health reflect the range of the WHO definition of health—physical, mental, and quality of life.

Table 7.1 Changes in freight transport by mode, UK, 1952, 1994, and 2003

	1952	1994	2003
Volume (million tonnes)			
Road	861	1689	1725
Rail	289	97	89
Distance (million tonne km)			
Road	31	144	n/a
Rail	37	13	n/a
Average length per haul (km)			
Road	n/a	85	92
Rail	n/a	133	213

Sources: Potter 1997 and Department of Transport 2004*b*.

7.5.1 Heart disease

Probably the most important contribution of transport to health is through encouraging exercise—either walking or cycling—which protects against heart disease. There is strong epidemiological evidence that regular exercise, a balanced diet, and not smoking, promote cardiovascular health. Walking, the most accessible form of regular moderate physical exercise, benefits people of all ages. Regular exercise probably has both short-term effects of cardiovascular fitness and long-term cumulative protective effects by limiting development of obesity, strengthening the heart muscle, and reducing blood pressure, and metabolic effects, including improving cholesterol and fibrinogen levels and insulin sensitivity (Morris and Hardman 1997).

Two major studies showing the protective effects of exercise are shown in Fig. 7.5 and Table 7.2. Beneficial exercise may be undertaken in bouts of continuous moderate activity, for example, daily 30-minute periods, or accumulated during the day in shorter periods. In other words, it is not necessary to create 'special' exercise, but instead exercise can be incorporated within a day's activities, including travel, gardening, leisure, and social visits.

A further benefit of exercise comes in limiting progression of osteoporosis (loss of bone density that develops in older people, especially women, and leads typically to hip and arm fractures). Regular exercise and weight-bearing ensure continued bone strength, and is probably more beneficial, on a population level, than current drug treatments for osteoporosis.

7.5.2 Mental health

Exercise is recognized to have mental health benefits (Morris and Hardman 1997) through stimulating thought and protecting from depression—there is probably a direct physiological causal path. A rather more complex, negative relationship to mental health is the effect of traffic through 'community severance' (the separation of geographical parts of a community because of traffic flows). Studies in the USA and Europe (British Medical Association 1997, pp. 38–43) have shown that streets with less traffic (speed and

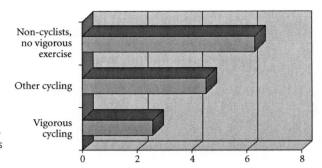

Fig. 7.5 Heart attack rates in male cyclists and non-cyclists, 1976–86, UK. (*Source*: Morris 1990).

Table 7.2 Risk of death, over 4 years, of older men (age range 56–75); related to regular daily walking

Regular daily walking (min/day)	Age-adjusted relative risk (men 60+)
0	1.00
<20	0.99
21–40	0.85
41–60	0.76
60+	0.52

Source: Wanamethee *et al.* 1998.

volume) have a better quality of life (measured, for example, by counts of street activities, open windows, flower boxes, and other signs of personal care), and are perceived by families to be more friendly and free from danger. In San Francisco, people living in three streets in a single neighbourhood with different intensities of traffic were shown to have a marked gradient in social contacts (Fig. 7.6). With heavy traffic density, there is a relative fall in land values, the houses are less desirable, and the streets are perceived as more stressful, especially for children and elderly people. While motor journeys can help social support for people who live at a distance from each other, the negative impacts are largely on other people who live close to the traffic routes. Increased social dispersion, supported by car transport, may thus be damaging health.

The link between traffic noise and health at population exposure levels (in contrast to higher noise industrial exposure) has been difficult to investigate (Berglund and Lindvall 1995; Stansfeld *et al.* 2000). Within limited studies, annoyance and loss of concentration have been shown, but no causal association with mental illness. Road traffic, neighbours, and aircraft are the most widespread noise nuisance (Fig. 7.7). The reduced quality of life from both airport and trunk road noise is demonstrated through lower house prices.

7.5.3 Respiratory disease

Most people in towns spend most of their lives indoors, and thus there are important effects of indoor air on respiratory diseases: coal fires contribute to respiratory diseases

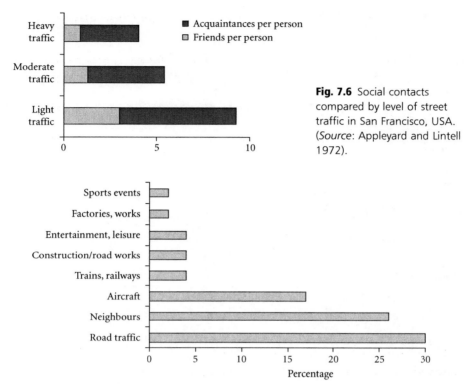

Fig. 7.6 Social contacts compared by level of street traffic in San Francisco, USA. (*Source*: Appleyard and Lintell 1972).

Fig. 7.7 People adversely affected by noise, by cause, England and Wales, 1999/2000. (*Source*: Department of Transport 2004*a*).

in childhood, while central heating or damp walls, creating environments suitable for house dust mites or mould respectively, may increase allergic asthma. Urban external air quality has improved considerably in recent decades, as a result of industrial zones and changing from coal to oil and gas domestic heating. Urban air pollution is now mainly due to road traffic—and air respects few boundaries. For example, ozone resulting from the interaction of sunlight with road traffic pollution in one country can affect a neighbouring country in the following days (Schwartz 1997).

Tables 7.3 and 7.4 indicate levels of air pollutant emissions from transport, and their proportion from transport compared with other sources. Air pollution can affect health in four ways: carcinogenic volatile organic compounds such as benzene and 1,3 butadiene; greenhouse gases, especially carbon dioxide, affecting the global climate; acid gases, including sulphur and nitrogen oxides, contributing to acute respiratory illnesses; and particulates, especially produced as diesel vehicles.

Pollutants act both through acute episodes and by long-term action (McMichael 1997). The former, especially as photochemical smog, catches public awareness, and has led governments, for example, to advise car drivers to leave their cars at home for

Table 7.3 Transport emissions of air pollutants

Year	Air pollutant (1000 tonnes)						
	Carbon monoxide	Nitrogen oxides	Particulates (PM$_{10}$)	Sulphur dioxide	Benzene	1,3 butadiene	Lead
1980	5842	1199	64	103			7537
1990	5836	1516	73	110	43	11	2176
2000	2975	995	50	38	8	4	3

Source: Department of Transport 2004a.

Table 7.4 Proportion of air pollution from transport, UK, 2002

Emissions	Percentage						
	Carbon monoxide	Nitrogen oxides	Particulates (PM$_{10}$)	Sulphur dioxide	Benzene	1,3,butadiene	Lead
Transport	92	72	54	48	29	3	1
Other	8	28	46	52	71	97	99

Source: Department of Transport 2004b.

the day. Short-term health impacts in 26 European cities have been estimated in an international comparative study (APHEIS 2004). The long-term impacts on chronic respiratory diseases and deaths has been inferred from epidemiological studies in the United States. These studies suggest that particulates, rather than acidic gases, are the primary cause of lung damage, and indicate a gradient between average particulates exposure and premature deaths, at population level. While acute smog episodes may temporarily increase asthma rates, the effects are primarily on people with previous respiratory disease (Anderson 1997)—suggesting the need for much broader policies than temporary car restriction. Current attention is being given to small particulates (PM$_{2.5}$) from vehicle exhausts which can penetrate the bronchiolar systems more deeply than soot particles (PM$_{10}$).

7.5.4 Accidents

Data on deaths are more reliable than on injuries because of more complete recording; however, countries use different approaches in applying coding rules, so that differences between countries should be interpreted with caution. Traveller injury rates vary by mode of transport, but there are different ways of presenting these data. Using distance travelled, long-distance modes, including rail and air, appear the most safe, with motor cyclists the highest risk. For individuals, however, it is probably the rate per journey that matters. Risks per journey show the greater risk from car travel.

The persistent differences between countries in road traffic accident death rates relate, in part, to cultural and technical characteristics. Countries appear to follow

Smeed's law (Adams 1985) in starting with high accident rates per driver, and these fall as drivers become more experienced. However, with increasing numbers of drivers, the total road accidents death rates may not fall: for example, the all-ages road accident death rates in Greece were 14.9 per 100,000 in 1981 and 17.1 in 2001.

However, safety is not represented by accident rates because it is mediated by human action and exposure (Adams 1988). Motorways are not safe to cross as a pedestrian, yet pedestrian deaths on motorways are very few because pedestrians recognize that they are very unsafe. Cyclist death rates per head of population are higher in the Netherlands than in most other European countries; but there are many more journeys made by bicycle in the Netherlands, so the risk per journey is lower. Moreover, there appears to be safety in numbers for both cyclists and walkers (Robinson 2005).

There is an exponential rise in risk to pedestrians with increasing traffic speed (Finch *et al.* 1994). At 30 km/h, only five per cent of pedestrians involved in road accidents are killed, and most injuries are slight. At 40 km/h, 45 per cent of pedestrians are killed; while in crashes at more than 50 km/h, up to 85 per cent of pedestrians struck by a car are killed. It is estimated that, in the UK, about 30 per cent of all road deaths are caused directly by speeding (British Medical Association 1997).

Different road users have different accident profiles: the cause of an accident should not be attributed to the victim. It is car driving that is 'unsafe' (it causes injuries because of velocity), while cycling is much safer (rarely causing deaths either to car drivers or cyclists). Much effort has been put into 'improving' roads to reduce accidents. However, the net effect, linked with higher car technical performance, has been increasing car speeds, fuller roads, and greater perceived risk for those not using cars. Few pedestrians would regard town roads in the 1990s as safer than in the 1950s, even if the accident rate per kilometre travelled is lower. 'Safety' improvements (apparently for other road users) have been converted into 'performance' improvements (for car drivers).

Road injuries occur to people of all ages, but there are different exposures by age. Pedestrian road deaths are highest in children and old people; young adults are particularly at risk as drivers and passengers of cars and motorbikes. Middle-aged male car drivers are at greater risk because of high exposure. Cyclists are at risk at all ages. Internationally, these rates differ country by country according to exposure, environment, and cultural habits. For example, in 2001, Sweden had 0.3 child (age 5–14 years) pedestrian deaths per 100,000 children, whereas the UK had 0.9 per 100,000 children.

Accidents characteristically show a social class gradient—in the UK, deaths from road traffic accidents to children from the poorest families (social class V) are more than four times greater than those in the richest (social class I) families (Jarvis *et al.* 1995). In the USA, accident rates for drivers from deprived areas are also higher than for those from rich areas (Abdalla *et al.* 1997). Fatal road accidents (pedestrians and vehicle occupants combined) are more frequent in socially deprived areas, but less frequent in urban than rural areas (Haynes *et al.* 2005).

Geographical variations are significantly associated with measures of exposure, including number of cars per capita, length of roads, and average measured volume of traffic in the location of the accident. Unfortunately, no analysis has been made of the socio-economic characteristics of the drivers, rather than the victims. Tennant (2005) investigated the socio-economic determinants of head injury admission in England, and found substantial geographical variations. As with fatal accidents, head injury admission rates are lower in urban than rural areas, independently of socio-economic factors. In regression analysis, the age 16–24 unemployment rate, proportion permanently sick of working age, and proportion of lone parent families, are associated with higher admission rates; using public transport to go to work is associated with lower admission rates.

7.6 Interventions

The focus of interventions proposed here is strategic and mainly within the responsibilities of national or municipal departments of transport. Engineering-based policies for road 'safety' continue to form the main approach by governments: transport policies should give higher priority to walking, cycling, and public transport—forms of travel that are health promoting, of low risk, and fulfil sustainability objectives. In many European cities, high levels of investment in cycling have contributed to an overall reduction in casualties and perceptions of safer environments (Transport for London 2004). However, increasing affluence, 'convenience', and commercial forces are all leading to greater use of motor vehicles.

7.6.1 Policies for walking

1 Changing thinking: in the past, pedestrians in towns have been physically separated from motor traffic, restrained by barriers, and detoured into underpasses, on the questionable grounds that this will improve 'safety'. Transport planning must prioritize pedestrians over cars in transport decisions, especially when crossing roads at junctions.

2 Increasing access: priority should be given to good interchange between pedestrians and public transport, with frequent access points.

3 Improving quality: walking should be an enjoyable environmental experience, with a good sense of safety. This can be encouraged by 'greening' towns, widening footways, narrowing roads, placing street furniture (traffic signs, barriers) in roads rather than on footways, ensuring good lighting, reducing traffic volumes and road parking to increase the pleasantness of journeys.

4 Creating clearly linked pedestrian networks for important routes; for example, for shopping, to schools, to libraries, and to hospitals.

5 Ensuring that there are good local facilities for all neighbourhoods within convenient walking/cycling distance.

7.6.2 **Policies for cycling**

1 Changing thinking: cycling must be seen as *the* normal means of travelling short- to middle-length distances in towns, backed by local authority and police support (including ensuring that their own staff use bicycles regularly). Special attention to promote cycling is needed in cities with hills.

2 Provision must be made for all potential cycle journeys—it is estimated that cycling could replace at least half of all present car trips in Britain (Friends of the Earth 1992).

3 Until car traffic has been severely reduced and on-street parking abolished, there should be separate cycle lanes on all roads, as there are (already) pavements.

4 Cycle parking facilities should be widespread, well designed (for safety), and prioritized for interchange with public transport.

5 Many examples of good practice in promoting cycling exist across Europe; for example, those described by the European Cyclists Federation (*http://www.ecf.com*).

6 Sustrans—a sustainable transport charity in the UK—has created a national cycle network and supported a range of practical cycling projects (*http://www.sustrans.org.uk*)

7.6.3 **Improving public transport**

Public transport is the key to middle- and long-distance travel. Group travel saves energy and is both economical and more sustainable. People who rarely travel by public transport on land are willing to use communal passenger aeroplanes.

Debate about public transport sometimes gets caught in disagreement on the level of subsidies. There are few grounds for subsidies that retain inefficient practices and arguments in favour of prices reflecting true costs, especially environmental costs. However, direct subsidies of public transport may be an efficient way of redressing income and access inequalities. It is necessary to invest in, and maintain, public transport to ensure a strong alternative to individual car travel. It is more important for central and local governments to maintain good services (through contracts and subsidies) than it is for the public authority actually to operate the service—although some public authorities do provide excellent services.

Policies for public transport include:

1 Integration of all modes of public transport with each other (e.g. with transferable tickets) and with walking and cycling (e.g. cycle parking);

2 Good facilities for cycles on buses and trains;

3 Frequent and reliable services;

4 Routes that serve suburbs and rural areas—this may involve good interconnections rather than many long routes going through the city centre;

5 Innovation and responsiveness to consumer concerns.

7.6.4 **Policies for vehicle restraint**

It is now recognized, at European level, that the trend of increasing vehicle use in the twentieth century should be reversed in the twenty-first century (Expert Group on the Urban Environment 1996). The means to achieve traffic reduction, however, will vary from country to country and at different levels. National, regional, and local authorities need to set targets for traffic reduction based on realistic policies, and then assess the effectiveness of implementation against these targets.

Historical trends for transport growth in European countries in the twentieth century, except during wars, have been for annual increases in car ownership and use, and a shift from rail to road transport of goods. The trends have been interpreted by planners as requiring more roads to be built—a process mockingly called 'predict and provide' by critics. But there are almost always advocates of road building—the construction companies, the landowners, the people living in a town that will be 'bypassed', and the motoring organizations. Instead, the new approach to sustainable transport must actively seek to restrain car journeys and road transport. Car use declines when people choose a nearer destination (shorter car trips), switch from car to an alternative mode (walking, cycling, or public transport), or decide not to travel (alternative modes of communication). Car reduction policies will need all three choices.

Strategies for reducing traffic have to be comprehensive:

1 Reducing traffic in one area must not lead to its diversion into another area.

2 All members of society must contribute (including, for example, politicians, professionals, and executives).

3 Incentives for change are needed—change must not depend just on goodwill from a minority.

4 Traffic reduction should be integrated with other priorities—increasing cycling and walking, improving public transport and urban environments, reducing 'car-dependent' urban facilities (for example, those using car parking, such as supermarkets and large leisure facilities).

Some of the strategies currently used for traffic reduction include:

1 Traffic calming: for example, chicanes that narrow streets, road 'humps' and raised tables at intersections and crossways, moving 'street furniture' (parking meters and notices, road signs) off pavements and into the road.

2 Closing roads: roads that are pedestrianized, and cul-de-sacs, whilst reducing the numbers of vehicles, can sustain the same number of journeys by other means of transport if planned effectively.

3 Bans and permit schemes: closing areas of cities to traffic, requiring vehicles to have at least three passengers, limiting the total number of vehicles licensed.

4 Substantial taxation of vehicles: on parking spaces (public and private), on licences, on buying and selling vehicles, on fuel.

5 Reducing demand: providing school buses and promoting children walking to school, working from home, and local sourcing of food and other goods.

Some cities have kept their historic centres entirely car-free (Venice and Fez (in Morocco) are two important examples); others have reduced the use of cars substantially in their ancient streets (e.g. Rome). Even cities built during the days of carriages and trams (e.g. Zurich) have achieved major reductions in vehicle use through integrated policies of limiting car access while promoting walking and cycling and good public transport.

Pedestrianizing city centres is now a normal policy in many cities to stem the otherwise inexorable increase of traffic and consequent traffic jams; but car reduction is a much larger concern. It must address the increasing car ownership across a wider range of the population—retired people, young people in their first job, parents with young families. Cars are exceedingly cheap to buy and run because their costs to other people are not properly paid. The marginal cost of commuting or leisure trips can be significantly less than that of public transport when there is more than one person in the car. Raising the price of car travel to reflect environmental costs can be achieved by road pricing (e.g. car mileage meters) and capital taxes (Singapore levies a high tax on buying a new car unless an old car is concurrently destroyed). Congestion charging, at eight euros per day, introduced in London in 2003, produced an immediate reduction of 15% in traffic volume.

Car reduction must also address the increasing use of cars across outer parts of cities, or as transport in from the countryside to the town. The predictions of car use over the next decades are not for more city-centre traffic, but for more rural driving. Having saturated the city centres, cars are now increasing in the emptier suburban and rural roads, assisted by peri-urban road building. More than ever before, rich people want to live in the countryside and use cars for access to towns and rural facilities. There is a further challenge—that the rural car owner claims more 'need' for a car since public transport is less available than in towns because it is less economic. But the number of people who work in farming is falling across Europe: people are making choices to live in the countryside (and work in the town) because of its physical and social environmental advantages. Land-use planning, which is under the direct control of central and local governments, is crucial in reversing the trend to rural commuting and expanding 'dormitory' villages.

Changes in the transport of goods are also needed. Some of these are national policies: for example, governments should concern themselves to maintain local production of natural local products (where skills and/or resources exist) and resist the commercial trends of globalization, where transport external costs are significant. International trade in buses, for example, makes little sense if a country has a sufficiently developed home market for local production; on the other hand, electronic goods and services can be traded with less environmental damage (e.g. through the Internet). Local governments need to pay special attention to local distribution of goods. A study of cyclists' deaths in London (Gilbert and McCarthy 1994) showed that more than half were killed by heavy (more than three-tonne) lorries. Leiden is introducing a system of transferring goods from large vehicles to small vans for city distribution: it is estimated that 70 per cent of the goods and 80 per cent of the journeys can be converted in this way (Expert Group on the Urban Environment 1996).

7.7 The politics of change

The three integrated policies needed for transport and health—beyond improving 'safety'—are therefore: promoting walking and cycling, improving public transport, and reducing motor vehicle transport (both passenger and goods). In the oil 'crisis' of the 1970s, the cartel of oil-producing countries raised their prices dramatically and generated the first major understanding of the international dependence on oil. Many countries introduced energy-saving regulations including, for example, 80 km/h speed limits on main roads and improved insulation in housing. However, as the oil supply stabilized, road speed limits were raised again: neither health nor environmental arguments were as strong as the pressure from road-user organizations to allow increased speeds.

The forces working politically for private transport have been described collectively as the 'road lobby' (Hamer 1987). The lobby includes motoring organizations (with millions of members subscribing to receive insurance and emergency services); road construction companies (some of the richest public building contracts have been for motorway construction); car manufacturers (most European countries build and sell cars at home and abroad); oil companies (with points of sale across the country); and advertisers (working to portfolios for all the previous groups). That many journeys are made by foot is not reflected in the relative lobbying power of pedestrians against the road lobby. Getting a bypass built around 'his' or 'her' town can be a major local success for a politician; improving facilities for cyclists gains few votes.

The difficulty of implementing change was described in detail in a study of the northern Danish city of Aalborg (Flyvbjerg 1998). This town was one of the first to take traffic restriction seriously, and sought to implement an inner-city scheme of improved bus services, partial pedestrianization, and improved cycle access. The study describes how these objectives of the city planners were thwarted by local coalitions—especially the Chamber of Commerce (worried about any change in journeys to local shops), the police (preferring car users to bus passengers or cyclists), and the local press (using the scheme to attack the political majority). Despite acclaim of the scheme by the Danish professional planning association, the actual results were modest: indeed, over a 10-year period, car traffic had increased.

Yet Aalborg was a pioneer. The innovative ideas of that time have now become more commonplace, and have been shown to be successful in a number of towns and cities. At the same time, Copenhagen, the capital of Denmark, introduced city policies to limit cars that were far more successful, and travel in Copenhagen now—by bus, metro, or cycle—is one of the pleasantest of experiences. A city council that is convinced of its course can have a considerable impact. Car Free Cities (Eurocities 1998) is a group of local authorities across Europe sharing experience on traffic-reduction policies and practice. Through publications and conferences, they are developing and demonstrating integrated local transport policies and promotion of walking and cycling.

Different attitudes towards transport across Europe were shown by a 'Eurobarometer' survey of the (then) 12 countries of the European Community. Respondents were asked to rate their perceptions of urban car traffic. Responses for 'unbearable' ranged from 14 per cent in Denmark and 18 per cent in the Netherlands to over 40 per cent in Italy and Greece, with the European mean as 22 per cent (European Commission 1996, Fig. 4.2.6). There is also strong support—a Europe-wide average of 71 per cent—for actions to limit car traffic in town centres, although 65 per cent said increasing charges would be ineffective in limiting car use (International Research Associates 1991).

7.8 **Conclusions**

National Ministries of Transport need to have greater understanding of the health benefits of transport through closer contact with health agencies. Equally, Ministries of Health need to improve their understanding of transport and health. European Ministers of Environment and Health, at a WHO summit in London, in 1999, jointly signed a Protocol on Transport and Health. WHO has continued this initiative through a pan-European programme on transport, health, and environment (THE PEP) and a research project modelling exposures and health effects of transport (HEARTS), as well as providing a range of resources (*http://www.euro.who.int/transport*).

National governments, which regulate choices for transport, are also responsible for the health to their people. Walking and cycling need to be prioritized in transport planning; compact cities that minimize vehicle journeys need to be prioritized in economic and land-use planning; public transport must be significantly improved, and car travel reduced; and leadership is needed from politicians, industry, and civil society (non-government organizations including unions, community groups, interest associations).

References

APHEIS (2004). Air pollution and health: a European information system. Health impact assessment of air pollution and communication strategy. *http://www.apheis.net/Apheis3NEW1.pdf*

Abdalla, I., Barker, D., and Raeside, R. (1997). Road accident characteristics and socio-economic deprivation. *Traff. Engin. Control* **38**, 672–6.

Adams, J. (1985). *Risk and freedom: the record of road safety regulation*. Transport Publishing Projects, Cardiff.

Adams, J. (1988). Risk homeostasis and the purpose of safety regulation. *Ergonomics* **31**, 407–28.

Anderson, R. (1997). Health effects of air pollution from traffic: discussion. In: *Health at the crossroads: transport policy and urban health* (ed. T. Fletcher and A.J. McMichael), pp. 82–5. John Wiley and Sons, London.

Appleyard, D. and Lintell, M. (1972). The environmental quality of city streets: the residents' viewpoint. *American Institute of Planners Journal* **38**, 84–101.

Berglund, B. and Lindvall, T. (ed.) (1995). *Community noise*. Centre for Sensory Research, Department of Psychology, Stockholm University, Stockholm.

British Medical Association (1997). *Road transport and health*. British Medical Association, London.

Davis, R. (1993). *Death on the streets: cars and the mythology of road safety*. Leading Edge Press, Hawes, North Yorkshire, UK.

Department of Transport (2004*a*). *National travel survey*. Department of Transport, London.

Department of Transport (2004*b*). *Transport trends, Great Britain*. Department of Transport, London.

Economic Commission for Europe (1994). *Annual bulletin of transport statistics for Europe*. United Nations, Geneva.

Eurocities (1998). *Car free cities magazine*. Eurocities, Brussels (cfc@eurocities.be)

Expert Group on the Urban Environment (1996). *European sustainable cities*. European Commission Directorate General XI, Brussels.

Finch, D., Kompfner, P., and Maycock, G. (1994). *Speed, speed limits and accidents*. Transport Research Laboratory, Crowthorne.

Flyvbjerg, B. (1998). *Rationality and power: democracy in practice*. University of Chicago Press, London.

Friends of the Earth (1992). *Less traffic, better towns*. Friends of the Earth, London.

Gilbert, K. and McCarthy, M. (1994). Cycling deaths in London 1985–92: the hazards of traffic. *BMJ* **308**, 1534–7.

Hamer, M. (1987). *Wheels within wheels: a study of the road lobby*. Routledge and Kegan Paul, London.

Haynes, R., Jones, A., Harvey, I., Jewell, T., and Lea, D. (2005). Geographical distribution of road traffic deaths in England and Wales: place of accident compared with place of residence. *Journal of Public Health* **27**, 107–11.

International Research Associates (1991). European attitudes towards urban traffic problems and public transport. INRA (Europe), Brussels.

Jarvis, S., Towner, E., and Walsh, S. (1995). Accidents. In: *The health of our children* (ed. B Botting for the Office of Population Censuses and Surveys). HMSO, London.

McMichael, A.J. (1997). Transport and health: assessing the risks. In: *Health at the crossroads: transport policy and urban health* (ed. T. Fletcher and A.J. McMichael), pp. 9–26. John Wiley and Sons, London.

Morris, J.N. (1990). Exercise in leisure time: coronary attack and death rates. *Br. Heart J.* **63**, 325–34.

Morris, J.N. and Hardman, A.E. (1997). Walking to health. *Sports Med.* **23**, 306–32.

Peden, M., *et al* (eds) (2004). *The world report on road traffic injury prevention*. Geneva, World Health Organization.

Potter, S. (1997). *Vital travel statistics*. Landor Publishing, London.

Robinson, D.L. (2003) Helmet laws and cycle use. *Inj. Prev.* **9**, 380–1.

Robinson, D.L. (2005). Safety in numbers in Australia: more walkers and bicyclists, safer walking and bicycling. *Health Promotion Journal of Australia* **16**, 47–51.

Schwartz, J. (1997). Health effects of air pollution from traffic: ozone and particulate matter. In: *Health at the crossroads: transport policy and urban health* (ed. T. Fletcher and A.J. McMichael), pp. 61–82. John Wiley and Sons, London.

Stansfeld, S.A., Haines, M.M., Burr, M., Berry, B., and Lercher, P. (2000). A review of environmental noise and mental health. *Noise and Health* **2**, 1–8.

Tennant, A. (2005). Admission to hospital following head injury in England: incidence and socio-economic associations. *BMC Public Health* **5**, 21.

Transport for London (2004). *A business case and evaluation of the impacts of cycling in London.* London, Transport for London Cycling Centre of Excellence.

Wanamethee, S.G., Shaper, A.G., and Walker, M. (1998). Changes in physical activity, mortality and incidence of coronary heart disease in older men. *Lancet* **351**, 1603–8.

World Health Organization (2005). *http://www.euro.who.int/transport*

Chapter 8

Social support and social cohesion

Stephen A. Stansfeld

8.1 Introduction

The evidence that social support is beneficial to health and that social isolation leads to ill health is now considerable. Social support has a positive effect on many different aspects of both physical and mental health. Yet the exact nature of the positive influence of social support on health remains elusive and definitions of support vary widely across the literature (Pahl 2003). As a concept, social support is used in many different ways and, in order to evaluate the evidence that social support influences health, it is important to be clear about its definition.

Social support has been defined as 'resources provided by other persons' (Cohen and Syme 1985). It has been seen as 'information leading the subject to believe that he is cared for and loved, is esteemed and valued and belongs to a social network of communication and mutual obligation' (Cobb 1976). Much of the theoretical work on social support is derived from the study of attachment and separation in early life (Bowlby 1969)—in other words, the effects of loss of relationships. Personal relationships are diverse in nature and have behavioural, cognitive, and affective components. The behavioural aspects include episodes of social interaction whose quality and content need to be assessed as part of social support. The cognitive aspects include the type of exchanges and rewards implicit in support transactions and how these are perceived by the participants.

8.2 Measurement of support

One of the most important distinctions is between social networks and the functional aspects of support—that is, the quality and type of support that is provided by the network member. Social networks refer to the social contacts of a group of persons. Such contact can be described in terms of the number of contacts and frequency of contacts (Table 8.1). These measures can be further refined by separating them into the number of contacts from the primary group, or group of persons to whom the subject is most attached, and from more distant contacts, less likely to provide meaningful support. Other useful measures include 'density' of the network, where it is estimated how much each network member is in contact with each other—this gives some idea of how integrated network members are.

Table 8.1 Measures of social support and social networks

Social networks	Contacts
	Number of contacts
	Frequency of contacts
	Density of network
Social support	Types of support
	Emotional—informational; self-appraisal
	Instrumental or practical
	Negative interaction

The great advantage of network measures to research on social relations is that they are relatively easy to measure, easy for respondents to recall reliably in surveys, and fairly easily verifiable by an external assessment. Such measures are also probably less susceptible to reporting socially desirable responses. These measures can provide an index of social integration, how much the individual is part of a community of mutual obligation and exchange—thus linking the needs of the individual with those of wider society. However, the major disadvantage of network measures is that they do not provide any indication of the quality of the interaction taking place in social contacts. Although sources of support may be identified, the type of support is not. This means that whereas a gross lack of social support, such as social isolation, may be identified, a more finely graded appreciation of social support transactions is not available.

A much greater richness of analysis may be achieved by examining the quality of support as well as the social network. In general, types of support may be divided into 'emotional' and 'practical' (or 'instrumental'). In some studies, other aspects of support have been identified which may be allied to emotional support. These include 'informational' support, where support sources provide information which may help the respondent in problem solving. A further important component of emotional support is related to self-appraisal, providing support that boosts self-esteem and encourages positive self-appraisal. Practical support is manifest in many forms, including practical help and financial support.

In assessing the impact of support on health it is important also to acknowledge the source of the support, as the impact of, say, emotional support from different sources may have a different meaning, dependent on closeness of that source to the respondent. In recent years, social support research has recognized that close relationships can have negative, as well as positive, aspects. There is increasing evidence to suggest that these negative aspects of close relationships may have a very powerful effect on ill health (Coyne and Downey 1991), perhaps rather greater than the positive effect on health.

There are methodological differences in the way questions about support are asked. The 'availability' of support is tapped by questions that ask the respondent whether there is someone available to provide support should the respondent need it. This has the advantage of assessing how supported people feel, but is somewhat abstract.

'Perceived' support indicates how much support the respondent feels and reports they have been given. The advantage of this measure is that it may indicate more accurately how much support the person has actually received. However, in cross-sectional studies of health causation, there is a risk that it may be measuring support elicited as a result of ill health rather than support, or the lack of it, leading to ill health.

It is easy, but misleading, to view social support as unidirectional. Social support involves both interactions and transactions between people. Hence, what a person gives in a relationship may also be important for their health, as well as what they receive from someone else—so-called 'reciprocity'. Reciprocity may have implications for the maintenance of good social relations. For instance, relations in which there is a mutual balance of give and take may be easier to sustain than those where there is an imbalance. However, there are likely to be structural prerogatives which guide these patterns of reciprocity. For example, the relationships between parents and young children will involve greater provision of practical support by parents. Both biological and social structural conditions shape the expectation of reciprocity in today's society, where social roles are much less fixed. The expectations of reciprocity in social relationships are also much less clearly defined and may lead to conflict where occupational and domestic roles collide.

8.3 **Social support and personality**

One difficulty in evaluating the evidence for the effect of social support on health is in distinguishing between the health-giving effects of the content of transactions in social relations from the inherent ability to develop and maintain relationships. It is likely that the ability to develop positive social relations is dependent on satisfactory early relationships with both mother and father (Fig. 8.1). Conversely, unhappy or disruptive early relationships may lead to patterns of anxious attachment, or dissociation from attachments, which may persist into adult life. These disturbed patterns of early relationships may, in themselves, be related to ill health, either through the development of abnormal or excessive responses to stress or through the adoption of unhealthy behaviours such as excessive eating, drinking, or smoking as a partial substitution for satisfactory emotional relationships. Thus it may be that part of the explanation for the relationship between social support and health is related to underlying personality factors which determine whether relationships are established. It is also likely that underlying personality factors influence the ability to maintain, nurture, and develop relationships.

Of course, that personality factors could contribute to the relationship between social support and health does not rule out the likelihood that social interactions themselves can promote health. Indeed, it is likely that the effects of social support on health include both the aspects of personality, which encourage the development and maintenance of relationships, as well as the health-giving effects of those interactions and transactions. Indeed, it is almost a prerequisite for social support to occur in any

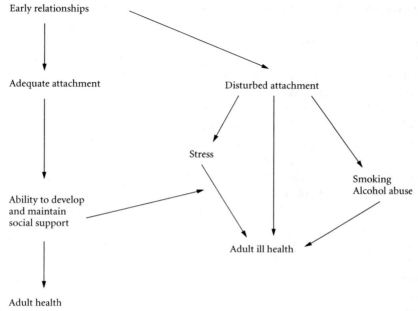

Fig. 8.1 Personality, social support, and adult health.

effective long-term manner that the personality characteristics are available to develop and sustain it. Curiously, it is the negative aspects of personality which provide this evidence, for there are some aspects of personality which work against the development of positive social relations. For instance, hostility, which has been shown in several studies to be predictive of future coronary heart disease (Barefoot *et al.* 1995), tends to have an inverse relationship with measures of social support. In some circumstances, social support may reduce the association of hostility with adverse health behaviours (Allen *et al.* 2001).

8.4 **Mechanisms for the action of social support on health**

Two types of mechanisms have been described for the action of social support on health. The first mechanism is that of direct effects of support on health. According to this mechanism, positive effects of support, or the lack of support resulting from social isolation, have direct effects on people's health. The second mechanism operates through the so-called 'buffering effect'. According to this mechanism, support does not have any direct effect on health but helps to moderate the impact of acute and chronic stressors on health (Fig. 8.2). It has long been recognized that the experience of a stressor, such as an acute life event, leads to ill health in some people but not others. It is hypothesized that this is explained by the causal impact of the life event on the development of illness being moderated by protective factors such as support, although it is more likely that 'vulnerability factors', such as lack of support, predispose the person to the development of ill health following the experience of a life event. There is evidence for both direct and buffering mechanisms.

How does a largely psychologically perceived set of processes, such as social relations, directly influence bodily physiology? There are a number of pathways through which social support may affect health. For instance, direct effects on health may be mediated through health-related behaviours. Support from others may encourage healthier behaviours, such as reducing fat in the diet, taking exercise, or giving up smoking. Thus, the effects of social support on health may be partially mediated by social control (Cohen *et al.* 2000). But this seems to explain only part of the direct effect of support on health, and support from other people may only be health inducing if they practice healthy behaviours themselves. If your spouse continues to smoke, it is less likely that you will be able to give up smoking than if he or she does not smoke. Direct effects of support on health may also result from support increasing perceptions of control over the environment, and giving an assurance of self-worth, which in turn may improve well-being and immunity to disease (Bisconti and Bergeman 1999).

There are several ways in which the buffering effects of social support may act. First, discussion of a potential threat with a supportive person may help to reappraise the threat implicit in a stressor, perhaps thus making it more manageable or even avoiding it. Secondly, practical aid or emotional consolation may help to moderate the impact of the stressor and help the person deal with the consequences of the stressor, which might otherwise be damaging for health.

There is also evidence that the association between social support and health works in the opposite direction—that is, the effects of health selection where poor health might be a barrier to maintaining or participating in social relationships (Ren *et al.* 1999), especially in the elderly (Cornman *et al.* 2003).

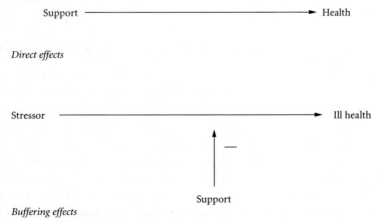

Fig. 8.2 Direct and buffering effects of social support.

8.5 **Hormonal pathways for the effects of support**

Environmental stressors may have direct effects on bodily systems. Acute stressors may stimulate the adrenal system, resulting in the classic 'fight-or-flight response' in which adrenal medullary hormones, such as adrenaline and noradrenaline, are secreted to prepare bodily metabolic systems for action by increasing levels of lipids and glucose (see Chapter 2). While this may be adaptive in the short term, if stressors are excessive or prolonged, the cumulative strain on the body (the allostatic load) may lead to illness. Similarly, stimulation of the hypothalamic–pituitary–adrenal (HPA) axis will lead to raised cortisol secretion, often also found in severe depressive illness, and may cause suppression of immune functioning and, thus, increase the susceptibility to infection.

Social relationships may act to modulate or damp down neuroendocrine reactivity (Seeman and McEwen 1996). This may be the mechanism for a common pathway for the effects of both social status and social support on health, as is illustrated by studies of primates. Dominant male primates in stable social situations have lower levels of adrenocorticotrophic hormone (secreted by the pituitary gland to stimulate the production of cortisol by the adrenal gland) and cortisol (Sapolsky 1989), and hence seem to show less stress response. Interestingly, however, dominant social status in an unstable social environment, associated with greater competition and hostility—the antithesis of a supportive environment—is associated, in male primates, with raised cortisol, sympathetic nervous system activity, and the development of atherosclerosis (Williams *et al.* 1991). Similarly, social isolation in primates contributes to increased activity of the HPA axis and the development of atherosclerosis. It was interesting that this biochemical response was attenuated by the presence of other adult primates.

There have also been a small number of human studies which have found that high levels of social support have been associated with lower heart rate, lower blood pressure, and lower levels of cortisol, adrenaline, and noradrenaline (Seeman *et al.* 1994). Hence, it is possible that social support has a direct effect on the neurohumoral responses of the body to environmental stress.

8.6 **Social support and mortality**

Evidence suggests that social support influences both mental and physical health. Perhaps the most striking evidence for the effect of social support on health, which is also some of the earliest evidence, relates to the effect of social support on mortality. The evidence that social networks influence mortality has come from a number of large prospective community studies. In the Alameda County Study, a social network index was constructed of marital status, number of contacts with friends and relatives, church and group membership. Low scores on this index were related to 1.9–3 times greater mortality over a nine-year period (Berkman and Syme 1979). Those with the fewest social connections had the highest mortality rate. A major strength of this study was to adjust for potential confounding factors such as health-related behaviour, and particularly prior ill health, which might have led to a reduction in social contacts and give a spurious relationship between social networks and subsequent ill health.

These early findings have been confirmed in a number of subsequent studies of community-based samples, including the Tecumseh Study (House *et al.* 1982), and in older people in the Durham County Study (Blazer 1982). Although in the Evans County, Georgia Study (Schoenbach *et al.* 1986), social network interaction was only found to have a protective effect on morbidity in white males. In Europe, studies from Sweden and Finland have provided further evidence for the positive effects of social integration on mortality. Social integration has been related to longevity in a Swedish cohort study of 50-year-old men (Welin *et al.* 1985) and lack of social ties was associated with considerably high risk in the North Karelia Study (Kaplan *et al.* 1988). Similarly, by linking social network interactions and Swedish national mortality data in 17,433 Swedish men and women, and comparing the lowest with the highest network group, an increased total mortality risk of 3.3 was found. This was reduced to a relative risk of 1.34 after adjustment for smoking, exercise, and chronic illness (Orth–Gomér and Johnson 1987).

Most studies of social support and mortality have measured social networks but not the functional aspects of support. Kaplan *et al.* (1994) reported from the Kuopio Study in eastern Finland that, among 2682 men followed-up for just under six years, those at increased risk of death reported few persons to whom they gave, or from whom they received, support, and a low quality of social relationships. Lack of participation in organizations, few friends, and not currently being married were also associated with greater overall mortality risk. These findings were not confounded by baseline health status, smoking, alcohol intake, coffee consumption, physical activity, body mass index, or income.

Functional aspects of social support are likely to have a stronger association with mortality than social networks because they capture more of the social interaction, as is shown in the results of the Kuopio Study as opposed to the Swedish National Study (Orth–Gomér and Johnson 1987). Frequency of interaction and use of emotional support when troubled were not associated with mortality risk in the Kuopio Study, although use of instrumental or practical support when troubled was associated with increased risk. It may be the case that the heavy use of instrumental support is associated with existing illness, loss of functioning in everyday activities, and, hence, additional need of support. Overall, Kaplan *et al.* (1994) argue that social support does not appear to be a proxy for baseline health status; in fact, associations between social support and mortality appeared to be stronger in the healthy subgroup at baseline.

One question which remains to be answered conclusively is whether social support has a non-specific protective effect across all causes of death. This has implications for the type of biological mechanism underlying its effects and would be in keeping with support showing an effect on general susceptibility to disease. Most studies in Western populations have examined cardiovascular mortality (unsurprisingly, in view of its importance as a cause of death in both men and women) and have consistently found an effect. In a study of 32,624 US male health professionals, Kawachi *et al.* (1996) confirmed that social isolation was related to increased cardiovascular disease mortality, and deaths from accident and suicide, but was not related to other causes of death, namely cancer, although the study yielded fairly few cases of cancer. A previous study had found a link between social isolation and smoking-related cancers (Reynolds and Kaplan 1990) but this was not confirmed by Kawachi and co-workers.

Different studies have tended to use different measures of social networks and the findings have not been uniform across all the studies. Nevertheless, the general pattern of an association between social integration and lower mortality remains. Certain of these studies have suggested that the protective effect of social networks seems to be greater in men than women but, as Seeman (1996) has pointed out, many of the middle-aged women in these samples have not reached the period of highest risk and, hence, the smaller number of events among women may have reduced the power of these studies to detect differences in risk by level of social integration. In comparative analysis of men and women aged 65 years or older in the National Institute on Ageing's established populations for epidemiological study of the elderly, social integration was found to be significantly associated with a lower five-year mortality risk for both women and men.

8.7 Social support and physical morbidity

In terms of physical illness and morbidity, the relationship between social support and cardiovascular disease—particularly coronary heart disease and stroke—has been studied most. Social isolation has been linked to stroke incidence in a large study of US male health professionals (Kawachi *et al.* 1996). A longitudinal community-based study from Sweden, examining men aged 50, found a significant protective effect of social integration on the incidence of non-fatal myocardial infarction in those found to be free of heart disease at baseline (Welin *et al.* 1985). One other study (Vogt *et al.* 1992) has also found a protective effect of social integration, measured by a range of different ties, on the 15-year incidence of myocardial infarction. However, not all measures of social network based on network size or frequency of contacts showed this association (Kawachi *et al.* 1996) and other studies, such as the Japanese American Study in Hawaii, did not find a relationship between social ties (marital status and ties with children and parents, social activities, and co-workers and group memberships) and the incidence of coronary heart disease (Reed *et al.* 1983).

The lack of consistent association between social support and incidence of CHD might be explained by the results of an Israeli study which reported that high levels of family problems were related to an increased risk of developing angina (Medalie and Goldbourt 1976). As Seeman (1996) points out, 'greater social integration, to the extent that it is accompanied by greater interpersonal conflict or other interpersonal problems, may not be uniformly associated with health benefits, including reduced risk of heart disease (or other health outcomes)'.

There have been several studies of patients undergoing coronary angiography to examine the association between social support and severity of progression of coronary atherosclerosis. In general, social network membership does not seem to have been related to degree of atherosclerosis (Seeman and Syme 1987). However, a significant inverse association was found between levels of instrumental support provided by others and atherosclerosis. A significant inverse association has been found between levels of emotional support and the extent of atherosclerosis, particularly among those patients classified as showing the type A behaviour pattern (Blumental et al. 1987). Thus, although more structural features of social integration, as indicated by social network measures, do not appear to be associated with disease severity, more qualitative features, such as levels of social support, do exhibit a negative association with disease severity and favour a role for social support in the development of CHD. However, the results of angiography studies need to be viewed cautiously because of the possibility of selection bias in such samples, on the basis of how people are referred for angiography.

8.8 **Social support and prognosis**

Social support may not only have a protective effect in preventing or decreasing the risk of development of illness but may also be helpful for people who have to adjust to, or cope with, the stress of a chronic illness (Lindsay et al. 2001).

The association between social support and the prognosis of post-myocardial infarction patients is strong and consistent. Socially isolated men are at increased risk of death post-myocardial infarction (Ruberman et al. 1984). Williams et al. (1992) found that individuals who were not married and had no confidant had significantly poorer survival post-myocardial infarction over a five-year follow-up period. Berkman et al. (1992) suggested that low levels of emotional support may be the reason why social isolation conveys greater mortality risk in post-myocardial infarction patients. In her study, emotional support was measured prior to the myocardial infarction, as all subjects were part of a longitudinal study in New Haven. Diagnosis of myocardial infarction was identified through hospital monitoring and chart review for all cohort members. In analyses adjusting for age, the severity of the myocardial infarction and other morbidity, subjects who reported no sources of emotional support experienced a nearly threefold higher mortality rate at six months than those reporting one or more sources of support. Lack of a confidant has also been associated with adverse outcomes after myocardial infarction in a UK sample (Dickens et al. 2004).

It is possible that the effects of lack of social support on mortality post-myocardial infarction are mediated through the development of depression, although this may be mediated by neuroticism (Pedersen et al. 2002). Depression, and especially recurrent depression, has been associated with increased mortality risk post-myocardial infarction (Lespérance *et al.* 1996). It is possible that depression could increase the risk of sudden death from ventricular arrhythmias via increased sympathetic activation influencing a susceptible, damaged heart (Cameron 1996). A randomized control study (Frasure–Smith and Prince 1985) suggested that monthly supportive and educational interventions by a nurse-therapist, to patients post-myocardial infarction who were identified by questionnaire to be under stress, was associated with greater longevity than in subjects who did not receive this intervention. In addition, stress scores were also reduced in the intervention group. However, in a subsequent intervention this favourable response was not replicated and, if anything, women fared less well in the intervention group (Frasure–Smith *et al.* 1997).

An ambitious randomized controlled trial of 2841 myocardial infarction patients (ENRICHD), using a cognitive behaviour therapy-based intervention with SSRI drug therapy, found no differences in recurrent myocardial infarction rates or mortality between the intervention group and the control group after an average 29-month follow-up (Berkman *et al.* 2003). The intervention improved social isolation and depression, but the findings are not in keeping with an effect of social support on mortality in post-myocardial infarction patients. Such interventions are difficult to design and may not easily replicate 'real life' support. Nevertheless, there is a disparity here between the results of observational and intervention studies that is unexplained.

Amongst subjects who experienced a stroke, those who were more socially isolated exhibited significantly worse functional status six months post stroke, as measured by impairment of activities of daily living and more frequent nursing home placement. Other studies have also found that levels of emotional support post stroke are predictive of better recovery, suggesting that greater available emotional support may be one reason why social integration predicts better outcome post stroke.

Less dramatically, but no less importantly, social support has been shown to be helpful in dealing with chronic disabling and painful diseases such as rheumatoid arthritis, preventing the onset of secondary depression and limiting disability (Fitzpatrick *et al.* 1991). In this way, social support may not only be contributing practical help to people who are restricted in activities of everyday living, but also providing crucial emotional support to maintain morale in the face of chronic illness. It is also possible that emotional support has a beneficial effect on the immune system in chronic illness. Social support has also been shown to be influential in some studies of cancer survival. Group therapy in melanoma patients was associated with increased survival time and reduced psychological distress (Kiecolt–Glaser and Glaser 1995). It may be that social support is operating here to strengthen the immune response to the illness. This certainly seems to be the case in AIDS, where the bereavement of an AIDS patient is associated with a fall in the CD4 lymphocyte count, while increases in social support have been associated with an improvement in this index of immune function (Kiecolt–Glaser and Glaser 1995).

8.9 **Social support and mental health**

The fact that social support influences psychiatric disorder has been known since the nineteenth century, when Durkheim (1897/1951) showed that social isolation was associated with higher rates of suicide. It has also long been known that bereaved adults experience high and unexpected levels of illness and mortality in the year following the death of their spouse (Parkes *et al.* 1969). Bereaved persons without a network of friends or relatives to whom they could turn for consolation were also at greater risk of developing lasting psychiatric problems.

Cross-sectional studies show a clear negative association between levels of support and psychiatric disorder (largely depression), although it is not clear that this is necessarily aetiological (Paykel 1994). The association appears in both community and patient samples, and in both men and women. There is, however, a consensus that emotional support buffers the effects of life events on minor psychiatric disorder (Aneshensel and Stone 1982; Kessler and McLeod 1985). A similar effect has also been found in studies examining chronic as well as acute stressors (Brown and Harris 1978). Alloway and Bebbington (1987), in a cautious review of buffering studies in minor affective disorder, suggest that, overall, Brown's vulnerability model of low emotional support as a risk factor for depression in women experiencing life events does receive appreciable support.

There have been fewer longitudinal studies of social support where questions of causation can be better addressed. Several community studies have been completely prospective, identifying deficiencies in social support prior to the onset of psychiatric disorder and relating this to the onset of disorder. Two studies found a buffering or interactive effect (Brown *et al.* 1986; Bolton and Oatley 1987), and a third (Henderson 1981) found some evidence for direct effects. The study by Brown *et al.* (1986) found little predictive effect on mental health of 17 measures of emotional support, measured at baseline in an inner-city sample of married mothers. However, they did find a greater risk of depression in women who received little 'crisis support'—that is, little support when it was needed to cope with a life event. A negative response from a partner in a crisis was also associated with a greater subsequent risk of depression. On the other hand, among single mothers, report of a close relationship at baseline was protective against the development of depression following a subsequent life event. They also found that women who reported the availability of adequate emotional support at baseline, but who were subsequently 'let down' and found that support was not forthcoming when they needed it, were at much greater risk of developing depression.

In Henderson's community study in Canberra (1981), a modest negative association was found between the availability of attachment and social integration, on the one hand, and neurotic symptoms on the other. However, measures of perceived adequacy of support showed a much stronger negative relationship with neurotic symptoms: perceived adequacy of close relationships was important for women, while that of more diffuse relationships was important for men. This was interpreted as indicating that those who view their social relationships as inadequate were substantially more at risk of developing neurotic symptoms. There is debate as to whether this reflects mainly the relationship between aspects of personality and psychiatric disorder, or whether it indicates the quality of the social support provided. A North American study, in 1982, also measured perceived adequacy of emotional and tangible support, and found that they predicted depressive symptoms at follow-up interview in 1985 in a sample of non-institutionalized elderly persons (Oxman *et al.* 1992).

A further longitudinal study of British, middle-aged civil servants (Whitehall II Study) showed a protective effect on mental health of emotional support from the closest person, in men (Stansfeld *et al.* 1998a, 1998b), and from the primary group, in women (Fuhrer *et al.* 1999), which was not abolished by adjusting for either hostility, as a measure of personality, or psychiatric disorder at baseline. Moreover, this study showed, prospectively, that negative aspects of close relationships were associated with greater risk of future psychiatric disorder up to five years later. In certain psychiatric conditions, such as schizophrenia, critical comments, hostility, and overinvolvement from the patient's primary group are related to a higher risk of psychotic relapse (Bebbington and Kuipers 1994). This risk may be reduced by adequate medication, curtailing contact between the person and his or her primary group, and, more positively, by reducing the high 'expressed emotion' in the primary group, using educational and therapeutic techniques.

A few studies have followed up clinical samples of depressed patients to assess the effect of support on outcome of depression. Brugha *et al.* (1990) found that the number of primary-group members named and contacted, and satisfaction with support, predicted recovery in women. In men, negative interaction with the primary group and marriage were associated with recovery. Low perceived social support has also been shown to increase the use of mental health care in people with existing psychiatric disorder (Ten Have *et al.* 2002).

A study of women who had been 'in care' during childhood (Quinton *et al.* 1984) shows how social support in adulthood may exert a beneficial effect on parenting problems, marital difficulties, and psychiatric disorder. Many of these women returned from care to a discordant home environment from which they then tried to escape by early marriage. But their marital relationships also often turned out badly and resulted in these women becoming more vulnerable to further difficulties. Nevertheless, a third of those studied showed good parenting ability themselves. This seemed to relate to both positive school experiences, including examination success, and good relationships with peers, but also to the later presence of a supportive marital relationship, which prevented subsequent parenting difficulties and depression from occurring.

Provision of adequate support at various critical stages in the life cycle when support is required, where its lack may lead to depression, may be a good prevention strategy in mental illness. In particular, support for mothers with young children can help prevent social isolation from other adults, and patterns of socialization in many societies encourage this. Although prevention of life events that may lead to depression is not generally feasible, there are opportunities for prompt intervention in crises, which may prevent the development of psychiatric disorder from understandable distress (Paykel 1994). Voluntary agencies providing support to bereaved persons may be included in this type of intervention, although there has been little systematic study of the efficacy of these interventions.

8.10 Social support and sickness absence

We found that negative aspects of close relationships, material problems in terms of financial, household, and neighbourhood problems, and social support at work were important predictors of sickness absence for psychiatric disorder in the Whitehall II study, an occupational cohort study of civil servants (Fig. 8.3; Stansfeld *et al.* 1997). However, effects vary by gender and length of spell of sickness absence. The most marked finding relating to sickness absence was for negative aspects of close relationships. High levels of negative aspects of close relationships were followed by increased rates of long spells of psychiatric sickness absence (greater than seven days' duration) in men; while for women, intermediate levels of negative aspects of close relationships were followed by increased rates of short spells (less than seven days' duration) of sickness absence.

Negative aspects of close relationships are not synonymous with a lack of positive aspects of support, and have been recognized increasingly as risk factors for mental ill health (Coyne and Downey 1991; Lakey *et al.* 1994). Negative aspects of close relationships also predicted higher rates of sickness absence for physical illness (Rael *et al.* 1995). It seems likely that negative aspects of close relationships are part of the cause of

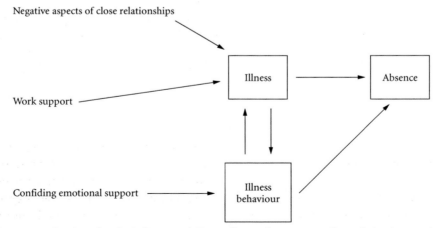

Fig. 8.3 Mechanisms for the influence of direct effects of support on illness behaviour and absence.

illness as they predicted psychiatric disorder scores on a screening questionnaire for anxiety and depression.

In women, medium and high levels of emotional support from the closest person were associated with higher risk of long spells of sickness absence. This is in keeping with findings for sickness absence for physical illness (Rael *et al.* 1995). This association was surprising in the light of findings that emotional support is protective against the development of depression in those exposed to life events (Brown and Harris 1978). However, the apparent contradiction could be explained if this were an effect on illness behaviour rather than illness. In this case, confiding/emotional support from the closest person may encourage empowerment, security, and perceptions of control in the employee, which legitimize taking leave from work when he/she is depressed or anxious (Stansfeld *et al.* 1997).

We also found that social support at work was protective against short spells of sickness absence for both men and women. Work support, as defined here, included support from colleagues, support from supervisors, and consistency and clarity of information from supervisors. Work support was also protective for those with high levels of negative aspects of close relationships, suggesting that support at work may help people cope with interpersonal stressors from home and, thus, not take short spells of absence.

8.11 Gender differences

Studies of cardiovascular morbidity and mortality suggest that being married is more beneficial to health for men than for women, and that women benefit as much from relationships with friends or relatives. Our own research suggests that for middle-aged civil servants, the most important support is provided for men by their spouse, whereas for women, there is a greater likelihood of support being provided by their immediate close network. We found that emotional support from the closest person was a predictor of good mental health in men but not in women (Stansfeld *et al.* 1998*b*). On the other hand, for women, there was a beneficial effect of emotional support on mental health when support from up to four close persons was included (Fuhrer *et al.* 1999).

8.12 Ethnic differences

There is increasing interest in ethnic differences in social support, especially as a possible explanation for differential prevalence rates of illness between ethnic groups. In a national UK study, EMPIRIC, patterns of social support differed between ethnic groups but did not explain differences in the prevalence of common mental disorders by ethnicity in any straightforward way (Stansfeld and Sproston 2002). With increasing population mobility, there is a risk of fragmentation of social networks that may have implications for ill health. Changes in health associated with migration have been associated with a decrease in social support. Puerto Rican women who migrated to the USA had less social support than non-migrants, around pregnancy, reported more stress, and had a higher risk of poor health behaviour and potentially compromised infant health (Landale and Oropesa 2001).

8.13 Society, social integration, and health

Social support operates at both an individual and a societal level. Social integration may have a positive effect on the whole community. Social cohesion (the existence of mutual trust and respect between different sections of society) contributes to the way in which people and their health are cherished. There is increasing evidence that communities with high levels of social cohesion have better health than those with low levels of social cohesion. Social cohesion means cohesive community relationships with high levels of participation in communal activities and public affairs, and high levels of membership of community groups. This often goes together with an egalitarian ethos in local politics. Various pieces of evidence support the link between social cohesion and health (Wilkinson 1996). Cities with stronger civic communities have lower infant mortality. In Russia, during periods of immense social upheaval in the 1970s and 1980s, there were greatly increased levels of mortality. It was striking that this was especially the case amongst divorced men, who might be expected to be more socially isolated.

The inhabitants of the Pennsylvanian town of Roseto in the USA, settled by Italians who emigrated from the town of the same name in Italy, seemed to retain the low levels of coronary heart disease that their relatives in Italy enjoyed, as long as they kept their traditional family-oriented social structure. But as people became assimilated into the surrounding American culture, where the individual rather than the family and community was considered to be the dominant unit, the incidence of coronary heart disease rose. It seemed unlikely that the rise in CHD could be attributed to the conventional cardiac risk factors, as diet had improved and levels of smoking had fallen. It was the case that the inhabitants of Roseto had become more sedentary, but this did not seem to be enough to explain the large increase in CHD, which could be attributed to the loss of social cohesion. Societies in which there are high levels of income inequality and diminished social cohesion have higher levels of crime and violence and higher mortality rates (Kawachi and Kennedy 1997).

8.14 Social class and social support

Could the effect of social inequalities on health, such as those caused by income inequality, be partly mediated through an influence of social class on social support and thence on health? If this is the case, there should be evidence of social class gradients in social support.

Patterns of social network interaction have been described in different communities, but relatively little work has attempted to relate macro-social variables, such as social class, to social support. The evidence that individuals of lower socio-economic position (SEP) have relationships of lower quality is scattered and contradictory. The evidence for social networks is more consistent. Low perceived availability of support in adolescents has been associated with a range of SEP indicators (Geckova *et al.* 2003). Fischer (1982) found higher income and education to be associated with larger networks, more contact with network members, and more voluntary associations. Turner and Marino (1994), in a study of 1394 adults in metropolitan Toronto, found that higher levels of perceived social support (measured by a global score of support from spouses, relatives, friends, and co-workers) was related to higher socio-economic status.

We have found similar results in the Whitehall II Study (Stansfeld *et al.* 1998*c*). Perceived social support was measured by asking respondents to nominate up to four close persons; respondents then had to rate the amount of three types of support (confiding/emotional, practical, and negative aspects of close relationships) given by each of these persons. Confiding/emotional support from the person mentioned as closest was highest for both men and women in higher employment grades. Practical support was highest for men in the higher employment grades, although this effect was not found for women. Conversely, negative aspects of close relationships tended to be more common in those of lower employment grade for men, while there was no clear gradient for women. Unlike the Toronto study, among civil servants there were more contacts with friends among those of higher employment grade and more contact with relatives among those in lower employment grades. This is likely to reflect greater mobility amongst those of higher SEP, and perhaps also greater opportunities for making friends. On the other hand, those in lower employment grades may have restricted opportunities for mobility and may be more closely in touch with their families of origin.

Thus, there is some evidence for a differential distribution of social support by social class but, in general, social support does not seem to be a major influence in explaining employment grade differences in depression (Stansfeld *et al.* 1998*c*) or sickness absence (Rael *et al.* 1995).

8.15 Social support and the physical environment

Apart from the macro-social environment encapsulated by social cohesion, the arrangement of the physical built environment can also influence social support and, hence, health. The physical environment can, to some extent, determine the opportunities for social support among residents of a particular area. (For further discussion of area effects on health see Chapter 14.) In this context, social support from neighbours is especially important. That the relationship between support and the physical environment is influential is indicated by the fact that the quality of relationships with neighbours largely explains reports of residents' satisfaction with the area in which they live. Moreover, residents who are more involved in the local community tend to be happier where they live, regardless of the physical quality of their homes (Halpern 1995).

Various factors tend to increase friendliness between neighbours. Areas that have high social homogeneity tend to increase neighbourliness, although there is a danger of such areas becoming so different from adjacent areas that ghettos may develop. More intimate physical settings for housing, such as cul-de-sac roads, are related to a greater likelihood of making friends and neighbours and to generally higher levels of friendliness, as was found by Willmott in his studies of Dagenham in East London (Willmott 1963). The relationship of these physical factors to ill health is indirect and not always easy to trace. However, some findings are fairly consistent. For instance, the low group density of a minority group in any population relates to worse mental health (Halpern 1993). This may be because of the relative isolation felt by people of a minority group in areas where they are genuinely in a minority and have few of their own community around them.

Studies have looked at perceptions of helpfulness of neighbours and health and have found a negative association between helpfulness and symptom levels. In fact, Halpern (1995) suggests that the associations between the objective characteristics of the residential environment and symptoms may be mediated through the rated helpfulness of neighbours. Perceived support has been shown to buffer the effects of neighbourhood problems on male residents' feeling of anger, whereas giving support to others seems to make feelings of anger worse for women (Schieman and Meersman 2004). Giving support to others taps into the research on caring which is often associated with a negative impact on mental health.

It has been recognized that the design of buildings and groups of buildings, their layout, and the way in which buildings relate to each other, may help to encourage or discourage neighbourliness and, hence, may have effects on health. Buildings or housing estates that have little opportunity for informal social contact tend to be disliked by their residents. Yancey (1971) emphasized the importance of 'semi-private space' where people could make informal social contacts in a non-threatening communal setting. Thus shared space, specifically allocated to local residents, will encourage the development of potentially supportive relationships. Studies of residential living have suggested that bedrooms arranged as small clusters around a common area tend to be associated with greater social interaction than bedrooms arranged along corridors (Baum and Valins 1977). These studies illustrate a common theme that people generally prefer to have control over their social interactions. Frequent interactions with strangers not of the participants' choosing may paradoxically lead to social withdrawal and a feeling of intrusion on privacy, rather than the reverse.

Similarly, there may be adverse social effects on health which derive from physical living conditions. It has been suggested that the adverse effects of crowding on psychological health in a study of inner-city Indian households was related to the breakdown of social support systems (Evans and Palsane 1989). Thus, the design of the physical environment can have an impact on social integration and social support and, through this, may influence health.

8.16 **Intervening to improve social cohesion and health**

Another factor that needs to be taken into consideration is the fear of violence and crime. This fear may inhibit social interaction and tend to increase mistrust. Several studies have tested interventions in terms of making unsafe housing estates more safe, with a consequent improvement in health. A landmark study was described by Halpern (1995), who assessed the refurbishment of a housing estate called Eastlake. This relatively conventional estate of two-storey row houses in a British new town had become very unpopular and was developing a reputation as a high-crime area. Apart from signs of a run-down area, such as graffiti, broken windows, and dismantled cars, the estate was characterized by a strong sense of distrust related to a network of alleyways through which strangers could easily gain access to the estate. At the time of initial intervention, there was close consultation between the planners and the residents. Interventions to improve the estate included the introduction of measures to slow traffic on the estate, provision of more convenient parking, the fencing in of 'ambiguous semi-private space', and the closing of alleyways. Internally, house windows were replaced and kitchens and bathrooms were refitted. At the same time, the facilities for children in a play area were improved and access to this was also improved. As a result of this intervention, residents' concern about safety from traffic and about the danger of personal attack and car theft reduced considerably from baseline interview to follow-up interview after the intervention. At baseline, only 41 per cent of residents described the estate as 'safe or very safe' but, by the time this work was all completed, this had risen to 81 per cent of residents. At the same time, residents' perception of the friendliness of the area greatly increased. What was most striking was that the mental health of the residents improved in terms of a fall in measures of anxiety and depression and an improvement in terms of self-esteem on simple self-report questionnaire scales between the baseline and the final follow-up of the study. This simple but striking study illustrates how important the interaction between the physical and social environment is in terms of determining mental health. It certainly seems plausible that it might have similar effects on physical health.

In a follow-up study in Oslo, 503 persons were re-interviewed over a period of 10 years with the same questionnaire (Dalgard and Tambs 1997). Only one satellite town to Oslo showed marked social changes over time. At baseline, there were high levels of mental ill health and the town was characterized by a relative 'lack of services, recreational possibilities and other facilities, economic problems and qualitative poor social networks'. During the 10-year follow-up period, there were reported significant improvements in playgrounds, shops, kindergartens, youth activities, and 'in general' in the satellite town compared to the other areas studied. There was also an improvement in social support which was not statistically significant. These improvements in the social environment, which seem to include greater opportunities for social interaction, were associated with an improvement in mental health in those who continued to live there. Although there was no direct evidence that social support was the major factor in the mental health improvements, decreased environmental stress associated with the social changes seems a plausible explanation. As in the Eastlake study and Leighton's (1965) follow-up study of Stirling County in rural Nova Scotia:

> . . . increased trust and interaction between the residents, as well as increased feelings of community cohesion and empowerment, seemed to be of crucial importance for the improvement in mental health. Obviously this is related to the social organization as well as to the physical characteristics of the neighbourhood. (Dalgard and Tambs 1997)

8.17 Conclusions

Social support has a wide spectrum of action on health, from influencing mortality at one end, through physical morbidity to psychological morbidity at the other end. Social support is a very personal matter and yet research shows that it is influenced by social structural imperatives and becomes more than the sum of the individual links of networks in terms of social cohesion. At the level of society, social cohesion can have a powerful effect on health which transcends that available from individual social relationships. This has implications for improving the health of communities. In terms of improving the general health of the population, it is important to recognize that many economic and fiscal policies may influence the social cohesion of a society. Those policies that increase income inequalities are likely also to increase health inequalities. On a slightly smaller scale, the design of the built environment may also influence possibilities for social interaction which may subsequently influence health.

As methods of communication change, new opportunities arise for social interaction. For instance, the Internet can be a source of information for people with illness. Persons with HIV who used the Internet for health information were better informed about HIV and reported more active coping strategies and greater social support (Kalichman *et al.* 2003). Mobile phone use has revolutionized communication, not least in developing countries, but its impact on health has yet to be assessed.

At a specific level, it can be important to identify particular groups who might be at risk of illness through social isolation. There have been several projects to increase support for young women with children who may be at risk of depression. Programmes of targeted assistance do not seem to prevent low birth-weight babies in women who are at risk, but these programmes may reduce the likelihood of Caesarean births (Hodnett and Fredericks 2003). It may also be important to target parents, with the aim of improving parenting skills and, hence, giving children a better start in life. This has been especially effective in the Home Start Programme for high-risk children. Another possibility is to target support services for particular stressful life events that frequently occur throughout the life cycle, including school change, job entry, unemployment, bereavement, and retirement.

It does not seem likely that social networks can be artificially induced and remain long-lasting. However, conversely, it seems very possible that interventions at a population level could reduce social support and impair health. Policy makers need to be aware of the costs and benefits of their policies in social terms across a wide range of different policies, from economics and town-planning, to health services' distribution. Finally, there is considerable scope for giving support to those with existing illness, especially myocardial infarction and stroke, and chronic illnesses such as rheumatoid arthritis and depression, who may very well benefit from continuing support.

Acknowledgements

Dr Stansfeld's research was supported by the Department of Health in analyses of social support and mental health in the Whitehall II Study. Emily Klineberg and Lisa Kass helped enormously in revising this chapter.

References

Allen, J., Markovitz, J., Jacobs, D.R., Jr., and Knox, S.S. (2001). Social support and health behavior in hostile black and white men and women in CARDIA. *Psychosom. Med.* **63**, 609–18.

Alloway, R. and Bebbington, P. (1987). The buffer theory of social support: a review of the literature. *Psychol. Med.* **17**, 91–108.

Aneshensel, C.S. and Stone, J.D. (1982). Stress and depression: a test of the buffering model of social support. *Arch. Gen. Psychiat.* **39**, 1392–6.

Barefoot, J.C., Larsen, S., von der Lieth, L., and Schroll, M. (1995). Hostility, incidence of acute myocardial infarction, and mortality in a sample of older Danish men and women. *Am. J. Epidemiol.* **142**, 477–84.

Baum, A. and Valins, S. (1977). *Architecture and social behaviour: psychosocial studies of social density.* Laurence Erlbaum Associates, Hillsdale, NJ.

Bebbington, P. and Kuipers, L. (1994). The clinical utility of expressed emotion in schizophrenia. *Acta Psychiat. Scand.* **89**, 46–53.

Berkman, L.F. and Syme, S.L. (1979). Social networks, host resistance, and mortality: a nine-year follow-up study of Alameda County residents. *Am. J. Epidemiol.* **109**, 186–203.

Berkman, L.F., Blumenthal, J., Burg, M., Carney, R.M., Catellier, D., Cowan, M.J., *et al.* (2003). Effects of treating depression and low perceived social support on clinical events after myocardial infarction: the Enhancing Recovery in Coronary Heart Disease Patients (ENRICHD) Randomized Trial. *JAMA* **289**, 3106–16.

Berkman, L.F., Leo–Summers, L., and Horwitz, R.I. (1992). Emotional support and survival after myocardial infarction: a prospective, population-based study of the elderly. *Ann. Int. Med.* **117**, 1003–9.

Bisconti, T.L. and Bergeman, C.S. (1999). Perceived social control as a mediator of the relationships among social support, psychological well-being and perceived health. *The Gerontologist* **39**, 94–103.

Blazer, D.G. (1982). Social support and mortality in an elderly community population. *Am. J. Epidemiol.* **115**, 684–94.

Blumental, J.A., Burg, M.M., Barefoot, J., Williams, R.B., Haney, T., and Zimet, G. (1987). Social support, type A behaviour, and coronary artery disease. *Psychosom. Med.* **49**, 341–54.

Bolton, W. and Oatley, K. (1987). A longitudinal study of social support and depression in unemployed men. *Psychol. Med.* **17**, 453–60.

Bowlby, J. (1969). *Attachment and loss. Vol. 1: Attachment*. Hogarth Press, Institute of Psycho-Analysis, London.

Brown, G.W. and Harris, T. (1978). *The social origins of depression*. Tavistock Publications, London.

Brown, G.W., Andrews, B., Harris R., Adler, Z., and Bridge, L. (1986). Social support, self-esteem and depression. *Psychol. Med.* **16**, 813–31.

Brugha, T.S., Bebbington, P.E., MacCarthy B., Sturt, E., Wykes, T., and Potter, J. (1990). Gender, social support and recovery from depressive disorders: a prospective clinical study. *Psychol. Med.* **20**, 147–56.

Cameron, O. (1996). Depression increases post-MI mortality: how? *Psychosom. Med.* **58**, 111–12.

Cobb, S. (1976). Social support as a moderator of life stress. *Psychosom. Med.* **38**, 300–13.

Cohen, S. and Syme, S.L. (ed.) (1985). *Social support and health*. Academic Press, London.

Cohen, S., Underwood, L.G., and Gottlieb, B.H. (2000). *Social support, measurement and intervention: a guide for health and social scientists*. Oxford University Press, New York.

Cornman, J.C., Goldman, N., Glei, D.A., Weinstein, M., and Chang, M.C. (2003). Social ties and perceived support: two dimensions of social relationships and health among the elderly in Taiwan. *J. Aging Health* **15**, 616–44.

Coyne, J.C. and Downey, G. (1991). Social factors and psychopathology: stress, social support, and coping processes. *Ann. Rev. Psychol.* **42**, 401–5.

Dalgard, O.S. and Tambs, K. (1997). Urban environment and mental health: a longitudinal study. *Br. J. Psychiat.* **171**, 530–6.

Dickens, C.M., McGowan, L., Percival, C., Douglas, J., Tomenson, B., Cotter, L., *et al.* (2004). Lack of a close confidant, but not depression, predicts further cardiac events after myocardial infarction. *Heart* **90**, 518–22.

Durkheim, E. (1897). *Suicide*. (Reprinted in 1951 by The Free Press, New York.)

Evans, G.W. and Palsane, M.N. (1989). Residential density and psychological health: the mediating effects of social support. *J. Person. Soc. Psychol.* **6**, 994–9.

Fischer, C.S. (1982). *To dwell among friends*. University of Chicago Press, Chicago.

Fitzpatrick, R., Newman, S., Archer, R., and Shipley, M. (1991). Social support, disability and depression: a longitudinal study of rheumatoid arthritis. *Soc. Sci. Med.* **33**, 605–11.

Frasure–Smith, N. and Prince, R. (1985). The ischemic heart disease life stress monitoring program: impact and mortality. *Psychosom. Med.* **47**, 431–45.

Frasure–Smith, N., Lespérance, F., Prince, R.H., *et al.* (1997). Randomised trial of home-based psychosocial nursing intervention for the patients recovering from myocardial infarction. *Lancet* **350**, 473–9.

Fuhrer, R., Stansfeld, S.A., Hudry–Chemali, J., and Shipley, M.J. (1999). Gender, social relations and mental health: prospective findings from an occupational cohort (Whitehall II Study). *Soc. Sci. Med.* **48**, 77–87.

Geckova, A., Van Dijk, J.P., Stewart, R., Groothoff, J.W., and Post, D. (2003). Influence of social support on health among gender and socio-economic groups of adolescents. *Eur. J. Public Health* **13** 44–50.

Halpern, D.S. (1993). Minorities and mental health. *Soc. Sci. Med.* **36**, 597–607.

Halpern, D.S. (1995). *Mental health and the built environment. More than bricks and mortar?* Taylor and Francis, London.

Henderson, A.S. (1981). Social relationships, adversity and neurosis: an analysis of prospective observations. *Br. J. Psychiat.* **138**, 391–8.

Hodnett, E.D. and Fredericks, S. (2003). Support during pregnancy for women at increased risk of low birthweight babies. *Cochrane Database.Syst.Rev.* CD000198.

House, J.S., Robbins, C. and Metzner, H.L. (1982). The association of social relationships and activities with mortality: prospective evidence from the Tecumseh Community Health Study. *Am. J. Epidemiol.* **116**, 123–40.

Kalichman, S.C., Benotsch, E.G., Weinhardt, L., Austin, J., Luke, W., and Cherry, C. (2003). Health-related Internet use, coping, social support, and health indicators in people living with HIV/AIDS: preliminary results from a community survey. *Health Psychol.* **22**, 111–16.

Kaplan, G.A., Salonen J.T., Cohen R.D., Brand, R.J., Syme, L., and Puska, P. (1988). Social connections and mortality from all causes and cardiovascular disease: prospective evidence from eastern Finland. *Am. J. Epidemiol.* **128**, 370–80.

Kaplan, G.A., Wilson, T.W., Cohen, R.D., Kauhanen, J., Wu, M., and Salonen, J.T. (1994). Social functioning and overall mortality: prospective evidence from the Kuopio ischemic heart disease risk factor study. *Epidemiology* **5**, 495–500.

Kawachi, I. and Kennedy, B.P. (1997). Health and social cohesion: why care about income inequality? *BMJ* **314**, 1037–40.

Kawachi, I., Colditz, G.A., Ascherio, A., *et al.* (1996). A prospective study of social networks in relation to total mortality and cardiovascular disease in men in the USA. *J. Epidemiol. Commun. Hlth.* **50**, 245–51.

Kessler, R.C. and McLeod, J.D. (1985). Social support and mental health in community samples. In: *Social support and health,* (ed. S. Cohen and S.L. Syme), pp. 219–40. Academic Press, Orlando, F.L.

Kiecolt–Glaser, J. and Glaser, R. (1995). Psychoneuroimmunology and health consequences: data and shared mechanisms. *Psychosom. Med.* **57**, 269–74.

Lakey, B., Tardiff, R.A., and Drew, J.B. (1994). Negative social interactions: assessment and relations to social support, cognition, and psychological distress. *J. Soc. Clin. Psychol.* **13**, 63–85.

Landale, N.S. and Oropesa, R.S. (2001). Migration, social support and perinatal health: an origin-destination analysis of Puerto Rican women. *J. Health Soc.Behav.* **42**, 166–83.

Leighton, A.H. (1965). Poverty and social change. *Sci. Am.* **212**, 21–7.

Lespérance, F., Frasure–Smith, N., and Talajic, M. (1996). Major depression before and after myocardial infarction: its nature and consequences. *Psychosom. Med.* **58**, 99–110.

Lindsay, G.M., Smith, L.N., Hanlon, P., and Wheatley, D.J. (2001). The influence of general health status and social support on symptomatic outcome following coronary artery bypass grafting. *Heart* **85**, 80–6.

Medalie, J.H. and Goldbourt, U. (1976). Angina pectoris among 10,000 men: II. Psychosocial and other risk factors as evidenced by a multivariate analysis of a five-year incidence study. *Am. J. Med.* **60**, 910–21.

Orth–Gomér, K. and Johnson, J.V. (1987). Social network interaction and mortality. A six year follow-up study of a random sample of the Swedish population. *J. Chronic Dis.* **40**, 949–57.

Oxman, T.E., Berkman, L.F., Kasl, S., Freeman, D.H., and Barrett, J. (1992). Social support and depressive symptoms in the elderly. *Am. J. Epidemiol.* **135**, 356–68.

Pahl, R. (2003). Some sceptical comments on the relationship between social support and well-being. *Leisure Studies* **22**, 1–12.

Parkes, C.M., Benjamin, B., and Fitzgerald, R.G. (1969). Broken hearts: a statistical study of increased mortality among widowers. *BMJ* **1**, 740–3.

Paykel, E.S. (1994). Life events, social support and depression. *Acta Psychiat. Scand. Suppl.* **377**, 50–8.

Pedersen, S.S., Middel, B., and Larsen, M.L. (2002). The role of personality variables and social support in distress and perceived health in patients following myocardial infarction. *J. Psychosom. Res.* **53**, 1171–5.

Quinton, D., Rutter, M., and Liddle, C. (1984). Institutional rearing, parenting difficulties and marital support. *Psychol. Med.* **14**, 107–24.

Rael, E.G.S., Stansfeld, S.A., Shipley, M., *et al.* (1995). Sickness absence in the Whitehall II Study, London: the role of social support and material problems. *J. Epidemiol. Comm. Hlth.* **49**, 474–81.

Reed, D., McGee, D., Yano, K., and Feinleib, M. (1983). Social networks and coronary heart disease among Japanese men in Hawaii. *Am. J. Epidemiol.* **117**, 384–96.

Ren, X.S., Skinner, K., Lee, A., and Kazis, L. (1999). Social support, social selection and self-assessed health status: results from the veterans health study in the United States. *Soc. Sci. Med* **48**, 1721–34.

Reynolds, P. and Kaplan, G.A. (1990). Social connections and risk for cancer: prospective evidence from the Alameda County Study. *Behav. Med.* **16**, 101–10.

Ruberman, W., Weinblatt, E., Goldberg, J.D., and Chaudhary, B.S. (1984). Psychosocial influences on mortality after myocardial infarction. *N. Engl. J. Med.* **311**, 552–9.

Sapolsky, R.M. (1989). Hypercortisolism among socially subordinate wild baboons originates at the CNS level. *Arch. Gen. Psychiat.* **46**, 1047–51.

Schieman, S. and Meersman, S.C. (2004). Neighborhood problems and health among older adults: received and donated social support and the sense of mastery as effect modifiers. *J. Gerontol.* **59**, S89–S97.

Schoenbach, V., Kaplan, B.H., Fredman, L., and Kleinbaum, D.G. (1986). Social ties and mortality in Evans Country, Georgia. *Am. J. Epidemiol.* **123**, 577–91.

Seeman, T.E. (1996). Social ties and health: the benefits of social integration. *Ann. Epidemiol.* **6**, 442–51.

Seeman, T.E. and McEwen, B.S. (1996). Impact of social environment characteristics on neuroendocrine regulation. *Psychosom. Med.* **58**, 459–71.

Seeman, T.E. and Syme, S.L. (1987). Social networks and coronary artery disease: a comparative analysis of network structural and support characteristics. *Psychosom. Med.* **49**, 331–40.

Seeman, T.E., Berkman, L.F., Blazer, D., and Rowe, J.W. (1994). Social ties and support as modifiers of neuroendocrine function. MacArthur Studies of Successful Aging. *Ann. Behav. Med.* **16**, 95–106.

Stansfeld, S. and Sproston, K. (2002). Social Support and networks. In: *Ethnic minority psychiatric illness rates in the community (EMPIRIC)*, (ed. K. Sproston J. Nazroo). TSO, London.

Stansfeld, A.S., Bosma, H., Hemingway, H., and Marmot, M.G. (1998a). Psychosocial work characteristics and social support as predictors of SF36 health functioning: the Whitehall II Study. *Psychosom. Med.* **60**, 247–55.

Stansfeld, S.A, Fuhrer, R., and Shipley, M. (1998b). Types of social support as predictors of psychiatric morbidity in a cohort of British Civil Servants (Whitehall II Study). *Psychol. Med.* **28**, 881–92.

Stansfeld, S.A, Head, J., Marmot, M.G. (1998c). Explaining social class differences in depression and well being. *Social Psychiatric and Psychiatric Epidemiology* **33**, 1–9.

Stansfeld, S.A., Rael, E.G.A., Head, J., *et al.* (1997). Social support and psychiatric sickness absence: a prospective study of British civil servants. *Psychol. Med.* **27**, 35–48.

Ten Have, M., Vollebergh, W., Bijl, R., and Ormel, J. (2002). Combined effect of mental disorder and low social support on care service use for mental health problems in the Dutch general population. *Psychol. Med.* **32**, 311–23.

Turner, R.J. and Marino, F. (1994). Social support and social structure: a descriptive epidemiology of a central stress mediator. *J. Hlth. Soc. Behav.* **35**, 193–212.

Vogt, T.M., Mullooly, J.P., Ernst, D., Pope, C.R., and Hollis, J.F. (1992). Social networks as predictors of ischemic heart disease, cancer, stroke and hypertension: incidence, survival and mortality. *J. Clin. Epidemiol.* **45**, 659–66.

Welin, L., Tibblin, G., Tibblin, B., *et al.* (1985). Prospective study of social influences on mortality: the study of men born in 1913 and 1923. *Lancet* **1**, 915–18.

Wilkinson, R.G. (1996). *Unhealthy societies: from inequality to well-being.* Routledge, London.

Williams, J.K., Vita, J.A., and Manuck, S.B. (1991). Psychosocial factors impair vascular responses of coronary arteries. *Circulation* **84**, 2146–53.

Williams, R.B., Barefoot, J.C., Califf, R.M., *et al.* (1992). Prognostic importance of social and economic resources among medically treated patients with angiographically documented coronary artery disease. *JAMA* **267**, 520–4.

Willmott, P. (1963). *The evolution of a community.* Routledge and Keegan Paul, London.

Yancey, W. (1971). Architecture, interaction, and social control: the case of a large-scale public housing project. *Environ. Behav.* **3**, 3–21.

Chapter 9

Food is a political issue

Aileen Robertson, Eric Brunner, and Aubrey Sheiham

Diet is one of the principal determinants of common diseases leading to premature mortality and disability. Improvements in food production, availability, and access have the potential to reduce the burden of ill health, especially in low-income countries and among the relatively poor. Policy makers are recognizing that major gains in public health can be made by developing and implementing food and nutrition policies that address the needs of their respective populations.

9.1 Food as a determinant of health

The burden of disease varies widely within the WHO European Region and has changed dramatically in many countries over the last 20 years. A large proportion of these changes and differences can be traced to socio-economic determinants and cultural trends in eating and physical activity patterns.

Nutrition contributes substantially to the burden of disease in Europe (Robertson *et al.* 2004). A large proportion (41%) of total disability adjusted life years (DALYs) lost result from cardiovascular disease (CVD), type II diabetes, and cancers—all of which have nutrition as a major determinant (Fig. 9.1). Another 38% of DALYs lost result from lowered resistance to infection, oral diseases, and congenital abnormalities, in which nutrition also plays an important role. In 2000, 136 million years of healthy life were lost in the European Region; major nutritional risk factors caused the loss of over 56 million and other nutrition-related factors played a role in the loss of a further 52 million DALYs.

In terms of mortality in the European Region, CVD is the leading cause of death, causing over four million deaths per year, and diet-related risk factors are prominent causes of premature mortality. A recent estimate of the contribution of risk factors to mortality in the WHO European Region (Fig. 9.2) shows that, of the seven major risk factors, six are related to diet and physical activity patterns.

The leading risk factor is high blood pressure, which is directly linked to obesity and high salt intakes. The second risk factor is high serum cholesterol, which is directly linked to high intakes of saturated fat. The third is tobacco (see Chapter 11). The fourth risk factor is high body mass index, because overweight and obesity are strongly

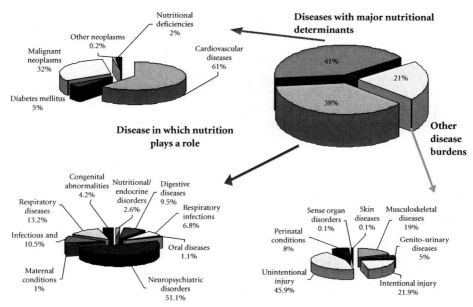

Fig. 9.1 Lost years[1] of healthy life in the European Region in 2000. (*Source*: WHO 2004, Fig. 1.1, p. 8).

linked to CVD, type II diabetes, and some cancers. Fifth, low fruit and vegetable intake is again closely correlated with a high prevalence of some cancers and CVD (Fig. 9.3). The sixth major risk factor is low levels of physical activity, and the seventh is high intakes of alcohol. This chapter focuses on the nutritional determinants of high blood pressure, high serum cholesterol, overweight and obesity, as well as low intake of fruit and vegetables. Less attention is given to excess alcohol intake and low levels of physical activity.

9.2 **Diet, nutrition, and the prevention of chronic diseases—WHO/FAO recommendations**

There is a wealth of evidence that inappropriate nutrition is a major factor contributing to diseases of public health importance (Brunner *et al.* 2001) as well as to the burden of disease as outlined above. The scientific evidence published after 1990 was reviewed by an Expert Consultation from the WHO and FAO (WHO 2003). This new technical report series (916) reinforced the nutritional goals recommended in the previous

---

[1] In the DALY approach, lost disability-adjusted life years (DALYs) combine information about morbidity and mortality in numbers of healthy years lost. Each state of health is assigned a disability weighting on a scale from '0' (perfect health) to '1' (death). The burden of a given disease is calculated by multiplying the number of years lived with that disease by its disability weighting and adding the number of years lost due to that disease. Only DALY represents the loss of one year of healthy life.

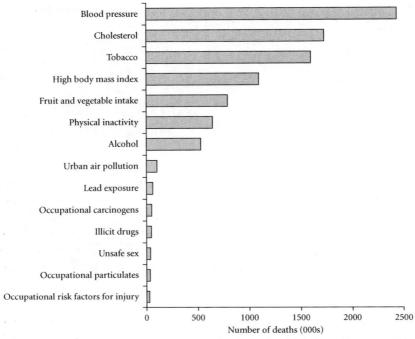

Fig. 9.2 Deaths in 2000, in Europe, attributable to major risk factors. (*Source*: WHO 2002).

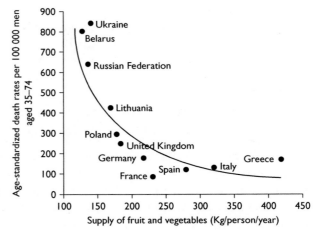

Fig. 9.3 Mortality from coronary heart disease in relation to fruit and vegetable supply in selected European countries.

WHO report (797) published in 1990 (WHO 1990). The updated nutrient goals (Table 9.1) differ only slightly and the main changes are:

1 **Fat.** The recommended goals for fatty acids are more detailed, in view of the growing evidence that the qualitative composition of dietary fats significantly modifies

CVD risk. In particular, there are findings concerning polyunsaturated fatty acids (PUFA) and hydrogenated fatty acids. To promote cardiovascular health, diets should provide very low intake (i.e. <1%) of *trans* fatty acids (hydrogenated fats). This recommendation is important in countries where low-cost hydrogenated fat is marketed. The diet should provide adequate intake of PUFA (6–10% of daily energy intake). Further, the goals specify an optimal balance between intake of *n*-6 PUFAs (5–8% of daily energy intake), derived largely from seed oils, and *n*-3 PUFAs (1–2% of daily energy intake), derived from marine and plant sources.

2 **Salt**. The recommended goal for salt (sodium chloride) was lowered by 1 g because of new evidence regarding the prevention of cardiovascular diseases. High blood pressure is a major risk factor for coronary heart disease and stroke (ischaemic and haemorrhagic stroke), and the distribution of sodium intake is an important influence on the distribution of blood pressure level in populations. Current evidence suggests that an intake of no more than 1.7 g (70 mmol) of sodium per day is beneficial in reducing blood pressure. This corresponds to a recommended salt intake of less than 5 g/day. Given the level of iodine deficiency disorders in some countries, the Expert Consultation emphasized the need to adjust salt iodization depending on salt intake and iodine status.

3 **Dietary fibre**. Adequate dietary fibre intake can be achieved through regular consumption of whole-grain cereals, legumes, fruit, and vegetables. The health benefits include protection from obesity, diabetes, CVD, colorectal and other cancers. The recommended intake of fruit and vegetables (>400 g/day) and consumption of whole-grain foods is likely to provide >20 g/day of non-starch polysaccharides, corresponding to >25 g/day of total dietary fibre.

4 **Sugar**. The Joint WHO/FAO Expert Consultation in 2003 were aware of the controversy surrounding a population goal for a sugar intake of <10% of total energy. However, studies suggesting that a high intake of sugar did not increase body weight were appraised, and considered to have significant scientific limitations. It was agreed that high intakes of sugar tend to undermine the nutrient quality of diets by providing significant amounts of energy without supplying nutrients. Restriction of sugar is likely to contribute to reducing the risk of unhealthy weight gain in several ways (Gross *et al.* 2004). Sugar promotes a positive energy balance. For example, reduction of food intake after the consumption of high-sugar drinks is less than when foods of equivalent energy content are consumed, and sweetened soft drinks thus increase overall energy intake (James *et al.* 2004). Children who consume large quantities of soft drinks rich in sugar are more likely to gain excess weight (Raben *et al.* 2002; Ludwig *et al.* 2001).

The Global Strategy on Diet, Physical Activity, and Health was endorsed by the World Health Assembly in 2004 (*http://www.who.int/dietphysicalactivity/en/*) and responds to member states' requests at the WHA, in 2002, for such a strategy to be

Table 9.1 Population nutrient goals

Dietary factor	2003 WHO/FAO recommendations[2]
Total fat	15–30%
Saturated fatty acids	<10%
Polyunsaturated fatty acids	6–10%
n-6 PUFAs	5–8%
n-3 PUFAs	1–2%
Trans fatty acids	<1%
Monosaturated fatty acids	By difference
Total carbohydrate	55–75%
Free sugars	<10%
Complex carbohydrate	No recommendation
Protein	10–15%
Cholesterol	<300 mg/day
Salt (sodium chloride)	<5 g/day
Fruit, vegetables, pulses, nuts, and seeds	>400 g/day
Total dietary fibre	From foods—see point 3 in text
Non-starch polysaccharides	From foods—see point 3 in text

Source: WHO 2003.

prepared. In 2000, 52 European health ministries endorsed the First Action Plan for Food and Nutrition Policy in the WHO European Region (2000–2005) (*http://www.euro.who.int/nutrition/FoodandNutActPlan/20010906_2*). This European initiative placed nutrition and prevention of non-communicable diseases on the WHO political agenda. Future implementation of the Global Strategy will largely depend on the six WHO Regions. It is planned that the relevant parts of the Global Strategy will be incorporated into the Second Action Plan for Food and Nutrition Policy in the WHO European Region 2006–2010, which will be discussed during a WHO ministerial conference on nutrition in 2006 in the European Region.

9.3 Designing a food supply to meet population nutrient goals

Population nutrient goals need to be translated into meaningful policy by determining how much food intake must change in order to reach the goals. One approach is to compare food supply statistics with the nutrient goals. If the actual food supply is different from the theoretical supplies (based on the goals), then changes in the food supply system should be investigated. In terms of change, the willingness of farmers, food processors and retailers to respond to a food and nutrition policy has to be negotiated.

Food intake patterns in Europe have already changed dramatically in the last decades. Trends were country-specific, and both positive and negative changes took place. For example, the population of Ireland was supplied with excess fat and sugar

---

[2] Recommended range of intake specified as % of total energy intake, unless otherwise stated.

Table 9.2 Comparison of dietary recommendations with food supplies to the populations of Ireland and Italy, 1965 and 1999

Food	Nutrient population goals	Theoretical food supplies required (per person/day)	Actual food supplies (per person/day)			
			Ireland		Italy	
			1965	1999	1965	1999
Total fat	<30% of total energy	<80 g fat	119 g	136 g	90 g	152 g
Saturated fat	<10% of total energy	<60 g fat from animal products	100 g	89 g	38 g	70 g
Sugar	<10% of total energy	<65 g raw sugar equivalent	146 g	116 g	73 g	81 g
Fruit and vegetables	>400 g/day	>600 g fruit and vegetables (>400 g edible)	245 g	390 g	720 g	858 g

Source: WHO 2004 (Table 3.10, p.187).

and insufficient fruit and vegetables in 1965 and 1999 (Table 9.2). However, dietary quality appeared to partly improve as supplies of saturated fat declined, while that of fruit and vegetables increased. Italy increased its fat supply well above the maximum recommended, but the amounts of fruit and vegetables remained high.

Trends in food supply, in comparison with nutrient goals, provide a good starting point for nutrition policy. However, such data do not take account of wide distribution of intakes within a population. Factors such as availability and access, inequalities between rich and poor communities and in rural versus urban areas are crucial. Income inequality, cultural preferences, and other influences such as pricing policies and catering practices will strongly influence consumption patterns in different sections of the population.

9.4 **Food poverty and inequality**

Some people in the European Region enjoy access to shops overflowing with food from all over the globe and have enough money to buy it. Others lack these advantages and endure days when they eat one meal or no meal at all; their food supplies are insecure and are likely to be deficient in essential nutrients. Such inequalities exist in every country in Europe. Poor people suffer from insecure income, lack of or low-quality food, and bad living standards. The United Nations Development Programme has estimated the proportion of the population living below locally defined poverty lines in selected countries in the European Region (Fig. 9.4), showing that more than 20% of the populations in the former Soviet countries are living below their national poverty lines compared with less than 10% in most EU countries.

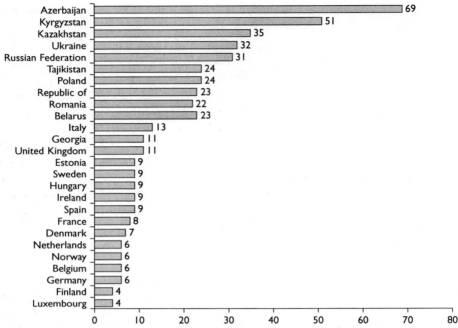

Fig. 9.4 Percentage of the population in selected European countries below the national poverty line (latest available years). (*Source*: WHO 2004, Fig. 3.3, p. 160).

The World Bank has estimated that more than 50 million children in the European Region live in low-income households, with nearly 20 million in extreme poverty (defined as less than US $2.15 per child per day). When poverty leads to suboptimal nutrition or outright hunger, the effects can harm both the individual and the community. Children cannot concentrate on their school lessons. Women may give birth to low birth-weight infants. Poorly fed men and women lack the ability to improve family income by seeking work, perpetuating their poverty. Agricultural workers have high poverty rates and also face declining employment prospects as farms are merged and food production is intensified.

9.4.1 Measuring food inequality

The proportion of household expenditure that has to be spent on food is a good proxy indicator of food inequalities. A high percentage of income spent on food means that households are likely to have trouble ensuring proper nourishment. A small percentage implies relatively easy access to food. For example, the percentage of total household expenditure on food in Tajikistan is on average 75%, and ranges from 60% to 79% in the richest fifth and poorest fifth of households respectively. In western European countries, the corresponding average percentages are 13% in Luxembourg to 36% in Greece. However, the national averages hide the fact that the range is broad and too many people in most European countries are struggling to afford a healthy diet.

The dietary patterns of socio-economic groups in European countries have been surveyed using a variety of indicators, such as household income, occupational class, and educational attainment (De Irala–Estevez *et al.* 2000). In general, lower socio-economic groups tend to consume less fruit and vegetables (Table 9.3) and more meat, fat, and sugar. Household food purchases may be insufficient for all family members to eat an optimum diet. The problem may be compounded by lack of kitchen appliances such as refrigerators or cookers. As a result, some—often the women—may get inadequate nourishment.

Although low-income households are usually very efficient purchasers of nutrients, considering how little money they have, such families spend less on micronutrient-rich foods such as fruit and vegetables and more on foods high in fat and sugar (Nelson 1999). In general, the cost per unit energy is lowest for fat, oil, white bread, and sugar. These cheap, high-energy foods are the main ones that the poor can afford. Such foods are unlikely to meet the nutrient recommendations, but they satisfy hunger by providing energy. For the poor, lack of money can, therefore, reduce the consumption of micronutrient-rich foods, such as fruit and vegetables, in favour of foods high in fat and sugar.

In the UK, household income is consistently related to certain dietary patterns. Families living on low incomes tend to consume less fruit and vegetables (Fig. 9.5), fish, and whole-grain cereal foods and more refined cereal foods, sweet foods, fat, and oil. As a result, the intake of essential nutrients shows a marked social gradient from poor to richer households.

Table 9.3 Difference in fruit and vegetable consumption between high and low education groups in selected western European countries and regions, 1980s and 1990s

Country or region	Difference (g/10 MJ/day)	
	Fruit	**Vegetables**
Finland	+55	+30
Sweden	+18	+23
Norway	+26	−3
Denmark	+46	+43
United Kingdom	+31	+33
Germany	+16	+14
Netherlands	+52	+19
Spain		
Navarra	+14	+9
Catalonia	+6	−19
Basque Country	−97	+31

Note: Figures are the excess in consumption of the high compared to the low education group.

Source: Roos *et al.* 2000.

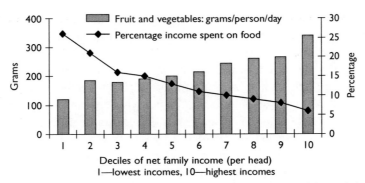

Fig. 9.5 Relationship of income to consumption of fresh fruit and vegetables and the share of income spent on food in the UK. (*Source*: WHO 2004, Fig. 3.3, p. 68).

Further surveys in the UK have shown that vulnerable groups—including older people, children from manual social classes, families claiming state benefits, and children from lone-parent families—have lower intake and lower blood levels of many vitamins and minerals than others in the population. Intakes of vitamin C, folate, iron, zinc, and magnesium are well below reference levels in households with incomes below £180 a week (the lowest income cut-off), in households with more than three children, and those headed by a lone parent. Among the poorest fifth of families, the intake of some nutrients declined over a period of 15 years: vitamin C by 23% and beta-carotene by 47% (Dowler and Leather 1997).

9.4.2 Inequality and diet-related diseases

The dietary patterns described above contribute to the different disease patterns experienced by different social groups. A national survey of more than 15,000 adults in the UK found significant inequalities in the prevalence of CVD and risk factors across social classes defined by occupation. Social gradients in health indices were particularly evident among women.

The environmental causes of health inequalities can be seen among individuals who change social class or migrate during their adult lives. A study in Oslo found that people who were upwardly or downwardly mobile showed mortality rates that approached, but did not equal, those of the class to which they had moved (Naess and Claussen 2000). Cancer rates can show similar patterns of change. Turkish migrants in Germany experience disease rates that approach those of native Germans (Razum and Zeeb 2000). It appears that changing lifestyle (including food and diet) is an important determinant of health, and that health inequalities are modifiable.

Lower-income groups in the UK tend to have higher CVD rates (Table 9.4), and many countries in northern Europe show a similar pattern. The causes are likely to be multifactorial, including smoking, physical inactivity, stress, occupational and psychosocial factors, in addition to nutrition. In contrast, the opposite association has been observed—higher CVD rates associated with higher income—in southern

Table 9.4 Social class and ill health: prevalence of disease and risk factors in adults in England & Wales, 1998

Diseases and risk factors	Registrar general social class					
	MEN			**WOMEN**		
	High	**Intermediate non-manual**	**Low**	**High**	**Intermediate non-manual**	**Low**
Ischaemic heart disease (%)	5.2	11.1	10.2	8.2	6.0	10.0
Stroke (%)	1.0	2.0	2.1	0.9	1.9	4.0
High blood pressure* (%)	34.3	37.2	40.2	31.4	34.4	35.9
Cholesterol ≥6.5 mmol/l (%)	14.5	21.2	19.8	22.2	21.2	22.6
HDL-C <0.9 mmol/l (%)	16.3	18.1	14.1	3.4	4.9	8.5
Obesity (BMI >30) (%)	11.6	16.4	17.7	14.4	18.2	28.1
High fat consumption**	19	23	38	7	12	17

Social class: High = I; intermediate non-manual = IIIN; low = V

* Systolic blood pressure ≥140 mmHg or systolic ≥90 mmHg or taking medication

** Semi-quantitative Dietary Instrument for Nutrition Education (DINE) questionnaire (fat score >40)

Source: Erens and Primatesta 1999.

European countries such as Portugal. A rapid transition among richer people from the traditional heart-protecting Mediterranean-type diets rich in fruit, vegetables, and fish to diets rich in animal products and sugar may account for this.

9.4.3 Reducing inequality in food and nutrition

The nutritional security of family members depends on many factors: macro-economics, local accessibility and affordability, influences on food choice, and individual preferences (Fig. 9.6).

Initiatives to help the poor by religious, voluntary, and neighbourhood organizations and food banks may be useful at the local level. However, comprehensive national food and nutrition policies must be developed (WHO 2000a). A review of national strategies for household food and nutrition security in the UK emphasized the need for a co-ordinated approach across government, including agriculture, environment and rural affairs, health, social welfare, education, employment and economic affairs. Problems identified included minimum wage legislation, unemployment support, child care, housing and fuel policies, and insufficient education on food topics in schools. In addition, a national food and nutrition policy requires integration of strategies concerning food distribution and retail planning. Food price data can be used for planning of legislation on minimum income, family budget standards, and welfare benefit levels.

National efforts are needed to monitor the food chain. A variety of types of data are needed to understand the influence of agricultural and other policies on individual nutrition security. The surveillance of dietary intake and nutritional status in households vulnerable to poverty and inequality is particularly important. National policies have

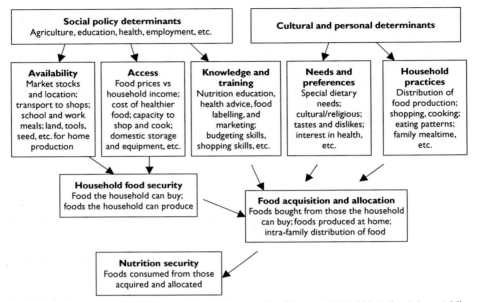

Fig. 9.6 Influences on food choice and nutrition security. (*Source*: WHO 2004, Fig. 3.5, p. 166).

a strong influence on the provision of food eaten outside the home, especially in institutions under government control, such as national and local government offices, schools, hospitals, prisons, and military bases. Policies can also influence catering in the high street, the workplace, and in private institutions. In these situations, decision makers should consider public health guidance on healthy diets and use pricing policies and other incentives to encourage good practices. For example, in Finland, mass catering has provided an excellent means of influencing food intake. The average Finn eats about 125 meals per year outside the home and the intake of fruit and vegetables more than doubled as a result of vegetables being included in the price of a meal.

9.5 **Twelve steps to healthy eating**

The first half of this chapter explained why policies are needed to reduce diet-related diseases and food and nutrition inequalities in Europe. Below we give some examples of problems, with emphasis on food and nutrition inequalities. The examples are organized according to the *WHO Dietary Guide* (WHO 2000b) which highlights 12 key recommendations for implementation of nutrition policy:

1 Eat a nutritious diet based on a variety of foods originating mainly from plants, rather than animals.

2 Eat bread, grains, pasta, rice, or potatoes several times a day.

3 Eat a variety of vegetables and fruits, preferably fresh and local, several times per day (>400 g per day).

4 Maintain a body weight between the recommended limits (BMI[3] of 18.5–25) by taking moderate levels of physical activity, preferably daily.

5 Control fat intake (not more than 30% of daily energy) and replace most saturated fats with unsaturated vegetable oils or soft margarines.

6 Replace fatty meat and meat products with beans, legumes, lentils, fish, poultry, or lean meat.

7 Use milk and dairy products (sour milk, yoghurt, and cheese) that are low in both fat and salt.

8 Select foods that are low in sugar, and eat refined sugar sparingly, limiting the frequency of sugary drinks and sweets (<10% energy).

9 Choose a low-salt diet. Total salt intake should not be more than one teaspoon (5 g) per day, including the salt in bread and processed, cured, and preserved foods. (Salt iodization should be universal where iodine deficiency is endemic.)

10 If alcohol is consumed, limit intake to no more than two drinks (each containing 10 g of alcohol) per day.

11 Prepare food in a safe and hygienic way. Steam, bake, boil, or microwave to help reduce the amount of added fat.

12 Promote exclusive breastfeeding and the introduction of safe and appropriate complementary foods from the age of six months while breastfeeding continues during the first years of life.

These recommendations should not be considered in isolation and are designed to be integrated within a food and nutrition policy based on existing cultures and eating patterns. Below each recommendation, there are examples of their policy implications to illustrate why 'healthy eating' is not just a question of individual personal choice but that policies are needed. Campaigns that provide nutrition information and health education tend to exacerbate the gap between the rich and poor and will not help much to change the eating patterns of the most disadvantaged in any society.

1. Eat a nutritious diet based on a variety of foods originating mainly from plants, rather than animals.

Food production and supply sectors are being driven against this recommendation in many countries. For example, considerable financial support for animal-derived products has led to a shift towards livestock rearing rather than horticulture. Three quarters of agricultural land in the EU is used for producing animal feed or grazing. In some EU countries, land devoted to fruit and vegetables has declined by over 20%, while that for animal feed has increased by 20% (Table 9.5) in the last four decades. The diet in these countries includes increasing quantities of animal products, resulting in more

---

[3] BMI (body mass index) is derived by dividing a person's weight (in kg) by height (in m^2). The recommended levels are adapted from the global WHO recommendation of 18.5–24.9 as a normal BMI.

Table 9.5 Land area devoted to production in France, Greece, Italy, Portugal, and Spain, 1961–2000

Crops	Land area (ha thousands)	
	1961	2000
Fruit and vegetables	8720	6680
Animal feed	7554	9063

Source: WHO 2004 (Table 3.8, p. 185).

Table 9.6 Meat and dairy supplies in France, Greece, Italy, Portugal, and Spain, 1961 and 1999

Country	Beef and veal (kg/person)		Milk (kg/person)		Animal fat (kg/person)	
	1961	1999	1961	1999	1961	1999
France	28.6	26.2	220	265	28.8	39.6
Greece	5.1	22.3	101	257	9.5	20.8
Italy	14.6	25.6	145	261	12.0	25.4
Portugal	6.4	16.8	62	207	8.6	28.0
Spain	6.0	14.0	83	165	14.5	23.0

Source: WHO 2004 (Table 3.9, p. 186).

animal fat being available (Table 9.6), and in direct contradiction with health recommendations.

2. Eat bread, grains, pasta, rice, or potatoes several times per day.

It is recommended that most (55–75%) of energy intake comes from these foods which should be the best possible quality and intrinsically rich in micronutrients. Greater dietary diversity is associated with reduced all-cause mortality (Kant *et al.* 2000) and reduced mortality from CVD and cancer. The available evidence 'indicates that, taking a week as a time frame, at least 20, and probably as many as 30 biologically distinct types of food, with the emphasis on plant food, are required' to ensure optimum health (Wahlqvist 1999). Therefore, in order to protect public health, biodiversity in food production should be protected. Biodiversity not only contributes to dietary diversity but also increases food security by safeguarding against climatic and pestilential disasters and the spread of invasive plants, pathogens, and toxins.

About 75% of the genetic diversity of agricultural crops worldwide was lost during the twentieth century. Previously, 10,000 plant species were used for food; now less than 120 cultivated species provide over 90% of human plant food. In Provence (France), the number of plant species in the diet fell from 250 to 30–60 in the twentieth century. Loss of agricultural biodiversity is seen across western Europe: recent data show that in France, 'Golden Delicious' accounted for 71% of apple production; in Holland, one variety accounted for 80% of land utilized in potato production; and in the UK, four varieties accounted for 71% of the land in wheat production (Robertson *et al.* 2004, p. 189)

3. **Eat a variety of vegetables and fruits, preferably fresh and local, several times per day (>400 g per day).**

The countries (Greece, Spain, Italy, France) who meet this recommendation (see Fig. 9.3) are also the largest producers of vegetables and fruit. Therefore, availability and access appear to be important for optimum consumption. However, the Common Agriculture Policy (CAP) reduces the availability of fruit and vegetables in order to maintain market prices. Fresh vegetables and fruit are highly perishable and cannot be put into European intervention stocks, like butter. Surplus produce is, therefore, processed or destroyed. In 2000/2001, 1 million tonnes of fruit and vegetables were composted, distilled, or fed to animals; a small amount was given as free fruit in schools. The amount destroyed was equivalent to 3300 g per person per year or 40 portions of fruit and vegetables for each person in the EU. This destruction process costs around 117 million Euros per year (National Institute of Public Health 2003).

Eliminating the destruction of fruit and vegetables is probably one of the most positive ways in which agricultural policy could contribute to nutrition policy in Europe. The Swedish National Institute of Public Health made recommendations that would lead to improvements regarding availability of fruit and vegetables:

> . . . withdrawal compensation should only be granted for produce used for human consumption; all classified fruit and vegetables should be marketed and prices allowed to fall; promotion of measures for fruit and vegetables should be based on scientific evidence and best practice; introduction of a school scheme similar to the school milk scheme. (NIPH 2003)

In addition to the health benefits of fresh produce being eaten as close as possible to where grown, there are also environmental benefits from rationalizing transport. Increasing distances adds to air pollution and road hazards. Food production and transport policies need to be analysed carefully to minimize both environmental and health damage.

As discussed earlier, poor and disadvantaged people often cannot afford to eat enough fruit and vegetables. Higher intake in populations in the Mediterranean countries compared with northern Europe (see Fig. 9.3) demonstrates that access and availability are key to increasing consumption. Authorities can develop partnerships with retailers and influence them to improve access and affordability. Some local authorities have successfully encouraged supermarkets to enter poorer areas of cities, leading to increased sales of fruit and vegetables.

4. **Maintain body weight between the recommended limits (BMI of 20–25[4]) by taking moderate levels of physical activity, preferably daily.**

> The poor do not eat what they want, or what they know they should eat, but what they can afford. Restrictions on access to food determine two simultaneous phenomena that are two sides of the same coin: the poor are malnourished because they do not have enough to feed

---

[4] Adapted from the global WHO recommendation of 18.5–24.9 kg/m^2 as normal values.

themselves and they are obese because they eat poorly, with significant energy imbalance. The foods available to them are industrialised, mass-produced, undifferentiated, and inexpensive products. (PAHO 2000).

In countries where undernutrition and poor child growth are still relatively common, obesity and underweight coexist. Evidence suggests that, the more rapid the nutrition transition, the more likely that both under- and overweight problems will coexist in the same household. The post-transition pattern is that poor people are more likely to eat less healthily and take less exercise. This unhealthy lifestyle in turn contributes to the inequality in morbidity and mortality from CVD and other diseases. Related risk factors, such as poor foetal nutrition, low birth weight, stunted child growth, and subsequent obesity, are shaped by circumstances that are beyond individual control. Efforts to improve health by exhorting the population to change their lifestyles tend to have negative impacts for complex reasons.

An inverse relationship between socio-economic status and obesity has often been observed in women. The relationship in men, although less clear in earlier reviews, seems now in Europe to be similar to that in women. A pan-EU consumer survey found a strong association between obesity and social class defined variously by household income, occupation, or educational level in both sexes (Table 9.7).

Inequality in BMI is also related to lack of physical activity. A survey of over 15,000 adults in the UK found that physical inactivity in both men and women increased as social class decreased. Surveys of physical activity rarely distinguish between leisure-related activity and work- or domestic-related activity. This can make the interpretation of inequalities in physical activity difficult. Less educated adults were more likely to have physically active jobs and, when not working, were more likely to spend time in

Table 9.7 Prevalence of obesity among men and women by social class and educational levels

	Men	Women
Economic status*		
Lower	11.1%	13.8%
Middle-lower	8.9%	12.6%
Middle	8.0%	8.0%
Middle-upper	7.8%	5.6%
Educational level		
Primary	12.1%	15.9%
Secondary	8.4%	8.5%
Tertiary	5.9%	4.4%

Obesity defined as BMI = 30 kg/m^2 based on self-reported weight and height

* Measured by household income or occupation

Source: Martinez et al. 1999.

sedentary leisure. Older people and those with only primary education were least likely to be physically active.

Local and national strategies need to be developed to improve levels of physical activity. Barriers include the lack of facilities, such as safe walking and cycling routes, unpleasant or hazardous environments, and the cost of using leisure facilities.

5. **Control fat intake (not more than 30% of daily energy) and replace most saturated fats with polyunsaturated vegetable oils or soft margarines.**

Consumers have very little control over the fatty acid composition of food products. For example, the rapid growth of cattle depends largely on the type of fodder (a combination of high-energy and high-protein), little exercise, and genetic selection. These factors combine to produce meat of a particular fat composition. Meat of farmed cattle contains 20–25% fat compared with less than 3% in free-living buffalo meats. Even so-called 'lean' farmed beef contains about 8% fat. In chicken, the carcass fat content has risen almost ten-fold over the past century (Crawford and Marsh 1989).

The fat of farmed, compared with free-living, animals has more saturated fatty acids. In cattle, nearly 50% of the fat content of free-living buffalo is polyunsaturated, compared with barely 2% from farmed beef cattle. Milk and butter from farmed cattle show a similarly low proportion of polyunsaturated fat: typically less than 3% of the fat. The nature of the polyunsaturates differs between free-living and farmed animals. Free-living animals have 10 times the amount of very long-chain derivatives of both linoleic and linolenic fatty acids and, correspondingly, smaller amounts of shorter-chain fatty acids. Human body fat and human milk tend to reflect the fat consumed in the diet. Clearly, more effort could be invested into producing fats with a healthier composition.

An EU directive on labelling meat in 2001 improves consumer information on pre-packed meat products. Nevertheless, concerns remain because this directive allows beef to contain up to 25% fat and still be called meat. It is hard for consumers to control their fat intake if they are neither informed how much fat meat contains, nor what the composition of the fat is. Honest labelling is indispensable (Hawkes 2004a).

6. **Replace fatty meat and meat products with beans, legumes, lentils, fish, poultry, or lean meat.**

Just as there are health benefits from replacing fatty meat products with beans and legumes, there are also significant environmental benefits. The Swedish Environmental Protection Agency examined food production implications of reducing land requirements, energy demands, and fertilizer input. The more ecologically sustainable results are compared with Sweden's current dietary pattern and illustrate the changes needed. They recommended a reduction in milk products and cheese, drastic reductions in meat, poultry and sausage, snacks, sweets, and soft drinks with concomitant increases in bread, cereal, potato, vegetables, fruit and a tenfold increase in legumes (Table 9.8).

Animal products are much more energy-dense than grains and vegetables, and a reduced intake of animal foods could result in more legumes and beans being eaten.

Table 9.8 Recommended daily consumption of various food groups, in Sweden, to reduce ecological impact

Food	Level of consumption (g/day)	
	Actual	Recommended for reduced ecological impact
Milk products	400	300
Cheese	45	20
Meat, poultry, sausage	145	35
Egg	25	10
Snacks/sweets	200	140
Soft drinks	150	80
Bread	100	200
Cereal	15	45
Potatoes	140	270
Vegetables	150	190
Root vegetables	25	100
Fruit	150	175
Dried legumes	5	50

Source: Swedish Environmental Agency 1999.

In addition, animal production requires a lot more land than growing legumes and pulses. The more ecologically sustainable results compare very favourably with the nutrient goals for health recommended by WHO. Reducing the environmental impact of food production can also help to meet health goals.

7. **Use milk and dairy products (sour milk, yoghurt, and cheese) that are low in both fat and salt.**

The analysis by Sweden's National Institute of Public Health (NIPH 2003) concluded that CAP has led to patterns of milk consumption that can harm health. For instance, CAP butter subsidies and the promotion of full-fat milk conflict with the health aim of reducing saturated fat intake.

Subsidized school milk is available to children in day care and in primary and secondary schools. The EC objective is 'a measure to help expand the market for milk products' and as a 'surplus disposal mechanism'. An important change happened in 2001 when skimmed milk and other low-fat products were entitled to support. However, full-fat products still received the highest subsidies (Table 9.9).

Considering the growing levels of obesity, giving subsidies in proportion to the fat content is counterproductive to health. A pupil who drinks 0.25 litres of full-fat milk (3.5% fat) every school day would consume 8.75 g of milk fat per day, amounting to 1750 g (1.75 kg) of milk fat per year. Skimmed milk (0.5% fat) would provide 1.25 g per day or 250 g (0.25 kg) per year. The difference is likely to reduce the risk of childhood obesity.

The aided consumption of milk fat costs EU citizens around 460 million Euros per year; promotion of high-fat milk products and wine costs 10 million Euros per year;

Table 9.9 School milk subsidies in 2001

Dairy product	Fat content	Subsidy (Euros/100 kg)
Whole milk and yoghurt	>3%	23.24
Standard milk	3%	21.82
Semi-skimmed milk	1.5%	17.58
Skimmed milk	<1.5%	13.34

and butter is sold at a 30% reduced price to industry to keep stockpiles low. These actions are in direct contradiction with nutrition and public health policies.

The National Institute of Public Health, Sweden, has put forward a number of specific recommendations that would lead to substantial improvements in the CAP from a public health point of view. Some important ones are:

1 Phase out all consumption aid to dairy products with a high fat content.

2 Abolish all milk fat disposal measures.

3 Adapt milk production in the EU to levels of unsubsidized consumption and exports.

4 Encourage farmers to produce milk with a lower fat content.

5 Promotion campaigns for milk and milk products should not include high-fat products.

6 Subsidize only skimmed milk and low-fat dairy products in schools.

8. Select foods that are low in sugar and eat refined sugar sparingly, limiting the frequency of sugary drinks and sweets (<10% energy).

An article in the *Financial Times* (27 February 2004) entitled 'Sweet deals: big sugar fights the threats to free trade and a global drive to limit consumption' describes how the sugar industry is fighting the WHO global strategy on diet, physical activity, and health, because industry perceives it as a threat to sugar consumption. The Sugar Association campaigned against the WHO/FAO sugar recommendations saying that it lacks proper scientific foundation. The President of the Sugar Association wrote to the WHO warning that his association would 'exercise every avenue available to expose the dubious nature' of the report. Funding of the USA's contributions to WHO were challenged. A World Bank report states that sugar is the most policy-distorted of all commodities. Sugar is the largest agricultural industry donor to political campaigns in the USA and donates 16.2% of funds, compared with 14.5% from tobacco.

Patterns of retailing and marketing are also important. For example, 60% of the direct foreign investment in the food sector in Central and Eastern Europe during the 1990s was in confectionery and soft drink production, compared with less than 6% in fruit and vegetables. Advertising influences food purchases and especially exposing children aged 2–6 years to 20-second commercials significantly influences their food preferences. The chapter 'Exploiting kids, corrupting schools' in Marion Nestle's book

(Nestle 2002) describes the creative marketing of the food industry. Consumers International (Consumers International 1996) found that candy, sweetened breakfast cereals and fast-food restaurants accounted for over half of all food advertisements, and so the most heavily advertised tend to be foods high in fat and sugar and low in micronutrients. A nutritional analysis of the advertised products found that 62% of advertisements were for products high in fat (>30% energy), 50% for products high in sugar (>20% energy), and 61% for products high in sodium. Food advertising dwarfs efforts for health education (Hawkes 2004b). The imbalance in information and power between the food industry, consumers, and governments results in the unprecedented promotion of energy-dense food.

It is difficult to see what hope consumers have to exercise their own personal choice and to reduce their sugar intake against such aggressive lobbying and marketing power. Promotional messages need to be more consistent with dietary guidelines.

9. Choose a low-salt diet. Total salt intake should not be more than one teaspoon (5 g) per day, including the salt in bread and processed, cured, and preserved foods. (Salt iodization should be universal where iodine deficiency is endemic.)

Salt added during food processing accounts for three quarters of the total consumed. The upper limit recommended is 5 g per day but most people eat much more than this because salt is added to processed foods. In many western countries, processed foods contribute around 80% of daily salt intake with only around 20% (only 1 g per day according to recommendations) added knowingly. Individuals have little possibility to lower their own salt intake voluntarily if the food industry does not reduce the amount of salt in processed foods, especially staple foods such as bread and cereals. Bread still accounts for nearly 25% of the salt in diets in the UK, although sodium levels in bread were reduced by up to 21% between 1998 and 2001. The Department of Health now wants to see all food industries follow the example set by the bread industry.

The policy for eliminating iodine deficiency is universal salt iodization: all salt used at the table, for cooking, and by food manufacturers, and all salt fed to animals, should be iodized. In some countries, only table salt is iodized. This may lead to the unintentional promotion of salt, adversely affecting blood pressure levels. In addition, if consumers succeed in reducing their salt intake to less than 5 g per day, prevalence of iodine deficiency may increase. Thus, iodine deficiency will only be eradicated if all salt (including fodder for milking cows) is iodized. Universal salt iodization is a good example of a policy warranting integrated intervention by nutritionists (both human and animal), food safety experts, the food industry, and farmers.

10. If alcohol is consumed, limit intake to no more than two drinks (each containing 10 g of alcohol) per day.

The major burden to society arising from alcohol-related problems is constituted by the negative social effects, such as problems within the family, with work, with money, and with the law. The 2002 World Health Report estimated the proportion of the total disease burden attributable to alcohol, excluding social effects, to be 14% in the European region for men and 3.3% for women. In addition, excessive alcohol consumption contributes to inequalities in health. Therefore, alcohol control policies are legitimate from a public health perspective and potentially cost-effective. Total wine consumption in the EU is on the decline, while production has not decreased to the same extent. These trends result in surplus production of about 20%. Of the entire wine budget of 1.2 billion Euros, 70% is used for managing surplus wine, while only 30% is utilized for the conversion of vineyards for other purposes.

11. Prepare food in a safe and hygienic way. Steam, bake, boil, or microwave to help reduce the amount of added fat.

Food policies are needed to reduce the spread of food-borne diseases and to reduce the level of health risks from unsafe food. Consumers are increasingly concerned about the microbiological and chemical safety of food, genetically modified foods, novel foods, and new processing techniques, and have lost trust in the food industry. Reports of antibiotic resistance, BSE, dioxins, and foot-and-mouth disease in animals have damaged their confidence. Many of the food-borne diseases are associated with intensive agriculture and mass-produced and widely distributed food. Producing more food nearer the consumer could improve ability to trace the source and perhaps reduce some of the risks.

Because many pesticides are persistent, they contaminate air, water, and soil. Nearly half (48%) of all fruit and vegetables tested in the UK in 1999 contained detectable pesticide residues. However, the real danger, from a public health point of view, is that the threat of pesticides discourages consumers from increasing their intake of fruit and vegetables. Convincing consumers is difficult if they fear ingesting high levels of pesticide residues. Similar public health dilemmas exist regarding dioxins in fish, *Salmonella* and *Campylobacter* in chicken, and *PCBs* in breast milk.

Clearly, integrated intervention by the nutrition, food safety, and environmental sectors is warranted. Nutritionists' advocacy of greater consumption of vegetables, fruits, poultry, and fish, and of breastfeeding must be backed by food safety measures to control pesticide levels, salmonella outbreaks, and dioxin contamination. Authorities should provide measured advice to citizens stressing the relative health benefits, along with the relatively small risk from food-borne disease, and how the latter can be avoided with better hygiene practices.

12. Promote exclusive breastfeeding and the introduction of safe and appropriate complementary foods from the age of about six months, while breastfeeding continues during the first years of life.[5]

Even although mothers make the personal choice to breastfeed and have a strong commitment to do so, they may find it hard. First, they may not get the necessary support

---

[5] Michaelsen *et al.* (2000)

Table 9.10 Breastfeeding rates in high and low socio-economic groups in the UK, 1999

Time	Breastfeeding rates (%)	
	Social class I	Social class V
At 1 week	84	40
At 6 weeks	73	23
At 4 months	56	13

Source: Nelson 1999.

from the health care facilities and, secondly, mothers of infants are very vulnerable to marketing and promotion from the industry. Infant formula milk companies are commercial enterprises which compete to survive.

In more affluent countries, frequency and duration of breastfeeding is greatest among higher-income groups. In the UK, mothers in the highest-income group are twice as likely to be breastfeeding during the first week after a baby's birth than mothers in the lowest group, and the social-class difference grows over subsequent weeks (Table 9.10).

Timely introduction of appropriate food promotes good health among infants. A newborn baby shows innate preferences for sweet tastes and innate dislike for sour or bitter ones, and young children have been shown to self-select a healthy diet. This points to the possibility that infants possess a biological control system that enables nutritionally adequate food choice if a variety of wholesome and natural foods is available. From the very beginning, these innate preferences are modified by learning processes, which play a major role in the development of food preferences and food rejection later. Three major processes have been described that modify the child's food acceptance patterns:

1 Mere exposure to unknown food—the repeated experience of tasting and eating it—reduces the tendency to reject it. Consequently, children's preference for vegetables, for example, increases with exposure.

2 Social influences modify food acceptance. Children learn to prefer food eaten by their peers; peer influence may be more influential than parental influence and has been shown to be effective in preschool children.

3 Children learn to associate the physiological consequences of food intake with taste.

If parents wish to give their children the best opportunity to develop a taste for healthy food, they need the correct information, skills, and support.

9.6 **Conclusion**

The relations between diet and health are of crucial social and economic significance. Policy questions have been dominated by agricultural interests. Marketing is guided by businesses' interests. Consequently, there have been quite dramatic changes in

EU diets over the past 40 years. There has been a:

> . . . considerable increase in the dietary energy supply for the EU as a whole and a particularly rapid catch-up process for many Mediterranean countries . . . In addition to higher calorie supply levels, there has been a shift in the composition of the diets. Nearly all country averages are above the recommended levels for cholesterol, saturated fats and sugar. (Schmidhuber and Traill 2004)

Local, national, and international government agencies, non-governmental organizations, and the food industry should ensure:

- The integration of public health perspectives into the food system to provide affordable and nutritious fresh food for all, especially the most vulnerable.
- Democratic, transparent decision making and accountability in all food regulation matters, with participation by all stakeholders, including consumers.
- Support for sustainable agriculture and food production methods that conserve natural resources and the environment.
- A stronger food culture for health, especially through schools, to foster people's knowledge of food and nutrition, cooking skills, growing food, and the social value of preparing food and eating together.
- The availability of useful information about food, diet, and health, especially aimed at children.
- The use of scientifically based nutrient reference values and food-based dietary guidelines to facilitate the development and implementation of policies on food and nutrition.

Public health policies are necessary to ensure that the choices required for a healthy lifestyle are readily accessible to all, especially the low-income and the most vulnerable. The healthy choices should be the easiest for everyone. Only when food and nutrition policies are in place can we truly say that 'healthy eating' is a matter of personal choice and individual responsibility.

Acknowledgements

Most of the material used in this chapter comes from the WHO European publication *Food and health in Europe: a new basis for action* (WHO 2004) which provides the scientific evidence to support the First Action Plan for Food and Nutrition Policy in the WHO European Region (2000–2005) (WHO 2000*a*). This chapter is based especially on the research carried out by and on inspiration from Tim Lobstein, one of the editors of the WHO publication. We are grateful for the expert editorial assistance of Gillian Holm.

References

Brunner, EJ., Rayner, M., Thorogood, M., Margetts, B., Hooper, L., Summerbell, C., *et al.* (2001). Making public health nutrition relevant to evidence-based action. *Public Health Nutrition*, 4:1297–9 (*http://www.nutritionreviews.org*)

Consumers International (1996). *A spoonful of sugar: television food advertising aimed at children—an International survey.* London, Consumers International.

Crawford, M.A. and Marsh, D. (1989). *The driving force.* London, Heinemann.

De Irala–Estevez, J., Groth, M., Johansson, L., Oltersdorf. U., Prattala, R., Martinez–Gonzalez, M.A. (2000). A systematic review of socio-economic differences in food habits in Europe: consumption of fruit and vegetables. *European Journal of Clinical Nutrition,* **54**:706–14.

Dowler, E. and Leather, S. (1997). Intake of micronutrients in Britain's poorest fifth has declined. *British Medical Journal,* **314**:1412.

Erens, H. and Primatesta, P. (1999). *Health Survey for England 1998, Vol.1 Findings.* London, The Stationery Office.

Gross, L.S., Li Li, E., Ford, S., and Liu., S. (2004). Increased consumption of refined carbohydrates and the epidemic of type 2 diabetes in the United States: an ecologic assessment. *American Journal of Clinical Nutrition,* **79**:774–9.

Hawkes, C. (2004a). *Nutrition labels and health claims: the global regulatory environment.* WHO, Geneva.

Hawkes, C. (2004b). *Marketing food to children: the global regulatory environment.* WHO, Geneva.

James, J., Thomas, P., Cavan, D., and Kerr, D. (2004). Preventing childhood obesity by reducing consumption of carbonated drinks: cluster randomized controlled trial. *British Medical Journal,* **328**:1237.

Kant, A.K., Schatzkin, A., Graubard, B.I., and Schairer, C. (2000). A prospective study of diet quality and mortality in women. *Journal of the American Medical Association,* **283**:2109–15.

Key, T.J., Schatzkin, A., Willett, W.C., Allen, N.E., Spencer, E.A., and Travis, R.C. (2004). Diet nutrition and the prevention of cancer. *Public Health Nutrition,* **7**:187–200.

Ludwig, D.S., Peterson, K.E., and Gortmaker, S.L. (2001). Relation between consumption of sugar-sweetened drinks and childhood obesity: a prospective, observational analysis. *Lancet,* **357**: 505–8.

Martinez, J.A., Kearney, J.M., Kafatos, A., Paquet, S., and Martinez–Gonzalez, M.A. (1999). Variables independently associated with self-reported obesity in the European Union. *Public Health Nutrition,* **2(1a)**:125–33.

Michaelsen, K.F. *et al.* (2000). *Feeding and nutrition of infants and young children: guidelines for the WHO European Region, with emphasis on former Soviet countries.* (WHO Regional Publications, European Series, No. 87) Copenhagen, WHO Regional Office for Europe.

Naess, O. and Claussen, B. (2000). Social inequalities in mortality in Oslo: is health-related selection the main cause? In: *Health inequalities in Europe,* p. 188. Paris, Societe Francaise de Sante Publique.

National Institute of Public Health, Stockholm (2003). Public health aspects of the EU CAP—developments and recommendations for change in four sectors: fruit and vegetables, dairy, wine and tobacco (*http://www.fhi.se/shop/material_pdf/eu_inlaga.pdf*).

Nelson, M. (1999). Nutrition and health inequalities. In: *Inequalities in health: studies in poverty, inequality and social exclusion* (ed. D. Gordon *et al.*). University of Bristol, Policy Press.

Nestle, M. (2002). *Food Politics—how the food industry influences nutrition and health.* London. University California Press.

PAHO (2000). *Obesity and poverty—a new public health challenge.* PAHO Sc. Publ. no. 576, Washington.

Raben, A., Vasilaras, T.H., Moller, A.C., and Astrup, A. (2002). Sucrose compared with artificial sweetners: different effects on ad libitum food intake and body weight after 10 weeks of supplementation in overweight subjects. *American Journal of Clinical Nutrition,* **76**:721–9.

Razum, O. and Zeeb, H. (2000). Risk of coronary heart disease among Turkish migrants to Germany: further epidemiological evidence. *Atherosclerosis,* **150**: 439–40.

Robertson, A., Tirado, C., Lobstein, T., Jermini, M., Knai, C., Højmark Jensen, J., *et al* (2004). *Food and health in Europe: a new basis for action.* European series, No. 96. Copenhagen, WHO European Regional Office.

Roos, G., Johansson, L., Kasmel, A., Klumbiene, J., and Prattala, R. (2000). Disparities in vegetable and fruit consumption: European cases from the north to the south. *Public Health Nutrition,* 4:35–43.

Schmidhuber, J. and Traill, W.B. (2004). *The changing structure of diets in the EU in relation to healthy eating guidelines* (in press).

Swedish Environmental Agency (1999). *A sustainable food supply chain.* (Report No. 4966) Stockholm, Swedish Environmental Agency.

Wahlqvist, M. (1999). *Prospects for the future: nutrition, environment and sustainable food production.* Conference on International Food Trade Beyond 2000: Science-Based Decisions, Harmonization, Equivalence and Mutual Recognition, Melbourne, Australia, 11–15 October 1999 (*http://www.fao.org/docrep/meeting/X2638e.htm*). Rome, Food and Agricultural Organization of the United Nations.

WHO (1990). *Diet, nutrition and the prevention of chronic diseases. Report of a WHO study group.* (WHO Technical Report Series, No. 797). Geneva, WHO.

WHO (2000a). *The First Action Plan for Food and Nutrition Policy, WHO European Region 2000–2005.* (*http://www.euro.who.int/nutrition/FoodandNutActPlan/20010906_2*). Copenhagen, WHO.

WHO (2000b). *CINDI Dietary Guide.* (*http://www.euro.who.int/Document/E70041.pdf*). Copenhagen, WHO Regional Office for Europe.

WHO (2002). *The World Health Report 2002.* Geneva, WHO.

WHO (2003). *Diet, nutrition and the prevention of chronic diseases. Report of a joint WHO/FAO expert consultation.* (*http://whqlibdoc.who.int/trs/WHO_TRS_916.pdf*). (WHO Technical Report Series, No. 916). Geneva, WHO.

WHO *(2004). Food and health in Europe: a new basis for action.* (*http://www.euro.who.int/eprise/main/ who/InformationSources/Publications/Catalogue/20040130_8*). Geneva, WHO.

Chapter 10

Poverty, social exclusion, and minorities

Mary Shaw, Danny Dorling, and
George Davey Smith

10.1 Introduction

Poverty, the extent of relative deprivation, and the processes of social exclusion in a society have a major impact on the health of its population. All over Europe, in richer countries as well as poorer ones, those people who are worse off in socio-economic terms have worse health outcomes and higher death rates than those who are better off. Particular 'minority' ethnic groups are often in poor socio-economic positions within particular countries and, hence, often experience poor health, which can be exacerbated by the additional effects of prejudice and racism. The harm to health comes not only from material deprivation but also from the social and psychological problems resulting from living in relative poverty.

This chapter first presents a small sample of the vast body of available evidence that shows a clear relationship between poverty, deprivation, and health, and then discusses briefly how and why poverty affects health. Evidence of the persisting incidence of poverty and social exclusion in western Europe and deepening poverty in eastern Europe, and the implications of this for health, are then presented. Following this, attention turns to the concept of 'social exclusion' in Europe and focuses on the evidence of the detrimental effect on health for particular 'minority' groups—the unemployed, refugees, poorer migrants, ethnic minorities, and homeless people. The chapter closes by offering short- and long-term policy suggestions for the reduction of health problems resulting from poverty, relative deprivation, and social exclusion.

10.2 Poverty and health

Whether we refer to mortality, morbidity, or self-reported health, and whichever indicator of socio-economic position we employ—income, class, housing tenure, deprivation, or education—we find that those who are worse off socio-economically have worse health. It is not only the case that the poorest in society have poor health, but a gradient of ill health and mortality spans all socio-economic strata. This gradient can be found across the industrialized world, although the strength of the relationship varies somewhat between different countries, for different age groups, by the health measures used, and for men and women (Kunst *et al.* 1995; Mackenbach *et al.* 2004).

Recent evidence from Britain, where there is a long tradition of research into inequalities in health (Davey Smith *et al.* 2001), shows that variations in life expectancy by social class continue to be found. Table 10.1 shows inequalities in all-cause mortality by social class in England, for males and females separately, for the period 1986 to 1999. Figures 10.1 and 10.2 show this in graphical form—the same scale is used for both males and females to emphasize the absolute differences in their respective death rates. These data show that while all-cause mortality fell in all classes over the study period, a consistent class gradient is apparent for both males and females. For males, the social class gap in mortality widened (see ratios in Table 10.1), whereas for females the social class gradient narrowed slightly. Occupational groups I and II include

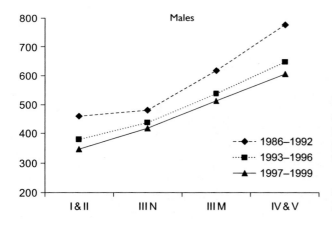

Fig. 10.1 Directly age-standardized all-cause mortality rates per 100,000 person years, England and Wales, males aged 35–64, 1986–1999. (*Source:* adapted from White *et al.* 2003).

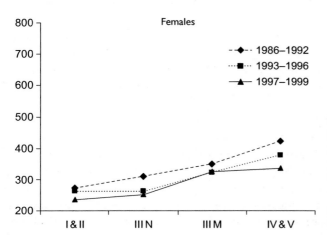

Fig. 10.2 Directly age-standardized all-cause mortality rates per 100,000 person years, England and Wales, females aged 35–64, 1986–1999. (*Source:* adapted from White *et al.* 2003).

Table 10.1 Trends in all-cause mortality in England and Wales, by social class, 1986–1999; males and females aged 35–64, directly age-standardized death rates (DSR) per 100,000 person years, with 95% confidence interval (CI)

	DSR (95% CI)			% change		
	1986–92	**1993–96**	**1997–99**	**1986–92 to 1993–96**	**1993–96 to 1997–99**	**1998–92 to 1997–99**
Males						
I & II	460 (427–494)	379 (338–426)	347 (302–399)	−17	−8	−24
IIIN	480 (431–533)	437 (377–506)	417 (352–494)	−9	−5	−13
IIIM	617 (587–649)	538 (502–577)	512 (472–556)	−13	−5	−17
IV & V	776 (731–823)	648 (593–707)	606 (546–672)	−16	−6	−21
Ratio IV & V: I & II	1.69	1.71	1.75			
Non-manual	466 (439–494)	396 (363–433)	371 (334–413)	−15	−6	−20
Manual	674 (649–700)	577 (546–610)	546 (512–582)	−14	−5	−19
Females						
I & II	274 (249–302)	262 (226–303)	237 (201–281)	−5	−9	−13
IIIN	310 (276–347)	262 (223–307)	253 (211–304)	−15	−3	−18
IIIM	350 (325–377)	324 (291–361)	327 (290–369)	−7	1	−7
IV & V	422 (388–459)	378 (335–427)	335 (289–388)	−10	−11	−21
Ratio IV & V: I & II	1.54	1.44	1.41			
Non-manual	289 (268–310)	257 (232–284)	246 (219–278)	−11	−4	−15
Manual	379 (358–401)	344 (317–373)	330 (301–362)	− 9	−4	−13

Source: adapted from White *et al.* 2003.

professionals, such as doctors and lawyers, as well as managerial occupations. Occupational groups IV and V include semi-skilled manual occupations, such as some coal miners and machine operators, and unskilled manual occupations, such as cleaners and labourers.

Similar findings of differences in mortality and life expectancy by social and occupational classes are reported for other European countries. For example, Kunst and Mackenbach (1992) compared mortality by occupational social class in six European countries (Denmark, England and Wales, Finland, France, Norway, and Sweden) and found that socio-economic gradients in mortality varied in each country and in different age groups, but that there were, nonetheless, gradients in each of these countries.

Kunst (1997) reports findings of socio-economic differences in mortality for a number of eastern and western European countries, in terms of occupational class and educational groups. Table 10.2 shows death rate ratios in the 1980s for males in manual versus non-manual occupational classes for various countries. Differences are particularly large for the former communist countries of the Czech Republic and Hungary, showing that socio-economic gradients in mortality were not the preserve of the capitalist countries of the West.

Table 10.2 Death rate ratios for males in manual versus non-manual occupational classes in the 1980s

Country	Death rate ratio	
	30–44years	45–59years
Czech Republic	2.25	1.83
Denmark	1.53	1.33
England and Wales	1.46	1.44
Finland	1.76	1.53
France	*	1.71
Hungary	2.89	2.65
Ireland	1.43	1.38
Italy	1.35	1.35
Norway	1.65	1.34
Portugal	1.5	1.36
Spain	*	1.37
Sweden	1.66	1.41
Switzerland	1.45	1.35

* Data not reported for this age group.

Source: adapted from Kunst 1997.

Table 10.3 Direct age-standardized rate ratios for deaths under 65, by housing tenure and car access: 1971 and 1981 census cohorts (Longitudinal Study data)

	Males		Females	
	1971–81	1981–89	1971–81	1981–89
Housing tenure				
Owner occupiers	1	1	1	1
Private renters	1.32	1.38	1.32	1.38
Social housing	1.35	1.62	1.42	1.44
Car access				
1 + cars	1	1	1	1
No cars	1.44	1.57	1.40	1.56

Source: adapted from Filakti and Fox 1995.

In Britain, alternative socio-economic measures, such as housing tenure and access to a car, are often used as indicators of social position; Table 10.3 presents data for England and Wales for the 1980s. Compared to owner occupiers, those who rented their home from a public or private landlord had increasingly higher death rates; similarly, compared to those who had access to one or more cars, those who did not have access to a car had increasingly higher death rates. Similar findings have been reported when education is used as the social indicator.

Some researchers have looked more specifically at the health effects of relative deprivation, a concept that refers to the disadvantaged position of an individual, family, or group relative to the society to which they belong, and focuses on the condition of deprivation as well as the lack of resources (Townsend *et al.* 1988). Using the Townsend index of deprivation, a composite indicator for areas (which includes unemployment, percentage of households with no car, the extent of overcrowding, and housing tenure), Eames *et al.* (1993) found that higher deprivation was associated with higher rates of premature death in every region in England and Wales, although the association was stronger in some regions than others.

There is also some evidence that living in a relatively deprived area can have a detrimental effect on an individual's health, even when the individual level of deprivation has been taken into account (i.e. that there is an area health effect over and above the effect of individual deprivation). This has been found in the USA (Haan *et al.* 1987) and in British studies of both mortality and morbidity (Langford and Bentham 1996; Shouls *et al.* 1996; Davey Smith 2003). However, when such area effects are found to exist, they tend to be small (see Chapter 14).

Suicide rates, in particular, have been found to be associated with deprivation (Hawton *et al.* 2001; Bartlett *et al.* 2004); Gunnell *et al.* (1995) report that socio-economic deprivation is an indicator and possible determinant of psychiatric morbidity and suicide. McLoone (1996) reported that the greatest rates of increase in suicide rates in Scotland between 1981 and 1993 were for deprived young people—their suicide rates being approximately twice those of young people in affluent areas. Similarly, in an ecological analysis, Crawford and Prince (1999) found increasing suicide rates among young men in Britain to be associated with social deprivation, unemployment, and living alone.

10.2.1 Why poverty is bad for health: the material, social, and psychological consequences of living in poverty

An understanding of why those who live in conditions of poverty and relative deprivation have poorer health is necessary in order to begin effectively to redress the issue. A number of different explanations for this relationship have been suggested, including living and working conditions, limitations on resources, and the subsequent effect on social relationships. Individual lifestyle factors, such as smoking, alcohol consumption, exercise, and diet, have been suggested by some as the main underlying causes. However, while such factors may indeed form a part of the explanation for inequalities in health, they should not be considered the exclusive cause, nor viewed as being distinct from the socio-economic environment.

The majority of the evidence suggests that material conditions are the underlying root of ill health, which includes being the determining factor for health-related behaviours (Davey Smith *et al.* 1994; Shaw *et al.* 1999). Poverty imposes constraints on the material conditions of everyday life—by limiting access to the fundamental building blocks of health such as adequate housing, good nutrition, and opportunities to participate in society (Black and Laughlin 1996). The concomitants of poverty are often poor nutrition; overcrowded, damp, and inadequately heated housing; increased risk of infections; and inability to maintain optimal hygiene practices (Davey Smith 2003). Poor housing, for example, can be damp, cold, and contain mould—conditions which are associated with wheezing, breathlessness, cough, phlegm, meningococcal infection, and respiratory diseases and asthma (Ineichen 1993; Shaw 2004). Poor housing conditions can also bring a risk of fire and accidents; and overcrowded housing not only increases the risk of infection but impacts upon mental health through factors such as high noise levels and lack of privacy (Shaw 2004).

Blackburn (1991) asserted that poverty affects health through not only nutrition and housing, but also in terms of the effect on mental health and caring for children. Income levels affect the way parents are able to care for their own and their children's health. As well as affecting other aspects of their lives—where they live, where their children go to school—living on a low income makes it difficult to exercise control over family health and, as a result, the health needs of parents, particularly women, are often compromised for those of children. For example, Graham (1995) found that smoking rates in young women in manual households were related to the strains of caring responsibilities as well as to greater material disadvantages—it was a combination of the psychological and material difficulties of life that led to their greater smoking prevalence. By compromising their own health, women thus felt better equipped to cope with the care of their children and families. It is therefore necessary to understand how material restrictions operate through a number of processes: 'unhealthy' behaviours need to be understood in the context of the constraints on everyday life which accompany them.

It is important to recognize that the experience of poverty is rarely static and unchanging and that it has a cumulative effect. A body of evidence is now emerging which shows that health outcomes in adulthood reflect the accumulating influence of poor socio-economic circumstances throughout life (Davey Smith 2003). Adverse socio-economic conditions in early life can produce lasting increases in the risk of cardiovascular disease, respiratory disease, and some cancers late in life. Adverse socio-economic conditions in adulthood compound these earlier-life influences, resulting in health differentials in adulthood which reflect the social patterning of exposure acting across the life course (Davey Smith 2003). The particular influence of deprivation in childhood should focus attention on social policies concerned with reducing poverty in households with young children.

10.2.2 Increasing poverty, unemployment, and inequality

What we know about the relationship between poverty and health should be cause for great concern, given that the proportion of people living in relative poverty has increased in many European countries in recent years in both western and eastern Europe.

The extent of poverty and relative deprivation increased in European countries in the 1980s and 1990s; while the incomes of the richest groups rose significantly, the incomes of the poor have hardly grown in real terms, or have even fallen (Gordon and Townsend 2000). Between 1980 and 1988, poverty rates increased in all European Community countries, with the exceptions of the Netherlands, Portugal, and Spain (Oppenheim and Harker 1996). The sharpest rises were seen in Italy, Germany, and the UK. In terms of income inequality, the UK, Sweden, Denmark, Norway, the Netherlands, and Belgium have all experienced increases over the time period 1967–92; the UK, Norway, the Netherlands, Belgium, and Germany all experienced increases in child poverty (Goodman *et al.* 1997).

Vogel (1997) points to economic developments underlying these increases in relative poverty and inequality which can be seen across the European Union—mass unemployment, reductions in welfare transfer systems, and cuts in public services. Sociodemographic changes, ageing populations, increasing divorce rates, and increasing numbers of lone parents also contribute to the increased proportion of people living in poverty. Vogel reported a clear tendency towards growing relative poverty rates in 9 of the 12 European countries he considered (increased poverty in the Netherlands, Denmark, Belgium, Luxembourg, Spain, Ireland, UK, Greece, and Portugal).

Although there is wide variation in the unemployment rates of European countries and methodological problems of comparing rates (Green 1998), most countries experienced mass unemployment in the 1980s and 1990s. Approximately half of the unemployment rate consists of long-term unemployed (those unemployed for more than 12 months), and the youth unemployment rate is higher than the general rate (Vogel 1997). This growth in unemployment and insecure employment, as well as rises in the numbers on welfare, rising debts and arrears, increase in the number of lone parents, and increasing numbers of homeless people is referred to by Room (1991) as the 'new poverty' of the European Community. This is in addition to, and not replacing, older forms of poverty among the elderly, sick, and children.

Examining the case in Britain, where much data is available, in the post-war period there have been considerable improvements in terms of living standards, and this has been reflected in falling overall mortality rates. However, despite this overall growth in prosperity, there has also been an increase in relative poverty and inequality. The case of housing provides an example. Home ownership in Britain increased from 57 per cent in 1981 to 68 per cent in 1991 (Dorling 1995) to 71 per cent in 2001 (Dorling and Thomas 2004). The proportion of households with central heating increased from 37 per cent in 1972 to 83 per cent in 1992 (Wadsworth 1996) and over 90 per cent in 2001 (Census 2001); the proportion of households with more than one car, from 9 per cent in 1972 to 24 per cent in 1992 (Wadsworth 1996) and 29 per cent in 2001 (Census 2001). However, the number of households in insecure housing tenures rose during the 1980s and 1990s, reflected in increases in the number of mortgage repossessions and households in temporary accommodation—the number of which rose from over 10,000 in 1982 to over 67,000 in 1992 (Wadsworth 1996). While the number of households in temporary accommodation fell in the early to mid-1990s, it subsequently rose steadily and, in 2002, stood at 85,000 (Social Trends 34). Thus, in the context of increased overall prosperity, relative poverty has been increased.

The situation regarding the distribution of wealth and income in Britain has been examined in detail by Hills (1995*a,b*, 1998). He reported (Hills 1995*a*) that income inequality grew between 1970 and 1990, and that while income inequality also grew in a number of other advanced industrialized countries, the rate of increase in Britain was faster than in any other country except New Zealand. Using the series of data on 'households below half average income' for Britain also shows this trend and takes it into the twenty-first century (Fig. 10.3). From this can be seen that the proportion of the population with less than half the average income rose from 7 per cent in the 1970s to 24 per cent in the 1990s, and that this high level has since been sustained (Department for Work and Pensions 2003). The extent of inequality is thus such that the lowest-income groups have not benefited from economic growth. As a result of high unemployment and economic activity (such as early retirement and invalidity), more people became dependent on state benefits. Those particularly vulnerable to low income are pensioners, lone parents, households with no earners, and families with children.

At the same time that economic inequality has increased in Britain, so too has the gap between the death rates of the better off and the deprived (McLoone and Boddy 1994; Phillimore *et al.* 1994; Shaw *et al.* 1999; Davey Smith *et al.* 2002). For example, Raleigh and Kiri (1997) looked at life expectancy and deprivation in district health authorities in England and Wales between 1984 and 1994. Those areas with the greatest gains in prosperity had the greatest gains in life expectancy, whereas in deprived areas, improvements in life expectancy were negligible. They report a difference in life expectancy of 6.7 years for men and 4.7 years for women between the most and least deprived areas. Davey Smith *et al.* (2002) looked at age–sex standardized mortality ratios for deaths under the age of 75 for poverty deciles in Britain for the period 1990–99. They found that inequality increased steadily across the decade; the chance of premature mortality polarized between richer and poorer areas of Britain over this decade.

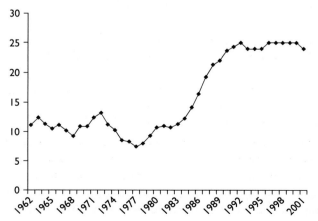

Fig. 10.3 Percentage of the population with below half average incomes after housing costs, Britain, 1961–2001. (*Source:* Department for Work and Pensions 2003).

Table 10.4 Annual age-adjusted rate of years of potential life lost, per 1000 population, for all causes of death, in men aged 20–64 in England and Wales for 1970–72, 1979–80 and 1982–83, and 1991–93 (standardized to population of England and Wales 1981)

Social class	1970–2	1979–80, 1982–83	1991–93
I	48.7	36.5	28.0
II	51.9	42.2	31.6
III non-manual	65.0	53.9	45.7
III manual	66.0	58.0	50.5
IV	75.6	67.7	52.8
V	103.0	105.8	93.3
Ratio V: I	2.1	2.9	3.3

Source: Blane and Drever 1998.

Blane and Drever (1998) have calculated this widening gap of health in terms of years of potential life lost. While standardized mortality ratios have the advantage of taking into account the different age structures of the social class groups, they are heavily influenced by the number of deaths occurring in the oldest age category. However, the largest relative class differences in absolute mortality are at younger ages, and so it is also worth considering the relative number of years of productive life which are lost through premature mortality (Davey Smith *et al.* 1994). As Table 10.4 shows, the ratio of years of life lost for social class V as compared to social class I between the early 1970s and early 1990s rose from 2.1 to 3.3. Thus, increasing poverty and income inequality are mirrored by increasing health inequalities.

Similar polarization can be seen on a larger scale. Shaw *et al.* (1998) have analysed changing all-cause standardized mortality ratios (SMRs) for deaths under the age of 65 for 160 regions of the European Union. Data were analysed at the NUTS 2 (Nomenclature of Statistical Territorial Units) level, which are generally provinces, *Regierungsbezike* (German regions), or groups of counties (for example, Herefordshire and Worcester and Warwickshire in the UK). Regions were amalgamated into population deciles according to their SMRs in 1990. Table 10.5 indicates that, while a number of the deciles had decreasing SMRs, including those that already had relatively low SMRs in 1990, deciles 5, 6, 7, and 10 have experienced increasing SMRs over the study period. Most notably, the SMR of the population decile with the highest death rates was 130.1 in 1990 but, by 1994, the SMR of this population decile was 134.9. Thus, the difference between the regions with the highest and the lowest SMRs is becoming greater. A cursory inspection of the geographical patterning of this polarization of mortality across Europe suggests that it reflects, to a large extent, the European geography of polarizing wealth and employment.

As further evidence of this trend of growing socio-economic and health inequality, a specific disease which traditionally has been associated with poverty, tuberculosis, rose

Table 10.5 SMRs, all causes, under 65, by population deciles, 1990 and 1994 (standardized to the European average)

Decile	1	2	3	4	5	6	7	8	9	10
1990	75.0	85.1	90.6	94.6	97.4	100.6	105.1	109.0	116.3	130.1
1994	73.5	84.0	89.4	94.4	97.8	102.2	105.9	108.7	113.7	134.9
Change	−1.5	−1.1	−1.2	−0.2	+0.4	+1.6	+0.8	−0.3	−2.6	+4.8

Source: Shaw *et al.* 2000.

in eastern Europe in the 1990s. Raviglione *et al.* (1994) reported increases in Romania, Armenia, Kyrgystan, Latvia, Lithuania, Moldova, and Turkmenistan, and no further decline in other countries. Likewise, recent rises in Britain have been linked with increased poverty, deprivation, and unemployment (Darbyshire 1995; Kumar *et al.* 1995) and incidence has become increasingly concentrated among non-white groups (Regan *et al.* 2003).

10.3 **Central and eastern Europe**

Increases in inequalities in health can thus be interpreted as a result of increases in poverty and inequality, and this phenomenon can be also seen in the former communist countries of eastern and central Europe. While overall death rates fell throughout the twentieth century in western Europe, in eastern and central Europe, mortality has been rising since the mid-1960s (Shkolnikov *et al.* 1998). In the years after the collapse of communism, death rates rose sharply. Between 1989 and 1994, life expectancy in Russia fell by 6.5 years for men and 3.5 years for women (Shkolnikov *et al.* 1998); similar changes have been seen in other former Soviet countries (Dennis *et al.* 1993). By 1993, death rates had risen substantially in all of the former Warsaw Pact countries with the exception of Hungary (UNICEF 1993). These changes have not been spread evenly throughout the population; for example, in Russia, death rates have risen fastest among those with lower levels of education (Shkolnikov *et al.* 1998).

As well as increasing rates of tuberculosis, Davis (1993) has noted that, in eastern Europe, morbidity as a result of diseases such as diphtheria, measles, whooping cough, and syphilis has also increased; nutritional, infectious, and degenerative diseases have all become more widespread. In terms of mortality, a great proportion of the increase is due to male deaths from accidents and homicide, and many of these deaths are alcohol-related (Ellman 1994; Leon *et al.* 1997; Shkolnikov *et al.* 2001). For example, Ellman states that for males aged 15–59, between 1987 and 1991, 77 per cent of the total increase in mortality was accounted for by accidents and homicide. These increases in morbidity and mortality all occurred within the context of a ravaged health care system:

> Medical facilities are underfunded and afflicted by shortages of all categories of supplies . . . The quality of medical care in state facilities has almost certainly fallen. These negative trends have not been offset by the increase in sophisticated treatment in private facilities, which only a small minority can afford. (Davis 1993, p. 34)

Severe environmental pollution has also been suggested as a possible contributory factor (Feshbach and Friendly 1992; Antunes *et al.* 2003). However, as increases in mortality rates have particularly affected certain groups—young men of working age in particular—it has been argued that this is unlikely to be a predominant cause of the overall increases (Watson 1995). Similarly, Hertzman (1995) argues that pockets of pollution tend to affect health at the local level and this effect is not enough to influence, significantly, national mortality rates.

Others point to behavioural changes as a major factor in these poorer health outcomes, particularly increased alcohol consumption. For example, Cockerham (1997) argues that lifestyle factors—alcohol consumption, smoking, poor diet, and lack of exercise—account for this increase in mortality. Bobak and Marmot (1996) also point to the role of unhealthy behaviours and lifestyles, arguing that smoking has probably had the largest impact; Leon *et al.* (1997) highlight alcohol consumption. However, these authors also emphasize that individual behaviours need to be understood in their broader social context: we must look to the far-reaching changes in socio-economic conditions for explanations as to why large groups of people behave as they do. Local considerations may also need to be borne in mind. For example, in a paper reporting mortality in a cohort of the Nova Huta steelworkers in Poland, Watson (1998) suggested that the results needed to be understood not only in the context of broader political and economic circumstances, but also regarding the history and experience of employment at that particular steelworks. Similarly, Phillimore and Morris (1991) have argued that, in order to understand geographical patterns in mortality, we need an understanding of what constitutes a 'place', and this may include looking not only at levels of deprivation but also examining closely the social and economic histories of particular localities, such as the provision of housing and the pattern of deprivation over a number of decades. Others have also addressed the issue of *how* places affect health (Pickett and Pearl 2001; Macintyre *et al.* 2002; Tunstall *et al.* 2004).

An understanding of place-specific factors, cultures, and societies is also needed at the international level. In virtually all states of central and eastern Europe and the former Soviet Union, political and economic changes were accompanied by drastic reductions in production output and in real wages, and living standards fell (Davis 1993). As a consequence, many people found themselves in a condition of sudden impoverishment (Cornia and Paniccia 1995); income inequalities widened. Many people took on two jobs and worked very long hours in order to provide for themselves and their families. For example, Ellman (1994) reported that, in Russia in 1992, 37 per cent of the Russian population were below the poverty line (defined in this study as an income which would allow a level of food consumption adequate to maintain a normal body weight at an average level of activity), and 47 per cent of children below the age of 15 were living below the poverty line.

Such conditions have direct effects, such as on food consumption (due to both lack of availability and lack of purchasing power), and also lead to social stress (Shapiro

1995). During the same period, marriage rates also declined and crime rates soared. People lost not only their incomes, but also a sense of pride, power, and participation, in relation to both work and national identity. Watson (1995) argued that it is likely that rising mortality rates in eastern European countries were not only associated with falling absolute standards of living for the majority of the population, but were also related to increased social and economic inequalities, a sense of hopelessness and disenfranchisement with the political process, and higher levels of insecurity and uncertainty, particularly in employment.

There are, thus, psychosocial implications (Davey Smith and Egger 1996) of social and economic stress, which may influence rates of murder, depression, suicide, and alcohol consumption. As Ellman says:

> ... someone whose job is insecure and who may become unemployed (or who has actually become unemployed), who is living on a low and uncertain income (which may frequently not be paid when due) under conditions of very high inflation and very high crime, and whose access to meat, vegetables, fruit and medical care has sharply worsened, may die in a brawl, car crash or of alcohol poisoning. (Ellman 1994, p. 343)

Economic conditions can so have a knock-on effect. Increased poverty, and the difficulties that accompany it, affect health in terms of morbidity and mortality, and it is those who are worse off whose health suffers most. This is the case in established market economies as well as societies in the process of transition.

10.4 **Social exclusion**

In many areas, the terminology of social exclusion is superseding poverty or deprivation in popularity. 'Poverty' emphasizes lack of economic resources, and the term 'relative deprivation' stresses the conditions of living. 'Social exclusion' refers not only to the economic hardship of relative economic poverty, but also incorporates the notion of the *process* of marginalization—how individuals come, through their lives, to be excluded and marginalized from various aspects of social and community life.

There is no European-wide definition of social exclusion, but it is generally considered to include a number of dimensions:

> Exclusion processes are dynamic and multidimensional in nature. They are linked not only to unemployment and/or to low income, but also to housing conditions, levels of education and opportunities, health, discrimination, citizenship and integration in the local community. (European Social Policy White Paper (1994), cited in Oppenheim and Harker 1996, p. 156).

As the Social Exclusion Unit in England has stated, the term is:

> ... a shorthand label for what can happen when individuals or areas suffer from a combination of linked problems such as unemployment, poor skills, low incomes, poor housing, high crime environments, bad health and family breakdowns. (Social Exclusion Unit (1997), cited in Levitas 2000)

The term 'social exclusion' also relates to cultural aspects of exclusion and discrimination and refers to the relationship between the included and excluded, the meaning and identity of the excluded. Social exclusion is about multidimensional disadvantage—there is not one 'social exclusion' but many 'social exclusions' (Room 1995) and, as with social class and relative economic deprivation, there are degrees of exclusion. The term 'socially excluded' can refer to those who may be stigmatized and marginalized, such as people with HIV/AIDS, who might not be considered in traditional analyses of economic deprivation. Those who are more socially included have greater access to resources, not only in economic terms but also resources which come from living within a society—such as educational opportunities, social networks, and support; those who are excluded are denied these (see Chapter 8). As Wilkinson has powerfully said:

> To feel depressed, cheated, bitter, desperate, vulnerable, frightened, angry, worried about debts or job and housing insecurity; to feel devalued, useless, helpless, uncared for, hopeless, isolated, anxious and a failure: these feelings can dominate people's whole experience of life . . . The material environment is merely the indelible mark and constant reminder of the oppressive fact of one's failure, of the atrophy of any sense of having a place in a community, and of one's social exclusion and devaluation as a human being. (Wilkinson 1996, p. 215)

The processes leading to social exclusion in Europe include economic change (increased unemployment and widespread job insecurity), demographic change (increased proportions of single households, lone parents, and elderly), changes to welfare regimes (cuts and withdrawal), and specific spatial processes of segregation and separation (stigmatization and marginalization of certain groups, often leading to spatial segregation of minorities) (White 1998). White (1998) refers to four aspects of social exclusion (Fig. 10.4). First, there is exclusion from civil society through legal constraint or regulation. This is particularly relevant to migrants; for example, the children born to foreign immigrants (with no German ancestry) in Germany, who remain foreigners in legal terms. Secondly, there is the failure to supply social goods to a group with particular needs; for example, facilities for the disabled, language services, or accommodation for the homeless. Thirdly, there is exclusion from social production—not being able to be an active contributor to society. Certain groups may be labelled as undesirable, unacceptable, or in need of control; for example, gypsies and travellers. Finally, there is economic exclusion from normal social consumption—not having access to the normal perequisites, routines, and experiences of everyday life.

Social exclusion can refer to individuals, but it is not just individuals who manifest conditions of exclusion and accompanying stress and insecurity. Spatial concentration and segregation can mean that areas can become deprived, disadvantaged, or stigmatized; this may affect all of those in the area, and their potential for mobility. For instance, living in an area where factories are closing and where there are no job vacancies increases an individual's chance of unemployment. An area which has high unemployment and high levels of deprivation is also likely to have poor schools—an individual's circumstances depend very much on his or her geographical setting.

The health-damaging and health-promoting features of local areas in Glasgow, Scotland's largest city, have been investigated in work by Sooman and Macintyre

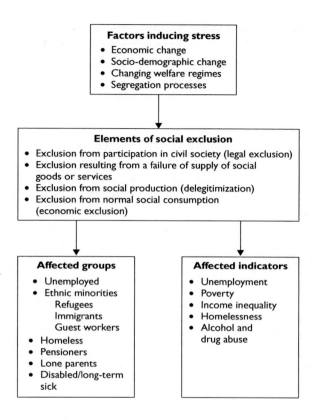

Factors inducing stress
- Economic change
- Socio-demographic change
- Changing welfare regimes
- Segregation processes

Elements of social exclusion
- Exclusion from participation in civil society (legal exclusion)
- Exclusion resulting from a failure of supply of social goods or services
- Exclusion from social production (delegitimization)
- Exclusion from normal social consumption (economic exclusion)

Affected groups
- Unemployed
- Ethnic minorities
  Refugees
  Immigrants
  Guest workers
- Homeless
- Pensioners
- Lone parents
- Disabled/long-term sick

Affected indicators
- Unemployment
- Poverty
- Income inequality
- Homelessness
- Alcohol and drug abuse

Fig. 10.4 The process and outcome of social exclusion in Europe. (*Source*: adapted from White 1998).

(1995). They found that not only were there differences in self-reported health between local areas, with those in more advantaged areas reporting fewer health problems, but there was also an association between the respondents' perceptions of their local social and physical environment which could not be explained by social class differences. Important factors were local amenities and problems, area reputation, neighbourliness, fear of crime, and area satisfaction. Later work by these authors on a similar theme has also reported on the role of the living environment for health (Macintyre *et al.* 2003) and, particularly, the role of social cohesion (Macintyre and Ellaway 2000). These findings highlight that social exclusion is not just about individuals, but that there is also a spatial dimension.

10.4.1 **Unemployment**

The groups of people who are socially excluded, and their characteristics, vary from state to state. They can include elderly people, people with disabilities (especially disabled children), lone parents and their children, as well as those with certain health conditions (e.g. the mentally ill and the long-term sick). However, here we concentrate on the evidence showing that unemployed people, refugees, poorer migrants and ethnic minorities, and homeless people have adverse health outcomes. As noted above, high unemployment rates (also termed mass unemployment) have become a permanent feature of developed economies, as the European postwar social contract has been reformulated (Korpi 2003). This unemployment tends to be concentrated in certain groups—there are growing numbers of long-term unemployed and youth unemployment is also widespread; increasing numbers of young people in Europe have never worked.

Unemployment is essentially a spatial process, because people are limited in how far they can travel to work in a day; they rely on the supply of work in their local area and when this supply falls, unemployment rises. Unemployment in Europe is also concentrated disproportionately among immigrants, particularly female migrants (Model 2002). For example, in the mid 1990s, in the Netherlands, unemployment was 7 per cent for the Dutch themselves, but for non-Dutch workers, it was 20 per cent; for those from Turkey and Morocco, it was even higher (Pinder 1998).

The research showing that unemployment carries a risk of premature mortality is discussed in Chapter 5 of this volume. The effect operates over and above pre-existing health and social class position. According to Drever and Whitehead (1997), after adjusting for social class, the excess mortality for the unemployed is 25 per cent for men and 21 per cent for women. Nor is this increased mortality due solely to behavioural factors. Data from the British Regional Heart Study have shown that differences in mortality between employed and unemployed men remain after adjustment for factors including smoking and alcohol consumption (Morris *et al.* 1994). Furthermore, evidence suggests that the negative health effects of unemployment are cumulative—the longer someone experiences unemployment, the more likely their health will suffer as a result (Bartley and Plewis 2002).

It is, therefore, not just the economic hardship which accompanies unemployment which has repercussions for health, but the psychosocial condition of unemployment appears also to have an effect. Consistent with this, job insecurity and the anticipation of job loss have been found to be associated with poorer health outcomes (Ferrie *et al.* 1995; Bartley *et al.* 1996). The health of temporary employees has also been found to be worse than permanent employees (Kivimaki *et al.* 2003) (see also Chapter 6).

10.4.2 Refugees, migrants, and ethnic minorities

Refugees and internationally displaced persons experience elevated risks of mortality in the period following their migration. For people fleeing from countries which have recently experienced conflict in Europe (the former Yugoslavia, Georgia, Azerbaijan, Chechnia, and Kosovo), this includes not only war-related injuries but also communicable diseases, neonatal problems, and nutritional deficiencies (Toole and Waldman 1997). The stresses accompanying this process—past traumatic experiences, the loss of family and friends and disruption of social support networks, and problems of settling in a new environment—will also have an impact upon a number of dimensions of

Table 10.6 SMRs by country of birth, for men aged 20–64, all causes (England and Wales 1991–93)

	All countries	Caribbean	West/South Africa	East Africa	Indian subcontinent	Scotland	Ireland (all parts)
SMR	100	89	126	123	107	129	135
SMR adjusted for social class	100	82	135	137	117	132	129

Source: Drever and Whitehead 1997.

physical and mental health. Migration can also impact upon mental health due to the effect of having to renegotiate cultural identities (Bhugra 2004) (see also Chapter 8).

People also migrate in order to find work, unemployment being a spatial phenomenon. Some migrants and guest workers will experience similar problems to those of refugees (although perhaps to a lesser degree). There is a range of evidence that poorer migrants and ethnic minorities have different health outcomes to those of the general population of the society in which they are living. In terms of all-cause mortality, Drever and Whitehead (1997) report raised rates for most ethnic groups in Britain (Table 10.6).

Table 10.6 shows that migrants from the Indian subcontinent, East, West, and southern Africa, as well as from Scotland and Ireland, have significantly higher SMRs than the average population in England and Wales, and that this is the case even after social class is taken into account. Only those who were born in the Caribbean have lower SMRs. This is likely to be explained by a healthy migrant effect, with only the healthiest from the Caribbean migrating to Britain (Marmot *et al.* 1984), or may possibly be due to the fact that many migrants return to the Caribbean shortly before their death and, thus, have not been included in these mortality data.

This elevated mortality has also been found to extend to the children of migrants. Harding and Balarajan (1996) found that the mortality of second-generation Irish migrants living in England and Wales was significantly higher for most causes of death than that of all men and women, and this was only partially explained by socio-economic variables (social class, car access, and housing tenure). In the Netherlands, the mortality rate of Turkish and Moroccan children under 15 is two to three times higher than that for Dutch children—the main causes of death responsible for this elevated rate being perinatal death (including congenital malformations), accidents (including drowning), and infectious diseases (Schulpen 1996).

There is also evidence in terms of particular health outcomes. Evidence from Australia suggests that migrant workers may be more prone to work-related accidents, as Corvalan *et al.* (1994) found that language and duration of stay were related to occupation-related fatalities. In Canada, the stress of resettlement after migration has been linked to higher suicide rates (Trovato 1992). Harding (2003) has reported that for South Asian migrants resident in England and Wales, longer duration of residence was associated with increased cardiovascular and cancer mortality.

Etienne *et al.* (1994) report that tuberculosis is higher in immigrants in Belgium; Elender *et al.* (1998) showed the same in England and Wales, noting that this was accounted for by overcrowded living conditions and poverty. Circumstances in country of origin may also play a role. In Sweden, there is evidence of elevated morbidity in labour migrants and refugees (Sundquist 1995). That research found that migrants were more likely to live in rented housing and have low material standards of living; they were also more likely not to feel secure in everyday life and to have poor leisure opportunities—being an immigrant was a risk factor for poor health of equal significance to lifestyle risk factors.

Nazroo (1998) has highlighted the importance of social position in determining the health of migrants. He asserts that much of the variation in health by ethnicity can be explained by standards of living. The health of ethnic minorities may also be influenced by geographical concentration in certain areas, as well as the experience of harassment and discrimination. Nazroo warns:

> The ethnic classifications we use do not reflect unchangeable and natural divisions within groups. Also ethnicity does not exist in isolation, it is within a social context that ethnicity achieves its significance, and part of that social context is the ways in which those seen as members of ethnic minority groups are racialised. Indeed, one of the most important purposes for undertaking work on ethnicity and health is to extend our understanding of the nature and extent of the social disadvantage faced by ethnic minority groups. Not only is health part of the disadvantage, it is also a consequence. (Nazroo 1998, p. 8)

Methodological issues also need to be considered when looking at the health of migrant workers. Egger *et al.* (1990) report on health inequalities by occupational class in Switzerland, suggesting that class differences may be understated as large numbers of migrant workers (mostly from Yugoslavia, Italy, Spain, and Portugal), concentrated in partly skilled and unskilled manual occupations, are not routinely included in official statistics. Even within particular occupational groups, there is evidence that migrant workers experience worse conditions, and hence demonstrate unfavourable health outcomes, compared to the indigenous Swiss population. Studies have attempted to address this issue by using name-based searches for identifying migrants in records (Razum *et al.* 2001), but such as method is far from ideal.

10.4.3 Homeless people

Even in developed societies with relatively high gross domestic product (GDP) per capita and highly developed welfare systems, we see the problem of homelessness. There are many methodological problems with the definition and enumeration of homelessness (Pleace and Quilgars 1996). The European Federation of National Organisations Working with the Homeless states that 'it is not possible to provide a single reliable European statistic on the extent of homelessness in Europe'. (FEANTSA

2002, p7). However, FEANTSA say that some tentative comparisons can be made. Germany, with the largest population in the EU, also has the largest homeless population—around 390,000 (data for 2000)—of who almost a quarter of a million are homeless families. For the UK, an estimate can be derived from the figures for the number of people accepted by local authorities under the homelessness legislation, which stood at 165,000 people 'in priority need' in 2000/2001. Estimates for France suggest a homeless population (including people living in temporary accommodation) at around 200,000 (2001), and there are 70–80,000 'roofless' people in Italy (2000).

In terms of trends over time, homelessness increased in Germany from the late 1980s to the mid-1990s, and has since followed a sustained reduction (FEANTSA 2002). In the UK, the total number of people accepted by local authorities as homeless also declined over the 1990s, and the government has also claimed to have significantly reduced the number of people sleeping rough (although this is perhaps the most difficult manifestation of homelessness to enumerate). There is no reliable data to compare trends in France. In the Scandinavian countries, levels of homelessness remained steady, or fell slightly, during the 1990s. However, homelessness nonetheless remains a feature in industrialized, wealthy nations. Factors which have contributed to this are high unemployment and long-term unemployment, restrictions on emigration (due to worldwide economic trends), lack of availability of low-cost rented accommodation, and progressive disinvestment in local authority housing.

There is a great deal of evidence that homeless people have poor health outcomes, and this can be seen in terms of a range of both physical and mental health problems. A comprehensive study of the health problems of homeless people in Britain (Bines 1994) found that people using hostels, living in bed and breakfast accommodation, and those sleeping rough were not only more likely to have health problems than the general population, but were also more likely to have multiple health problems. Health data were collected from 1280 people living in hostels and bed and breakfast accommodation and 507 people sleeping rough and using day centres and soup runs. These were compared to data from the first wave of the British Household Panel Survey (BHPS), which is a representative sample of 10,264 individuals from over 5000 households (Buck et al. 1994). Bines calculated standardized *morbidity* ratios which take into account the age and sex structure of each group. This is a more accurate comparison than merely reporting rates of ill health, as the homeless group is, on average, much younger than the general population and so should 'expect' good health. The standardized morbidity ratios are presented in Table 10.7. As with standardized mortality ratios, the rate of the general population is set at 100. A number higher than 100 means that the group is more likely than the general population to experience that particular health problem.

We can see from Table 10.7 that homeless people have higher rates of morbidity than the general population. Those in hostels have rates higher than the general population (whose rates are set equal to 100) and those sleeping rough have even higher rates.

Table 10.7 Standardized morbidity ratios (SMorbRs) for reported health problems for hostel users and rough sleepers compared to the general population*

Health problem	Hostels and B&Bs	Sleeping rough	
		Day centres	Soup runs
Musculoskeletal problems	153	185	221
Wounds, skin ulcers, or other skin complaints	105	189	298
Chronic chest or other breathing problems	183	259	365
Fits or loss of consciousness	651	2109	1892
Frequent headaches	264	338	365

* SmorbRs for the general population (from the BHPS) are 100

B&B = bed and breakfast

Source: Bines 1994.

For example, those living in hostels and bed and breakfast accommodation have an SMorbR of 183 for 'chronic chest or other breathing problems'—meaning they are nearly twice as likely to report suffering from this health problem. Those using soup runs are almost four times as likely to report this problem, with an SMorbR of 365. Rates are highest, however, for 'fits or loss of consciousness', a result which is likely to be related to the high levels of drug and alcohol use amongst these groups, in conjunction with the deprivations of living on the streets.

Infectious diseases are also a problem for homeless people. Studies have found relatively high rates of tuberculosis amongst homeless people in England and Wales (Ramsden *et al.* 1988). In the mid-1990s, Darbyshire (1995) linked increases in tuberculosis in England and Wales with poverty, unemployment, and homelessness. Kumar *et al.* (1995) found that nearly one-quarter of 642 shelter users examined had abnormal chest radiographs and 5 per cent had active tuberculosis. As homelessness and injecting drug use often coincide, there are also increased risks of HIV and Hepatitis B and C infection (Raoult *et al.* 2001). Skin problems such as scabies, pediculosis, tinea infections, and impetigo are common reasons for homeless people to seek medical attention (Raoult *et al.* 2001).

Mental health problems are also an important issue for this vulnerable group. A survey by the (then) Office of Population Censuses and Surveys of psychiatric morbidity amongst homeless people is notable for its coverage and depth. It included hostel residents, residents of private-sector leased accommodation (used as a substitute for bed and breakfast accommodation by local authorities), adults staying in night shelters, and people sleeping rough (Gill *et al.* 1996). The results (Table 10.8) show high rates of physical and mental illness, and many individuals reporting both. A recent systematic review of studies of schizophrenia amongst homeless people included 33 studies from eight countries. In the ten methodologically superior studies, the weighted average

Table 10.8 Selected results of the OPCS survey of psychiatric morbidity (% self-reported items)

	Sample size*	Physical illness only	Physical and mental illness	Mental illness only	Alcohol dependence	Drug dependence	GP registration
Hostels	530	36	6	6	16	11	92
PSLA	268	33	2	3	3	7	95
Night shelters	187	26	9	12	44	29	71
Sleeping rough	181	39	14	7	50	24	58

* Not all respondents completed all parts of the questionnaire

PSLA = private-sector leased accommodation

Source: adapted from Gill *et al.* 1996.

prevalence of schizophrenia was 11%; rates were higher among young people, women, and the 'chronically homeless' (Folsom and Jeste 2002).

Table 10.8 also indicates high rates of alcohol and drug dependence, with half of the rough sleepers, alcohol-dependent, and one quarter, drug-dependent. This compared to rates for the general population of about 5 per cent and 2 per cent, respectively (Meltzer *et al.* 1995). This can lead to cirrhosis, overdoses, and accidents. Injecting drug use also brings problems such as thrombosis, abscesses, and infected injecting sites.

Another health issue associated with homelessness is suicide (Baker 1997). In a recent study (Desai *et al.* 2003), suicidal ideation was found to be common amongst a sample of homeless people in the US (66.2% lifetime prevalence). Half of the sample reported that they had at some time attempted suicide, and 8% reported an attempt in the previous 30 days. Suicide and suicidal feelings are likely to occur at all stages of homelessness—fear of losing one's home, sudden and unprepared moves, having no settled home, seeking accommodation, waiting for a home, and settling into a new home (in some ways similar to the challenges faced by migrants). As Baker notes, various emotions are associated with homelessness:

> . . . a sense of isolation and loneliness, feeling worthless, a failure and uncared for, lacking hope for the future, feeling trapped and powerless to change things, despised, rejected and marginalised by society, feeling frustrated, betrayed and misunderstood. (Baker 1997, p. 24)

In England, Keyes and Kennedy (1992) found that homeless people were 34 times more likely to kill themselves than the general population; similarly, Grenier (1997) reports that they are 35 times more likely to do so.

Violence from others is also an everyday threat faced by those without a home, especially homeless women and those sleeping on the streets. North *et al.* (1996), in a study of the use of accident and emergency departments by homeless people, found that their accidental injuries were four times as likely to be the result of assault as those of housed people. Keyes and Kennedy (1992) found that homeless people were 150 times more likely to be fatally assaulted and eight times more likely to die in an accident than the general population. An Australian study also reports that homeless people are likely to witness violence against others as well as to be victims themselves, and that half of homeless women and 10 per cent of homeless men, in a study in Sydney, reported being the victims of rape (Buhrich *et al.* 2000).

Homeless people have also been found to have much higher overall mortality rates than the housed population. In the US, Hwang *et al.* (1997) have reported the average age of death of homeless people in Boston to be 47 years. A study in Georgia reports an average age of death of 46 years; 42 per cent of deaths were from injuries (mostly accidental), nearly half of which were related to acute or chronic effects of alcohol (Hanzlick and Parrish 1993). A Danish study of two homeless hostels in Copenhagen has also reported a higher rate of mortality for homeless people, particularly young women (Nordentoft and Wandall–Holm, 2003). However, due to problems with estimating denominators (the number of homeless people in each age group), it is often difficult to compare death rates with those of the general population. In Britain, a study of deaths of rough sleepers found the average age of death to be 42 (Grenier 1997), which translates to a standardized mortality ratio of over 2500 (Shaw and Dorling 1998). Thus, the street homeless are 25 times more likely to die in any given period than the people who walk past them on the streets.

The direction of the relationship between health and homelessness, and particularly mental health, is unclear—the health problems of some homeless people may predate their homelessness (Pleace and Quilgars 1996). For example, Bines' study (1994) found that 12–20 per cent of homeless people had previously stayed in a psychiatric institution; 9–21 per cent had been in a young offenders' institution; and 15–24 per cent had been in a children's home—over half had been resident in some kind of institution before becoming homeless. Moreover, while some health problems may precede homelessness, it is certainly the case that the daily conditions of homelessness, both material and psychosocial, compound existing health problems, cause additional problems (such as problems with feet and respiratory illness), and make access to health care more problematic (Fisher and Collins 1993; Pleace and Quilgars 1996).

10.5 **Conclusion and implications for policy**

There is a well-established link between poverty and poor health—those who are socially excluded, such as the unemployed, refugees and other poorer migrants, and homeless people, experience worse or very much worse health outcomes than the general population. In the context of sustained or increasing relative poverty, inequality, and social exclusion in Europe, health inequalities are also polarizing.

In the long term, the way to address the poor health of the socially excluded is to pursue economic policies that lead to greater economic equality. A redistribution in wealth and income will have the greatest influence on improving the health of those who are worse off. There is evidence that societies that are more economically equal and socially cohesive have lower overall mortality than those that are more unequal (Wilkinson 1996).

However, in the short term, a number of specific actions can be taken to improve the health of those who are socially excluded. As social exclusion is dynamic and multidimensional, so too should be the policies to combat it and its effects. Policies include:

1 Legislation to protect the rights of minority and migrant groups, particularly concerning citizenship and employment rights, anti-discrimination, and protection of those seeking asylum.

2 Income support/welfare regimes to provide an adequate standard of living for the unemployed. Adequate minimum wages to protect those on low incomes.

3 Focusing on reducing the proportion of children born into and living in poverty (which will have short-term as well as long-term effects on health).

4 Aiming to reduce inequalities in income and wealth within populations; for example, through progressive taxation of income and inherited wealth.

5 Ensuring access to educational, training, and employment opportunities, especially for those such as the long-term unemployed.

6 Removing barriers to access to health and social services, which will involve understanding where and why such barriers exist.

7 Providing adequate follow-up support for those leaving institutional care.

8 Aiming to provide enough affordable housing of reasonable standard.

9 Employment policies that aim to preserve and create jobs.

10 Improving the health of migrants, which requires attention to the unfavourable socio-economic position of many migrant groups and also their particular difficulty of access to health and other care services.

Policies such as these, which are focused on the many dimensions of social exclusion and which aim to reduce inequality in a society, will have an effect on health. As Blane and colleagues have said:

> A society which nurtures people's skills and abilities throughout the population, which provides economic opportunities for all, and fosters a cohesive and integrated social environment, would do more for health than curative medical services are able to. (Blane *et al.* 1996, p. 12)

Acknowledgements

Mary Shaw is funded by the South West Public Health Observatory. Tables 10.1, 10.3, 10.6, and 10.8, and Figures 10.1 and 10.2 are Crown copyright material and reproduced with the permission of the controller of HMSO.

References

Antunes, J.L., Toporcov, T.N., de Andrade. F, P. (2003). Trends and patterns of cancer mortality in European countries. *Eur. J. Cancer Prevention* **12**, 367–72.

Baker, L. (1997). *Homelessness and suicide*. Shelter, London.

Bartlett, C.J., Gunnell, D., Harrison. G., and Moore, L. (2004). Neurotic symptoms, stress, or deprivation: which is most closely associated with incidence of suicide? An ecological study of English Health Authorities. *Psychol. Med.* **32**, 1131–6.

Bartley, M. and Plewis, I. (2002). Accumulated labour market disadvantage and limiting long-term illness: data from the 1971–1991 Office for National Statistics' Longitudinal Study. *Int. J. Epidemiol.* **31**, 336–41.

Bartley, M., Montgomery, S., Cook, D., and Wadsworth, M. (1996). Health and work insecurity in young men. In: *Health and social organization: towards a health policy for the 21st century* (ed. D. Blane, E. Brunner, and R. Wilkinson). Routledge, London.

Bhrugra, D. (2004). Migration, distress and cultural identity. In: *Cultures of health, cultures of illness* (ed. G. Davey Smith and M. Shaw). Oxford University Press, Oxford.

Bines, W. (1994). *The health of single homeless people.* Centre for Housing Policy, University of York, York.

Black, D. and Laughlin, S. (1996). Poverty and health: the old alliance needs new partners. *Benefits* Sept./Oct., 5–9.

Blackburn, C. (1991). *Poverty and health: working with families.* Open University Press, Buckingham.

Blane, D. and Drever, F. (1998). Inequality among men in standardised years of potential life lost, 1970–93. *BMJ* **317**, 255.

Blane, D., Brunner, E., and Wilkinson, R. (1996). The evolution of public health policy: an Anglocentric view of the last fifty years. In: *Health and social organization: towards a health policy for the 21st century* (ed. D. Blane, E. Brunner, and R. Wilkinson). Routledge, London.

Bobak, M. and Marmot, M. (1996). East–West mortality divide and its potential explanations: proposed research agenda. *BMJ* **312**, 421–5.

Buck, N., Gershuny, J., Rose, D., and Scott, J. (ed.) (1994). *Changing households. The British Household Panel Survey 1990–1992.* ESRC Centre for Micro-Social Change, Colchester.

Buhrich, N., Hodder, T., and Teesson, M. (2000). Lifetime prevalence of trauma among homeless people in Sydney. *Australian & New Zealand J. Psych.* **34**, 963–6.

Census (2001). see *www.statistics.gov.uk/census2001*

Cockerham, W.C. (1997). Life expectancy in Russia and Eastern Europe: a lifestyle explanation. *J. Hlth. Soc. Behav.* **38**, 117–30.

Cornia, A.G. and Paniccia, R. (1995). The demographic impact of sudden impoverishment: Eastern Europe during the 1989–94 transition. In: *UNICEF Innocenti Occasional Papers*, Economic Policy Studies, No. 49. UNICEF, Florence.

Corvalan, C.F., Driscoll, T.R., and Harrison, J.E. (1994). Role of migrant factors in work-related fatalities in Australia. *Scand. J. Work, Environ. Hlth.* **20 (5)**, 364–70.

Crawford, M.J. and Prince, M. (1999). Increasing rates of suicide in young men in England during the 1980s: the importance of social context. *Soc. Sci. Med.* **49**, 1419–23.

Darbyshire, J.H. (1995). Tuberculosis: old reasons for a new increase? *BMJ* **310**, 954–5.

Davey Smith, G. (ed.) (2003). *Health inequalities: lifecourse approaches.* The Policy Press, Bristol.

Davey Smith, G. and Egger, M. (1996). Commentary: understanding it all—health, meta-theories, and mortality trends. *BMJ* **313**, 1584–5.

Davey Smith, G., Blane, D., and Bartley, M. (1994). Explanations for socioeconomic differences in mortality: evidence from Britain and elsewhere. *Eur. J. Publ. Hlth.* **4 (2)**, 131–44.

Davey Smith, G., Dorling, D., and Shaw, M. (2001). *Poverty, inequality and health in Britain: 1800–2000—a reader.* The Policy Press, Bristol.

Davey Smith, G., Dorling, D., Mitchell, R., and Shaw, M. (2002). Health inequalities in Britain: continuing increases up to the end of the 20th century, *J. Epidemiol. Commun. Hlth.* **56**, 434–5.

Davis, C.M. (1993). *Eastern Europe and the former USSR: an overview*. RFE/RL Research Report, Vol.2, No. 40, 8 October.

Dennis, B.H., Zhukovsky, G.S., Shestov, D.B., *et al*. (1993). The association of education with coronary heart disease mortality in the USSR. Lipid Research Clinics Study. *Int. J. Epidemiol.* **22**, 420–7.

Department for Work and Pensions. (2003). *Households below average income* (series). London.

Desai, R.A., Liu–Mares, W., Dausey, D.J., and Rosenheck, R.A. (2003). Suicidal ideation and suicide attempts in a sample of homeless people with mental illness. *J. Nerv. Mental Dis.* **191**, 365–71.

Dorling, D. (1995). *A new social atlas of Britain*. Wiley, Chichester.

Dorling, D. and Thomas, B. (2004). *People and places: a 2001 census atlas of the UK*. The Policy Press, Bristol.

Drever, F. and Whitehead, M. (1997). *Health inequalities: decennial supplement*. ONS, The Stationery Office, London.

Eames, M., Ben–Shlomo, Y., and Marmot, M.G. (1993). Social deprivation and premature mortality: regional comparison across England. *BMJ* **307**, 1097–102.

Egger, M., Minder, C.E., and Davey Smith, G. (1990). Health inequalities and migrant workers in Switzerland. *Lancet* Sept. 29, 816.

Elender, F., Bentham, G., and Langford, I. (1998). Tuberculosis mortality in England and Wales during 1982–1992: its association with poverty, ethnicity and AIDS. *Soc. Sci. Med.* **46 (6)**, 673–81.

Ellman, M. (1994). The increase in death and disease under 'katastroika'. *Camb. J. Econ.* **18**, 329–55.

Etienne, T.J., Spiliopoulos, A., and Megevand, R. (1994). Surgery for lung tuberculosis and related lesions: change in clinical presentation as a consequence of migration of population. *Acta Chir. Belg.* **94 (2)**, 101–4.

FEANTSA (2002). *Review of statistics on homelessness in Europe*. European Federation of National Organisations Working with the Homeless.

Ferrie, J., Shipley M.J., Marmot, M.G., Stansfeld, S., and Davey Smith, G. (1995). Health effects of anticipation of job change and non-employment: longitudinal data from the Whitehall II study. *BMJ* **311**, 1264–9.

Feshbach, M. and Friendly, A. (1992). *Ecocide in the USSR*. Basic Books, New York.

Filakti, H. and Fox, J. (1995). Differences in mortality by housing tenure and by car access from the OPCS Longitudinal Study. *Popn. Trends* **81**, 27–30.

Fisher, K. and Collins, J. (1993). Access to health care. In: *Homelessness, health care and welfare provision* (ed. K. Fisher and J. Collins). Routledge, London.

Folsom, D. and Jeste, D.V. (2002). Schizophrenia in homeless persons: a systematic review of the literature. *Acta Psychiat. Scand.* **105**, 404–13.

Gill, B., Meltzer, H., Hinds, K., and Petticrew, M. (1996). *Psychiatric morbidity among homeless people*. OPCS Surveys of Psychiatric Morbidity in Great Britain. HMSO, London.

Goodman, A., Johnson, P., and Webb, S. (1997). *Inequality in the UK*. Oxford University Press, Oxford.

Gordon, D. and Townsend, P. (eds) (2000). *Breadline Europe: the measurement of poverty*. The Policy Press, Bristol.

Graham, H. (1995). Cigarette smoking: a light on gender and class inequality in Britain? *J. Soc. Policy* **24 (4)**, 509–27.

Green, A. (1998). Problems of measuring participation in the labour market. In: *Statistics in society* (ed. D. Dorling and S. Simpson). Arnold, London.

Grenier, P. (1997). *Still dying for a home: an update of Crisis' 1992 investigation into the links between homelessness, health and mortality*. Crisis, London.

Gunnell, D.J., Peters, T.J., Kammerling, R.M., and Brooks, J. (1995). Relation between parasuicide, suicide, psychiatric admissions, and socioeconomic deprivation. *BMJ* **311**, 226–30.

Haan, M., Kaplan, G., and Camacho, T. (1987). Poverty and health: prospective evidence from the Alameda County Study. *Am. J. Epidemiol.* **125 (6)**, 989–98.

Hanzlick, R. and Parrish, R.G. (1993). Death among the homeless in Fulton County, GA, 1988–90. *Publ. Hlth. Rep.* **108**, 488–91.

Harding, S. (2003). Mortality of migrants from the Indian subcontinent to England and Wales: effect of duration of residence. *Epidemiology* **14**, 287–92.

Harding, S. and Balarajan, R. (1996). Patterns of mortality in second generation Irish living in England and Wales: longitudinal study. *BMJ* **312**, 1389–92.

Hawton, K., Harriss, L., Hodder, K., Simkin, S., and Gunnell, D. (2001). The influence of the economic and social environment on deliberate self-harm and suicide: an ecological and person-based study. *Psychol. Med.* **31**, 827–36.

Hertzman, C. (1995). *Environment and health in central and eastern Europe.* World Bank, Washington DC.

Hills, J. (1995*a*). *Joseph Rowntree Foundation inquiry into income and wealth*, Vol. I. Joseph Rowntree Foundation, York.

Hills, J. (1995*b*). *Joseph Rowntree Foundation inquiry into income and wealth*, Vol. II. Joseph Rowntree Foundation, York.

Hills, J. (1998). *Income and wealth: the latest evidence.* Joseph Rowntree Foundation, York.

Hwang, S.W., Orav, E.J., O'Connell, J.J., Lebow, J.M., and Brennan, T.A. (1997). Causes of death in homeless adults in Boston. *Ann. Int. Med.* **126**, 625–8.

Ineichen, B. (1993). *Homes and health: how housing and health interact.* Chapman and Hall, London.

Keyes, S. and Kennedy, M. (1992). *Sick to death of homelessness.* Crisis, London.

Kivimaki, M., Vahtera, J., Virtanen, M., Elovainio, M. Pentti, J., and Ferrie, J.E. (2003). Temporary employment and risk of overall and cause-specific mortality. *Am. J. Epidemiol.* **158**, 663–8.

Korpi, W. (2003). Welfare-state regress in Western Europe: politics, institutions, globalization, and Europeanization. *Ann. Rev. Sociol.* **29**, 589–609.

Kumar, D., Citron, K.M., Leese, J., and Watson, J.M. (1995). Tuberculosis among the homeless at a temporary shelter in London: report of a chest X-ray screening programme. *J. Epidemiol. Commun. Hlth.* **49**, 629–33.

Kunst, A. (1997). *Cross-national comparison of socio-economic differences in mortality.* Ph.D. Thesis, Erasmus University, Rotterdam.

Kunst, A.E. and Mackenbach, J.P. (1992). *An international comparison of socio-economic inequalities in mortality.* Erasmus University, Rotterdam.

Kunst, A.E., Guerts, J.J.M., and van der Berg, J. (1995). International variation in socioeconomic inequalities in self reported health. *J. Epidemiol. Commun. Hlth.* **49**, 117–23.

Langford, I.H. and Bentham, G. (1996). Regional variations in mortality rates in England and Wales: an analysis using multilevel modelling. *Soc. Sci. Med.* **42 (6)**, 897–908.

Leon, D.A., Chenet, L., Shkolnikov, V.M., *et al.* (1997). Huge variation in Russian mortality rates 1984–1994: artefact or alcohol or what? *Lancet* **350**, 383–8.

Levitas, R. (2000). What is social exclusion? In: *Breadline Europe: the measurement of poverty* (ed. D. Gordon and P. Townsend). The Policy Press, Bristol.

McLoone, P. (1996). Suicide and deprivation in Scotland. *BMJ* **312**, 543–4.

McLoone, P. and Boddy, F.A. (1994). Deprivation and mortality in Scotland, 1981 and 1991. *BMJ* **309**, 1465–70.

Macintyre, S. and Ellaway, A. (2000). Neighbourhood cohesion and health in socially contrasting neighbourhoods: implications for the social exclusion and public health agendas. *Hlth. Bull.* **58**, 450–6.

Macintyre, S., Ellaway, A., and Cummins, S. (2002) Place effects on health: how can we conceptualise, operationalise and measure them?. *Soc. Sci. Med.* **55**, 125–39.

Macintyre, S., Ellaway, A., Hiscock, R., Kearns, A., Der, G., and McKay, L. (2003). What features of the home and the area might help to explain observed relationships between housing tenure and health? Evidence from the west of Scotland. *Health & Place* **9**, 207–18.

Mackenbach, J.P., Huisman, M., Andersen, O., Bopp, M., Borgan, J.K., Borrell, C., *et al.* (2004). Inequalities in lung cancer mortality by the educational level in 10 European populations. *Eur. J. Cancer* **40**, 126–35.

Marmot, M.G., Adelstein, A.M., and Bulusu, L. (1984). *Immigrant mortality in England and Wales, 1970–78: causes of death by country of birth.* Studies on medical and population subjects, No. 47. HMSO, London.

Meltzer, H., Gill, B., Petticrew, M., and Hinds, K. (1995). *The prevalence of psychiatric morbidity among adults living in private households.* HMSO, London.

Model, S. (2002). Immigrants' social class in three global cities. In: *Globalization and the new city* (ed. Cross, Malcolm, and Moore). Palgrave, Hampshire.

Morris, J.K., Cook, D.G., and Shaper, A.G. (1994). Loss of employment and mortality. *BMJ* **308**, 1135–9.

Nazroo, J. (1998). The racialisation of ethnic inequalities in health. In: *Statistics in society* (ed. D. Dorling and S. Simpson). Arnold, London.

Nordentoft, M. and Wandall-Holm, N. (2003). 10 year follow up study of mortality among users of hostels for homeless people in Copenhagen. *BMJ* **327**: 81–3.

North, C., Moore, H., and Owens, C. (1996). *Go home and rest? The use of an accident and emergency department by homeless people.* Shelter, London.

Oppenheim, C. and Harker, L. (1996). *Poverty: the facts.* Child Poverty Action Group, London.

Phillimore, P.K. and Morris, D. (1991). Discrepant legacies: premature mortality in two industrial towns. *Soc. Sci. Med.* **33** (2), 139–52.

Phillimore, P., Beattie, A., and Townsend, P. (1994). Widening inequality of health in northern England, 1981–1991. *BMJ* **308**, 1125–8.

Pickett, K.E. and Pearl, M. (2001). Multilevel analysis of neighbourhood socioeconomic context and health outcomes: a critical review. *J. Epidemiol. Commun. Hlth.* **55**, 111–22.

Pinder, D. (1998). New Europe or New Europes? East–West development dynamics in the twentieth century. In: *The New Europe: economy, society and environment* (ed. D. Pinder). Wiley, Chichester.

Pleace, N. and Quilgars, D. (1996). *Health and homelessness in London: a review.* King's Fund, London.

Raleigh, V.S. and Kiri, V.A. (1997). Life expectancy in England: variations and trends by gender, health authority, and level of deprivation. *J. Epidemiol. Commun. Hlth.* **51** (6), 649–58.

Ramsden, S.S., Baur, S., and el Kabir, D.J. (1988). Tuberculosis among the central London homeless. *J. R. Coll. Gen. Pract.* **22**, 16–17.

Raoult, D., Foucault, C., and Brouqui, P. (2001). Infections in the homeless. *The Lancet Infectious Diseases* **1**, 77–84.

Raviglione, M.C., Rieder, H.L., Styblo, K., Khomenko, A.G., Esteves, K., and Kochi, A. (1994). Tuberculosis trends in eastern Europe and the former USSR. *Tubercle and Lung Dis.* **75** (6), 400–16.

Razum, O., Zeeb, H., and Akgun, S. (2001). How useful is a name-based algorithm in health research among Turkish migrants in Germany? *Trop. Med. Intern. Hlth.* **6**, 654–61.

Regan, C.M., Coffey, E., Tocque, K., Ashton, M., and Syed, Q. (2003). Secular trends in the occurrence of tuberculosis in an urban community in north-west England, 1918–2001: implications for a local tuberculosis control programme. *Communicable Dis. Public Hlth.* **6**, 311–6.

Room, G. (1991). *New poverty in the European Community*. Macmillan, Oxford.

Room, G. (1995). Conclusions. In: *Beyond the threshold: the measurement and analysis of social exclusion* (ed. G. Room). The Policy Press, Bristol.

Schulpen, T.W. (1996). Migration and child health: the Dutch experience. *Europ. J. Pediat.* **155** (5), 351–6.

Shapiro, J. (1995). The Russian mortality crisis and its causes. In: *Russian economic reform at risk* (ed. A. Aslund). Pinter, London.

Shaw, M. (2004). Housing and public health. *Ann. Rev. Public Hlth.* **25**, 397–418.

Shaw, M. and Dorling, D. (1998). Mortality among street youth in the UK. *Lancet* **352**, 743.

Shaw, M., Dorling, D., Gordon, D., and Davey Smith, G. (1999). *The widening gap: health inequalities and policy in Britain*. The Policy Press: Bristol.

Shaw, M., Orford, S., Brimblecombe, N., and Dorling, D. (1998). *Widening inequality in mortality between 160 regions of 15 European countries in the early 1990s*. Proceedings of the 8th International Symposium in Medical Geography, Baltimore, USA, 13–17 July, pp. 371–90.

Shaw, M., Orford, S., Brimblecombe, N., and Dorling, D. (2000). Widening inequality in mortality between 160 regions of 15 European countries in the early 1990s. *Soc. Sci. Med.* **50**, 1047–58.

Shkolnikov, V.M., Leon, D.A., Adamets, S., Andreev, E., and Deev, A. (1998). Educational level and adult mortality in Russia: an analysis of routine data 1979 to 1994. *Soc. Sci. Med.* **47**, 357–69.

Shkolnikov, V., McKee, M., and Leon, D.A. (2001). Changes in life expectancy in Russia in the mid-1990s. *Lancet* **357**, 917–21.

Shouls, S., Congdon, P., and Curtis, S. (1996). Modelling inequality in reported long term illness in the UK: combining individual and area characteristics. *J. Epidemiol. Commun. Hlth.* **50**, 366–76.

Social Trends 34. *Households in temporary accommodation*. The Stationery Office, London.

Sooman, A. and Macintyre, S. (1995). Health and perceptions of the local environment in socially contrasting neighbourhoods in Glasgow. *Hlth. Place* **1**, 15–26.

Sundquist, J. (1995). Living conditions and health: a population-based study of labour migrants and Latin American refugees in Sweden and those who were repatriated. *Scand. J. Primary Hlth. Care* **13** (2), 128–34.

Toole, M.J. and Waldman, R.J. (1997). The public health aspects of complex emergencies and refugee situations. *Ann. Rev. Publ. Hlth* **18**, 283–312.

Townsend, P., Phillimore, P., and Beattie, A. (1988). *Health and deprivation: inequality in the north*. Croom Helm, London.

Trovato, F. (1992). Violent and accidental mortality among four immigrant groups in Canada. *Soc. Biol.* **39** (1), 82–101.

Tunstall, H., Shaw, M., and Dorling, D. (2004). Glossary: places and health. *J. Epidemiol. Commun. Hlth.* **58**, 6–10

UNICEF (1993). *Central and eastern Europe in transition: public policy and social conditions*. Regional Monitoring Report No. 1. International Child Development Centre, Florence.

Vogel, J. (1997). *Living conditions and inequality in the European Union 1997*. Eurostat Working Papers. University of Umea, Stockholm.

Wadsworth, M. (1996). Family and education as determinants of health. In: *Health and social organization: towards a health policy for the 21st century* (ed. D. Blane, E. Brunner, and R. Wilkinson). Routledge, London.

Watson, P. (1995). Explaining rising mortality among men in Eastern Europe. *Soc. Sci. Med.* **41** (7), 923–34.

Watson. P. (1998). Health differences in Eastern Europe: preliminary findings from the Nowa Huta study. *Soc. Sci. Med.* **46**, 549–58.

White, P. (1998). Urban life and social stress. In: *The New Europe: economy, society and environment* (ed. D. Pinder). Wiley, Chichester.

White, C., van Galen, F., and Chow, Y.H. (2003). Trends in social class differences in mortality by cause, 1986 to 2000. Hlth. Stat. Quart. **20**, 25–37.

Wilkinson, R.G. (1996). *Unhealthy societies: the afflictions of inequality*. Routledge, London.

Chapter 11

Social patterning of individual health behaviours: the case of cigarette smoking

Martin J. Jarvis and Jane Wardle

11.1 Introduction

Poverty is intimately linked to a variety of behaviours which impact on health. As illustrated in Table 11.1, poor people in a country such as the UK are less likely than those who are well off to eat a good diet, more likely to have a sedentary lifestyle, more likely to be obese, and more likely to be regularly drunk. These associations may be due to a variety of factors, including poverty itself, as well as poorer access to education and information, rather than reflecting a single invariant cause, and not all of these associations may be found in all societies. Nevertheless their consistency is impressive.

Nowhere are the links between deprivation and health behaviours stronger than in the case of drug use, both legal and illegal. Alcohol abuse is frequently a marker for acute social breakdown and, through accidents and violence induced by drunkenness, has a significant impact on death rates (Makela et al. 1997). Binge drinking, which is more common in deprived groups in the population, may lead directly to sudden cardiac death (Kauhanen et al. 1997). Drug users are differentially recruited from groups with disturbed family backgrounds, low self-esteem, and impaired psychological functioning. The costs to society through drug-related crime and social disruption are immense. Cigarette smoking stands out as somewhat different: nicotine is not a drug whose acute effects lead directly to disturbed behavior, crime, or violence, but it imposes the greatest costs of all in terms of premature death. It too shows a strong association with indicators of social disadvantage.

Smoking, drinking, and drug use are individual behaviours which involve an element of personal choice. It is perhaps for this reason that they have frequently been seen not in a broad social context but as a matter of individual responsibility: if smokers wish to avoid the adverse effects of tobacco on their health, it is for them to change their behaviour and quit. If they don't, they have brought ill health on themselves and it is no-one else's fault. Persistence in unhealthy behaviours is seen as simply fecklessness rather than as a response to social circumstances. This victim-blaming approach is

Table 11.1 Distribution of some health behaviours by level of socio-economic deprivation

	Level of socio-economic deprivation			
	0 Least deprived	1	2	3+ Most deprived
Men (%)				
Eat fruit less often than weekly	6.3	9.7	15.2	21.3
Sedentary lifestyle	14.3	14.5	21.0	28.9
Body mass index > 30	13.3	13.4	13.8	17.0
Drunk at least once per week	7.0	13.2	16.1	15.9
Women (%)				
Eat fruit less often than weekly	4.2	6.9	10.7	14.1
Sedentary lifestyle	14.5	17.3	24.6	31.5
Body mass index > 30	14.9	16.0	21.0	25.2
Drunk at least once per week	3.0	5.9	7.6	8.1

Source: Health Survey for England 1994.

unhelpful, in that it fails to address underlying questions of why disadvantaged people are drawn to these behaviours and the nature of the social and individual influences that maintain them. It has also been signally unsuccessful in leading to the development of effective interventions to achieve behaviour change in disadvantaged groups.

This chapter will focus on cigarette smoking, as the individual health behaviour with the single largest impact on health inequalities. As a legal, widespread and, until recently at least, little stigmatized behaviour, there is a wealth of detailed data available documenting its natural history, social patterning, and impact on health. Drawing on data from the UK, a country where the smoking epidemic is now mature, we consider first the nature and extent of the association of smoking with indicators of disadvantage, and trends in rates of current and ex-smoking by deprivation. We then briefly give estimates of the contribution of smoking to death rates in different social groups, before attempting to address the question of why poor people are more likely to smoke and why they find it harder to give up. The final section outlines possible policy options to reduce smoking-induced inequalities.

11.2 Rates of cigarette smoking by material and cultural disadvantage

The gradient in cigarette smoking prevalence by occupational class is well known, as is also the high rate of smoking by lone parents (Marsh and McKay 1994), the unemployed (Lee *et al.* 1991), and the mentally ill (Hughes *et al.* 1986). But these links by no means fully characterize the extent of smoking's association with disadvantage. Table 11.2, which draws on several years of recent data from the General Household Survey and closely replicates analyses of earlier data (Jarvis 1997), documents how a whole range of circumstances independently predict current cigarette smoking. Thus, the odds of being a smoker are substantially increased in those in lower occupational class groups, those living in rented housing, without access to a car, who are unemployed, and in crowded accommodation. Above and beyond this, there is a substantial gradient by educational level, and an increased risk in those who are divorced or separated or lone parents. With the exception of lone parenthood, which is uncommon in men and appears not to carry a risk of smoking for them, the magnitude of the associations is very similar in men and women.

These independent associations imply extreme differences in smoking prevalence between groups with different constellations of circumstances. For example, by comparison with professional owner-occupiers with degree-level education and owning a car, the predicted odds of smoking for unemployed, unskilled, manual workers living in rented, crowded accommodation and with no car are 17.8, corresponding to smoking prevalences in these groups of about 15% and 75%. It should be noted that these variables do not provide an exhaustive list of factors influencing smoking prevalence, as other work shows that smoking is more common in people suffering from mental illness or who are heavy drinkers or who are homeless. Indeed, groups who have an extreme clustering of deprivation indicators (such as prisoners in gaol and

Table 11.2 Predictors of current cigarette smoking among men and women

	Men		Women		All	
	OR	95%CI	OR	95%CI	OR	95%CI
Social class						
I	1.00		1.00		1.00	
II	1.43	1.19–1.70	1.61	1.28–2.04	1.48	1.29–1.71
III NM	1.35	1.12–1.64	1.51	1.20–1.91	1.40	1.21–1.62
III M	1.92	1.59–2.30	1.98	1.56–2.51	1.94	1.68–2.24
IV	1.56	1.28–1.91	2.07	1.63–2.63	1.80	1.55–2.10
V	2.01	1.60–2.53	1.96	1.50–2.57	1.95	1.64–2.31
Rented tenure	1.81	1.67–1.97	1.78	1.64–1.94	1.81	1.70–1.92
No car	1.43	1.29–1.59	1.33	1.20–1.46	1.37	1.28–1.47
Unemployed	1.70	1.41–2.06	1.74	1.39–2.17	1.72	1.47–1.99
Crowding	1.07	0.94–1.23	0.92	0.80–1.05		
Education						
Degree level	1.00		1.00		1.00	
Higher < degree	1.50	1.30–1.74	1.36	1.18–1.57	1.42	1.29–1.58
A level	1.67	1.47–1.91	1.67	1.46–1.91	1.67	1.52–1.83
O level	1.89	1.66–2.15	2.03	1.78–2.31	1.96	1.79–2.15
CSE grade	2.28	1.95–2.67	2.03	1.74–2.36	2.14	1.92–2.39
No qualification	2.52	2.20–2.89	2.73	2.38–3.14	2.62	2.38–2.89
Lone parent	1.13	0.87–1.46	1.39	1.24–1.57	1.32	1.19–1.46
Divorced or separated	1.77	1.40–2.24	1.45	1.32–1.60	1.58	1.47–1.70

OR = odds ratio; CI—confidence interval.

Source: General Household Survey 2000–2003.

homeless people sleeping rough) have been observed to have rates of smoking prevalence of 80–90% (Bridgwood and Malbon 1995; Gill *et al.* 1996).

The factors which predict smoking include material circumstances, cultural deprivation, and indicators of stressful marital, personal, and household circumstances. This illustrates what might be proposed as a general law of western industrialized society—namely, that any marker of disadvantage that can be envisaged and measured, whether personal, material, or cultural, is likely to have an independent association with cigarette smoking. Of course, this may not be true of all societies, such as, for example, Asian countries where there is an overriding cultural prohibition on women's smoking and, in particular, may not be true of developing societies in which cigarette smoking is associated with images of glamour and western prosperity, rather than disadvantage and poverty. However, recent data suggest that smoking in India, as in Britain, is now associated with indicators of disadvantage (Sorensen *et al.* 2005).

11.3 Trends in cigarette smoking prevalence and rates of cessation by deprivation

Cigarette smoking prevalence has been on a declining trend in Britain for over 30 years, reducing overall from 53% in 1973 to 28% in 2003 in men, and from 42% to 25% in women. But over this same period, there has been a substantial widening of the gulf in prevalence between social groups. Figure 11.1 shows trends by a composite index of deprivation which incorporates several of the variables in Table 11.1. Respondents are assigned a score of 1 for each of the following: manual occupational class; rented housing; no car; unemployed; living in crowded conditions (one or more persons per room). The resulting index, with scores ranging from 0 among the affluent to 5 among the most deprived, is similar to the indices employed by Townsend (Townsend *et al.* 1988) and by Carstairs (Carstairs and Morris 1989), but is applied to

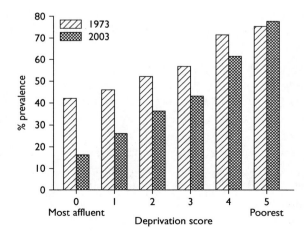

Fig. 11.1 Cigarette smoking by deprivation in the UK. (*Source*: General Household Survey 1973 and 2003).

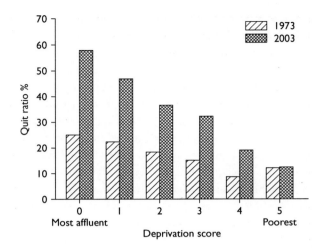

Fig. 11.2 Smoking cessation by deprivation in the UK. (*Source*: General Household Survey 1973 and 2003).

individuals rather than areas. In both 1973 and 2003, for both men and women, there was an approximately linear increase in cigarette smoking with increasing deprivation. Among the most affluent, smoking rates more than halved over the years, reaching a figure of 16% in 2003. Among the most deprived, on the other hand, about 70% were smokers in 1973, and that still remained the case 30 years later.

Figure 11.2 shows rates of smoking cessation by deprivation in 1973 and 2003 (Jarvis 1997). Mirroring the observations in Fig. 11.1, it indicates that while rates of cessation more than doubled in affluent people (from 25% to 58%), among the poorest groups, there was little or no change, with 10% of ever-regular smokers giving up.

11.4 **Contribution of smoking to differences in death rates by social group**

It has long been acknowledged that smoking has a major bearing on observed differences in death rates by social class. One in two of those who smoke are ultimately killed by the habit if they persist and do not give up (Doll *et al.* 1994; Thun *et al.* 1995), and in view of higher prevalence and lower rates of cessation, it would be anticipated that smoking-related disease would bear more heavily on poorer groups. Poorer diet and factors such as earlier age of starting to smoke (leading to longer duration of smoking at any given age) and higher levels of smoke intake in poorer smokers (see below) would act to amplify smoking risks.

Unsurprisingly, observed rates of death from smoking-related diseases show a gradient that parallels the gradient in smoking prevalence. Standardized mortality ratios in unskilled male workers are three times higher than in professionals for heart disease, five times higher for lung cancer, six times higher for emphysema, and 14 times higher for chronic airways obstruction (Drever and Whitehead 1997). Similar, but somewhat smaller, variations are seen in women. As would be expected from the preceding discussion, alternative indicators of socio-economic status such as housing tenure or access to a car are additionally predictive of death rates (Smith and Harding 1997; Goldblatt 1990).

Recently, the indirect methods developed by Peto and Lopez (Peto *et al.* 1992, 1994) to estimate deaths from smoking in different countries have been applied to deaths by socio-economic status within countries. For men aged 35–69, in England and Wales, estimates have been made of the proportion of deaths attributable to smoking by social class for the years since 1970. In 1970–1972, among men in social class I and II, the overall risk of dying in middle age was 36%, and just over one third of these deaths (13%) were estimated to be attributable to smoking. By 1996, the overall risk of dying had declined to 21%, and tobacco-attributable deaths were 4%. Thus, the reduction in deaths attributable to tobacco was responsible for over half of the overall reduction in risk of death. Men in social class V, by contrast, had an overall risk in 1970–1972 of dying in middle age of 47%, and over half of this (25%) was accounted for by tobacco. By 1996, the risk had declined only modestly to 43% and the estimated smoking-attributable element, to 19%.

Of course, the accuracy of these estimates depends on the adequacy of the data and of the assumptions underlying their calculation. The overall number of deaths attributed to tobacco is subject to considerable uncertainty, due to fairly approximate assumptions. For example, only half of the apparent excess of vascular deaths observed in smokers is attributed to tobacco. This somewhat arbitrary proportion, intended to be conservative, may either underestimate true smoking effects, or not be conservative enough. However, for the method to give seriously misleading results for differences in the proportions of deaths attributable to smoking in different social class groups, there would have to be major bias introduced in the calculations across different classes. It is difficult to see that any major bias could be present which would invalidate the estimates.

These findings carry a number of implications. First, the observed widening in overall risk of death between men in social classes I/II and V, that has been observed over the past 25 years, largely reflects changes in tobacco-attributable mortality. Deaths caused by tobacco have dropped far more steeply in social class I and II than in social class V, paralleling changes in smoking prevalence and cessation in these groups. Men in social class V have not experienced an absolute increase in risk of death: the widening of health inequalities that has occurred has been due to their failure to share, to the same extent, in the major overall reduction in risk of death consequent upon smoking cessation. This implies that further reductions in smoking prevalence, unless they are concentrated in poorer groups, may only serve to widen inequalities in death rates still further. The 1996 data indicate that somewhere around two thirds of the observed difference in risk of death across social class groups in middle age is caused by tobacco.

11.5 **Why do poor people smoke?**

The discussion so far has shown that disadvantaged groups in society are disproportionately likely to smoke and least likely to give up cigarettes. As a consequence, the burden of smoking-related disease also falls disproportionately on these groups. Those who can least afford to smoke smoke the most and suffer most from it. That nicotine is a powerful drug of addiction no doubt has much to do with this state of affairs, but we need to move beyond this to ask why it is that the poor are particularly drawn to this drug. The association could be mediated by higher rates of smoking initiation, stronger perceived rewarding effects (either positive or negative) leading to higher levels of dependence, or to greater difficulties in cessation through lower motivation, higher dependence, or fewer available coping resources. These influences are not mutually exclusive, and it could be that a variety of factors operate at each stage of the smoker's career to accentuate the link with disadvantage.

A particularly important distinction to be drawn is between ever becoming a regular cigarette smoker and persisting with the habit. Among those who take up smoking but give up before their early 30s, there is no detectable increase in risk of premature death in comparison with those who never smoke (Doll *et al.* 1994, 2004). As shown in Fig. 11.3, there exists a gradient between ever-regular cigarette smoking and deprivation in both men and women, but among those aged 35–64, the gradient with current smoking is far steeper. Thus, although poor people are somewhat more likely to become smokers, the strongest association is with persisting smoking. What we need to explain above all is not so much why poor people start smoking, but why they do not give it up.

11.5.1 **Disadvantage and smoking uptake**

A gradient in uptake of smoking by level of deprivation is not hard to explain. Children growing up in poverty experience social environments outside the home where most adults are smokers, and the vast majority, 80% or more, will live in households where one or both parents smoke. Thus, cigarette smoking is modelled as normal adult behaviour and cigarettes are readily available to experiment with. But in addition to this, there is evidence that smoking is a measure of smoking trajectory, with prevalence being more closely related to people's social destination than to their circumstances of origin (Glendinning *et al.* 1994). In the national cohort of all the babies born in one week in 1958, who have been followed up at regular intervals ever since (Ferri 1993), cigarette smoking at age 16 increased from 24% among those from the most affluent homes to 48% among the most deprived. But the gradient at age 16 was much sharper (80% among the most deprived) when cohort members were characterized by deprivation measured seven years later at age 23 by their own achieved social position rather than by the characteristics of the parental household. This implies that factors conferring an increased risk of smoking at age 16 (such as poorer

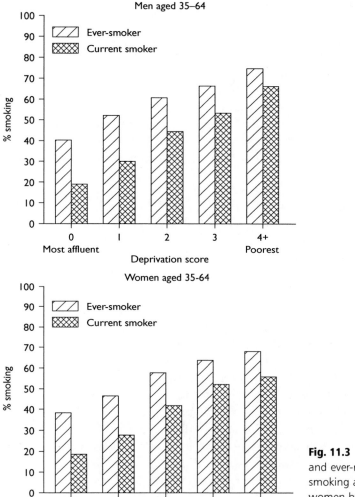

Fig. 11.3 Rates of current and ever-regular cigarette smoking among men and women by deprivation. (*Source*: General Household Survey 2000–2003).

school achievement and lower levels of self-esteem) also have a bearing on subsequent downward social mobility.

11.5.2 Motivation to give up smoking

A superficially attractive hypothesis to explain poor people's lower likelihood of quitting smoking is that they are less well informed and concerned about effects on health, leading to a lower probability of attempts at quitting. Taking this view, the problem is that the health education message simply isn't getting through. Motivation to quit is not an easy construct to measure reliably, as it can fluctuate greatly over time and in different situations (raised in the doctor's surgery, for example, but much lower when drinking in the pub with friends). At present, we are not able to do much better than ask people the question: how much they want to give up smoking altogether. Responses to this have been shown to have some validity by predicting future attempts to quit. In the General Household Survey, levels of expressed motivation to quit are essentially flat across deprivation categories—just over two thirds of cigarette smokers in each group saying that they want to give up. To the extent, therefore, that this measure can be taken at face value, there is no evidence that disadvantaged groups are any less likely than the more affluent to want to give up.

11.5.3 Nicotine dependence and deprivation

By contrast with the lack of variation in motivation to quit by disadvantage, there is strong emerging evidence that level of nicotine dependence increases systematically with deprivation. This is evident both from questionnaire indicators of dependence in the General Household Survey (for example, time to first cigarette of the day; perceived difficulty of going for a whole day without smoking) and from quantitative measures of smoke intake. Figure 11.4 shows levels of saliva cotinine (a measure of total nicotine intake) among smokers in the Health Survey for England (Bajekal *et al.* 2002) . Increasingly high levels of nicotine intake are seen with increasing deprivation, with average intake being 30% higher in the most deprived than in the most affluent smokers. Poor people achieve their higher intakes both by choosing to smoke more cigarettes and by smoking each cigarette more intensively. There are indications that this may turn out to be a phenomenon of wide generality, as similar observations have been made in the USA comparing black with white smokers (Caraballo *et al.* 1998; PerezStable *et al.* 1998; Wagenknecht *et al.* 1990; English *et al.* 1994) and a gradient in intake by level of education has been observed in Czech smokers (Bobak *et al.* 2000).

Since nicotine dependence is an important determinant of ease of quitting, these findings suggest one reason for lower rates of cessation in those who are disadvantaged. Since smoking- related disease bears a dose–response relation to intake, they have implications for higher risk of disease in poor rather than affluent smokers. They also raise the question of just why it should be that poor smokers seek higher nicotine doses.

11.5.4 Functional aspects of nicotine use: positive and negative rewards

Nicotine has a number of positively rewarding effects which could serve as the basis for cigarette use. Although euphoriant effects are not as prominent as with many drugs, they are reported for at least some cigarettes by smokers (Pomerleau and Pomerleau 1992) and could achieve a greater valence for people whose lives are generally deficient in rewards. It is difficult to think of evidence which would strongly support this hypothesis but, equally, it should not be ruled out either.

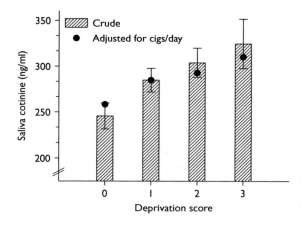

Fig. 11.4 Saliva cotinine by deprivation in adult smokers in UK. (*Source*: Health Survey for England 2001).

An alternate functional view of smoking is that it is self-medication. Cigarette smoking is seen as a means of regulating mood, of managing stress, and of coping with all the hassles and strain resulting from material deprivation (Graham 1987; Smith and Morris 1994). This account chimes with smokers' self-reports of the calming effects from cigarettes and with poor women's observation that smoking is the one thing they do for themselves, that gives them space from the difficult task of caring for children in poverty (Graham 1994). It also recalls soldiers' demands for cigarettes in the First World War to help them cope with the rigours of life in the trenches.

Attractive though the self-medication view of smoking is, it faces several major objections. The most serious of these is the nature of nicotine as a drug. Pharmacologically, nicotine is a stimulant, similar to drugs such as amphetamine. Sedative or anxiolytic effects, if they exist, are very hard to find either in animal models or in humans. Smoking is closely associated with adverse mood states, but there is no good evidence in humans that it ameliorates them other than through withdrawal relief (Schoenborn and Horm 1993; Anda *et al.* 1990). Smokers' self-reports of the calming effects from cigarettes could refer to relief of nicotine withdrawal by smoking. Onset of withdrawal symptoms is rapid and certainly occurs with overnight abstinence during sleep, and may, in a more subtle way, begin within an hour or two of the last cigarette. Stress modulation over the course of the day suggests that mood-elevating effects of cigarettes are attributable to relief of adverse mood from incipient withdrawal rather than to any absolute benefits (Parrott 1995).

Studies of the process of smoking cessation have found that successful quitting leads to lower, rather than to higher, levels of perceived stress, consistent with the idea that smoking may actually be a stressor rather than relieve stress (Cohen and Lichtenstein 1990).

11.5.5 Giving up smoking could be particularly difficult for poor people

If it is difficult to find unequivocal reasons why smoking should be more rewarding for the poor and disadvantaged, there are a number of identifiable factors which would tend to make it harder for them to give up. Even if poor people are as likely to make an attempt at quitting, higher levels of nicotine dependence would place a barrier between the attempt and success. Poor people's generally smokier environment and their much greater likelihood of having a smoking partner would further reduce their chances of succeeding (Jarvis 1997).

It is important to appreciate how hard it is for smokers to give up. Estimates of the chances of succeeding for at least a year in a serious unaided attempt to quite are no better than about 1 in 100 (Jarvis 1997; Cohen *et al.* 1989). When preparing themselves for an attempt at giving up smoking, smokers need to take a medium- to long-term view and be prepared to tolerate the discomfort of nicotine withdrawal and cravings for several weeks at least before things start to get easier. If this is difficult for every-body, it may be especially difficult for those whose lives are stressful and full of hassles to forego the certainty of short-term craving relief and elimination of withdrawal for longer-term gains in disposable income, health, and well-being. The logic of addiction, if not of economics, may win out and dictate buying the next pack of cigarettes.

11.6 **Implications for policies to promote cessation**

Two general kinds of approach can be identified which might reduce the association of smoking with disadvantage. Improvements in housing, education, and employment would target the underlying social conditions which foster high levels of smoking. There is little doubt that substantial progress in this direction would greatly facilitate reductions in smoking, as well as contributing to the wider adoption of other desirable health behaviours, such as an improved diet. But such change is not easy to achieve, and most government policy has sought instead to target the downstream factors which more proximally determine smoking behaviour.

The policies to reduce smoking that have been followed over the past decade or more have been successful in reducing overall prevalence, but have had the paradoxical effect of increasing health inequalities. The main planks of policy have been interventions designed to increase people's motivation to quit (for example, price and restrictions on smoking in public places) and health education campaigns. Addressing dependence has received less attention. While price increases are effective in reducing consumption, there is some uncertainty about their impact on the poor, for whom tobacco expenditure amounts to a high proportion of disposable income (Marsh and McKay 1994). Some economists have argued that poor smokers respond equally as much or more to price than do affluent smokers (Townsend *et al.* 1994), while others are less certain. The very low rates of cessation seen in disadvantaged groups are inconsistent with the idea that, for them, price is an effective means of promoting cessation. Price increases may influence poor people to switch to cheaper and higher yielding brands (Jarvis 1998), to roll their own cigarettes, and to cut down on the number of cigarettes they smoke, rather than to quit altogether. Because of the phenomenon of nicotine compensation, lowering cigarette consumption is unlikely to confer any benefit in lowering risk of smoking-related disease.

Restrictions on smoking in public places and the workplace carry an effective message about the social acceptability of cigarettes, and, as well as protecting non-smokers from other people's smoke, may enhance motivation and attempts to give up smoking. Legislative bans have recently been introduced in Ireland, Italy, Norway, and New Zealand with good acceptance and success. A complete ban is under consideration in Scotland but, in England, the government is planning a partial ban that will exempt pubs that do not serve food as well as private clubs (White Paper 2004). Since drink-only pubs are found disproportionately in poorer areas, a partial ban risks widening health inequalities by protecting affluent people from exposure to tobacco smoke, while leaving the culture of smoking in poor neighbourhoods unchallenged.

One key factor amenable to intervention would appear to be nicotine dependence. Nicotine replacement (NRT) and bupropion (Zyban) have been shown to be ueseful and cost-effective aids to cessation (Cromwell et al. 1997; Buck et al. 1997). NRT approximately doubles success rates from both brief and intensive treatments (Silagy et al. 2000) and there is evidence that its success is maintained in real-world settings (Shiffman et al. 1998). NRT and bupropion specifically target the dependence problem. The National Institute for Clinical Excellence reviewed these pharmacotherapies in 2002 and recommended that both should be reimbursed by the NHS as first-line treatments (National Institute for Clinical Excellence 2002). Now that smoking cessation services (including behavioural support as well as pharmacological aids) are provided by the NHS throughout the country, disadvantaged smokers have access to free and effective treatment. The challenge remains to ensure good uptake of these services by poor as well as by affluent smokers.

If the chances of achieving high rates of cessation in poor smokers are seen as questionable, an alternative, or complementary, approach, would be to take new initiatives in the area of product modification to make smoking less harmful. The advent of novel forms of nicotine delivery, as in NRT and some innovative products from the tobacco industry (Sutherland et al. 1993), is focusing attention on harm reduction as a potentially important new arm of policy (Warner et al. 1997; Bates et al. 1999; Royal College of Physicians Tobacco Advisory Group 2002) . There is compelling evidence that people smoke for nicotine, but much of the burden of smoking-related disease is attributable to other smoke components, particularly the tar fraction. Smoking cigarettes has been likened to injecting drugs through a dirty syringe. The potential benefit of shifting the market toward safer forms of nicotine delivery is illustrated by the case of Sweden, a country which has the lowest male rate of cigarette smoking in Europe (below 20%) and also the lowest rate of lung cancer. But its rate of tobacco dependence is not low, as 20% of adult males use moist oral snuff, a non-combustible form of nicotine delivery which carries considerably less risk than cigarettes (Bolinder 1997; Bates et al. 2003).

The risk is that an intensification of current smoking-control policies, without fresh thinking, may well succeed in further reducing prevalence, but only at the cost of still wider health inequalities.

References

Anda, R.F., Williamson, D.F., Escobedo, L.G., Mast, E.E., Giovino, G.A., and Remington, P.L. (1990). Depression and the dynamics of smoking: a national perspective. *Journal of the American Medical Association*, **264**, 1541–5.

Bajekal, M., Primatesta, P., and Prior, G. (2002) *Health Survey for England 2001*. The Stationery Office, London.

Bates, C., Fagerstrom, K., Jarvis, M.J., Kunze, M., McNeill, A., and Ramstrom, L. (2003). European Union policy on smokeless tobacco: a statement in favour of evidence based regulation for public health. *Tobacco Control*, **12**, 360–7.

Bates, C., McNeill, A., Jarvis, M., and Gray, N. (1999). The future of tobacco product regulation and labelling in Europe: implications for the forthcoming European Union directive. *Tobacco Control*, **8**, 225–35.

Bobak, M., Jarvis, M., Skpodova, Z., and Marmot, M. (2000). Smoke intake among smokers is higher in lower socioeconomic groups. *Tobacco Control*, **9**, 310–12.

Bolinder, G. (1997). Smokeless tobacco a less harmful alternative? In: *The tobacco epidemic*, Vol. 28 (ed. C.T. Bolliger and K.O. Fagerstrom). Karger, Basel.

Bridgwood, A. and Malbon, G. (1995) *Survey of the physical health of prisoners*. HMSO, London.

Buck, D., Godfrey, C., Parrott, S., and Raw, M. (1997) *Cost effectiveness of smoking cessation interventions*. Centre for Health Economics and Health Education Authority, York.

Caraballo, R.S., Giovino, G.A., Pechacek, T.F., Mowery, P.D., Richter, P.A., Strauss, W.J., et al. (1998). Racial and ethnic differences in serum cotinine levels of cigarette smokers. *Journal of the American Medical Association*, **280**, 135–9.

Carstairs, V. and Morris, R. (1989). Deprivation and mortality: An alternative to social class? *Community Medicine*, **11**, 210–19.

Cohen, S. and Lichtenstein, E. (1990). Perceived stress, quitting smoking, and smoking relapse. *Health Psychology*, **9**, 466–78.

Cohen, S., Lichtenstein, E., Prochaska, J.O., Rossi, J.S., Gritz, E.R., Carr, C.R., et al. (1989). Debunking myths about self-quitting. Evidence from 10 prospective studies of persons who attempt to quit smoking by themselves. *American Psychologist*, **44**, 1355–65.

Cromwell, J., Bartosch, W.J., Fiore, M.C., Hasselblad, V., and Baker, T. (1997). Cost-effectiveness of the clinical practice recommendations in the AHCPR guideline for smoking cessation. *Journal of the American Medical Association*, **278**, 1759–66.

Doll, R., Peto, R., Boreham, J., and Sutherland, I. (2004). Mortality in relation to smoking: 50 years' observations on male British doctors. *British Medical Journal*, **328**, 1519–20.

Doll, R., Peto, R., Wheatley, K., Gray, R., and Sutherland, I. (1994). Mortality in relation to smoking: 40 years' observations on male British doctors. *British Medical Journal*, **309**, 901–911.

Drever, F. and Whitehead, M. (eds.) (1997) *Health inequalities*. The Stationery Office, London.

English, P.B., Eskenazi, B., and Christianson, R.E. (1994). Black-White differences in serum cotinine levels among pregnant women and subsequent effects on infant birthweight. *American Journal of Public Health*, **84**, 1439–43.

Ferri, E. (ed.) (1993) *Life at 33: the fifth follow-up of the National Child Development Study*. National Children's Bureau, London.

Gill, B., Meltzer, H., Hinds, K., and Pettigrew, M. (1996) *Psychiatric morbidity among homeless people*. HMSO, London.

Glendinning, A., Shucksmith, J., and Hendry, L. (1994). Social class and adolescent smoking behaviour. *Social Science and Medicine*, **38**, 1449–60.

Goldblatt, P. (ed.) (1990) *Longitudinal study: mortality and social organization*. HMSO, London.

Graham, H. (1987). Women's Smoking and Family Health. *Social Science and Medicine*, **25**, 47–56.

Graham, H. (1994). Gender and class as dimensions of smoking-behavior in Britain—insights from a survey of mothers. *Social Science and Medicine*, **38**, 691–8.

Hughes, J.R., Hatsukami, D.K., Mitchell, J.E., and Dahlgren, L.A. (1986). Prevalence of smoking among psychiatric outpatients. *American Journal of Psychiatry*, **143**, 993–7.

Jarvis, M.J. (1997). Patterns and predictors of unaided smoking cessation in the general population. In: *The Tobacco Epidemic*, Vol. 28 (ed. C.T. Bolliger and K.O. Fagerstrom), pp. 151–64. Karger, Basel.

Jarvis, M.J. (1998). Supermarket cigarettes: the brands that dare not speak their name. *British Medical Journal*, **316**, 929–31.

Kauhanen, J., Kaplan, G.A., Goldberg, D.E., and Salonen, J.T. (1997). Beer binging and mortality: Results from the Kuopio ischaemic heart disease risk factor study, a prospective population based study. *British Medical Journal*, **315**, 846–51.

Lee, A.J., Crombie, I.K., Smith, W.C.S., and Tunstall–Pedoe, H.D. (1991). Cigarette smoking and employment status. *Social Science and Medicine*, **33**, 1309–12.

Makela, P., Valkonen, T., and Martelin, T. (1997). Contribution of deaths related to alcohol use of socioeconomic variation in mortality: register based follow up study. *British Medical Journal*, **315**, 211–6.

Marsh, A. and McKay, S. (1994) *Poor smokers*. Policy Studies Institute, London.

National Institute for Clinical Excellence (2002) *Guidance on the use of nicotine replacement therapy (NRT) and bupropion for smoking cessation*. Technology Appraisal Guidance No. 39. National Institute for Clinical Excellence, London.

Parrott, A.C. (1995). Stress modulation over the day in cigarette smokers. *Addiction*, **90**, 233–44.

Perez Stable, E.J., Herrera, B., Jacob, P., and Benowitz, N.L. (1998). Nicotine metabolism and intake in black and white smokers. *Journal of the American Medical Association*, **280**, 152–6.

Peto, R., Lopez, A.D., Boreham, J., Thun, M., and Heath C., Jr. (1992). Mortality from tobacco in developed countries: indirect estimation from national vital statistics. *Lancet*, **339**, 1268–78.

Peto, R., Lopez, A.D., Boreham, J., Thun, M., and Heath, C. (1994) *Mortality from smoking in developed countries 1950–2000: indirect estimates from national vital statistics*. Oxford University Press, Oxford.

Pomerleau, C.S. and Pomerleau, O.F. (1992). Euphoriant effects of nicotine in smokers. *Psychopharmacology*, **108**, 460–5.

Royal College of Physicians Tobacco Advisory Group (2002). *Protecting Smokers, Saving Lives*. Royal College of Physicians, London.

Schoenborn, C.A. and Horm, J. (1993) *Negative moods as correlates of smoking and heavier drinking: implications for health promotion*. National Center for Health Statistics, Hyattsville, Maryland.

Shiffman, S., Gitchell, J., Pinney, J.M., Burton, S.L., Kemper, K.E., and Lara, E.A. (1998). Public health benefit of over-the-counter nicotine medications. *Tobacco Control*, **6**.

Silagy, C., Lancaster, T., Stead, L., Mant, D., and Fowler, G. (2000). Nicotine replacement therapy for smoking cessation (Cochrane Review). In: *The Cochrane Library, Issue 1, 2003* (ed. T. Lancaster, C. Silagy, and D. Fullerton). Update Software, Oxford.

Smith, G.D. and Morris, J. (1994). Increasing inequalities in the health of the nation. *British Medical Journal*, **309**, 1453–4.

Smith, J. and Harding, S. (1997). Mortality of women and men using alternative social classifications. In: *Health inequalities: decennial supplement* (ed. F. Drever and M. Whitehead). The Stationery Office, London.

Sorensen, G., Gupta, P.C., and Pednekar, M.S. (2005). Social disparities in tobacco use in Mumbai, India: the roles of occupation, education, and gender. *American Journal of Public Health*, **95**, *1003–8*.

Sutherland, G., Russell, M.A.H., Stapleton, J.A., and Feyerabend, C. (1993). Glycerol particle cigarettes: a less harmful option for chronic smokers. *Thorax*, **48**, 385–7.

Thun, M.J., Day–Lally, C.A., Calle, E.E., Flanders, W.D., and Heath, C.W. (1995). Excess mortality among cigarette smokers: changes in a 20-year interval. *American Journal of Public Health*, **85**, 1223–30.

Townsend, J., Roderick, P., and Cooper, J. (1994). Cigarette smoking by socioeconomic group, sex, and age: Effects of price, income, and health publicity. *British Medical Journal*, **309**, 923–7.

Townsend, P., Phillimore, P., and Beattie, A. (1988). *Health and deprivation: inequality and the North*. Croom Helm, London.

Wagenknecht, L.E., Cutter, G.R., Haley, N.J., Sidney, S., Manolio, T.A., Hughes, G.H. *et al.* (1990). Racial differences in serum cotinine levels among smokers in the Coronary Artery Risk Development in (Young) Adults Study. *American Journal of Public Health*, **80**, 1053–6.

Warner, K.E., Slade, J., and Sweanor, D.T. (1997). The emerging market for long-term nicotine maintenance. *Journal of the American Medical Association*, **278**, 1087–92.

White Paper (2004) *Choosing health—making healthy choices easier*. The Stationery Office, London.

Chapter 12

The social determination of ethnic/racial inequalities in health

James Y. Nazroo and David R. Williams

12.1 Introduction

Differences in health across ethnic groups, in terms of both morbidity and mortality, have been repeatedly documented in the US (Department of Health and Human Services 1985; Rogers 1992; Sorlie *et al.* 1992, 1995; Rogot *et al.* 1993; Krieger *et al.* 1993; Davey Smith *et al.* 1998; Pamuk *et al.* 1998; Williams 2001), the UK (Marmot *et al.* 1984; Rudat 1994; Harding and Maxwell 1997; Nazroo 1997*a,b*, 2001; Erens *et al.* 2001), Latin America (Pan American Health Organization 2001), South Africa (Sidiropoulos *et al.* 1997), Australia (McLennan and Madden 1999), and elsewhere (Polednak 1989). However, the factors underlying such differences remain contested. In particular, the significance of social determinants, particularly the social inequalities that ethnic minority groups face, remains the subject of considerable debate. Some claim that social and economic inequalities make a minimal, or no, contribution to ethnic inequalities in health (Wild and McKeigue 1997); others suggest that even if they do contribute, the cultural and genetic elements of ethnicity must also play a role (Smaje 1996); and others argue that ethnic inequalities in health are predominantly determined by socio-economic inequalities (Navarro 1990; Sheldon and Parker 1992).

In part, the ongoing debate about the significance of social inequalities to ethnic differences in health is a consequence of the empirical complexity of the field, both in terms of the difficulties of undertaking research and the sometimes poor quality data that result, and in terms of the difficulty of interpreting findings. Take, for example, Table 12.1, which shows infant mortality rates for Black and White mothers in the US stratified by mother's educational status. The table shows that infant mortality rates are strongly patterned by education for both Black and White women, with increasing years of education predicting lower levels of infant mortality. However, there is an ethnic/racial difference in mortality rate at each educational level, with the Black/White ratio for infant mortality increasing with level of education. And, the most disadvantaged group of White women (those who have not completed high school) have a lower infant mortality rate than the most advantaged group of Black women (college graduates). How are such data to be interpreted? Which other explanations may be relevant?

Table 12.1 Infant mortality rates for mothers aged 20 years and over in the US, 1995

Maternal education	White	Black	Black/White ratio
Less than 12 years	9.9	17.3	1.74
12 years	6.5	14.8	2.28
13–15 years	5.1	12.3	2.41
16 years or more	4.2	11.4	2.71

Source: Pamuk *et al*. 1998.

Within the UK, similar data have been used to suggest that socio-economic inequalities do not contribute to ethnic inequalities in health (Marmot *et al*. 1984; Harding and Maxwell 1997). But such interpretations fail to account for the complexity of the social and economic inequalities faced by ethnic minority groups—a complexity that cannot be fully captured by simple measures of socio-economic position, such as class or education (Kaufman *et al*. 1997, 1998; Nazroo 1997*a*, 1998). It is likely that such findings in fact reflect:

1 The non-comparability of markers of socio-economic position across ethnic/racial groups (the social significance of a college education is different for White and Black women);

2 The importance of assessing socio-economic inequalities over the life course (a snapshot measure will fail to capture the full nature of the inequality faced by marginalized groups); and

3 The importance of assessing other risk factors related to ethnicity/race that may also affect health, such as racism and geographical segregation.

Indeed, in both the US and the UK, data limitations have greatly hampered investigations of ethnic inequalities in health and how they might be structured by social and economic disadvantages, particularly as obvious data limitations are often ignored by investigators. Given the growing sophistication of inequalities in health research generally, it is worrying, but perhaps not surprising, that such empirical difficulties lead to the persistence of crude explanations based on cultural stereotypes and claims of genetic difference (Soni Raleigh and Balarajan 1992; Gupta *et al*. 1995; Stewart *et al*. 1999), despite a lack of concrete evidence, more than 100 years of research exposing the limitations of the assumptions underlying such explanations (e.g. Bhopal 1997), and growing evidence that the obvious social and economic inequalities faced by ethnic minority groups are likely to be a fundamental explanation (Krieger *et al*. 1993; Williams *et al*. 1994; Williams 1999; Davey Smith *et al*. 1998; Krieger 2000; Nazroo 2001; Karlsen and Nazroo 2002*a*).

In this chapter, we will illustrate the impact of some of these limitations on how data are interpreted, and suggest that social and economic inequalities are fundamental causes of ethnic inequalities in health. We will then relate the socio-economic patterning of ethnic inequalities in health to the potential explanations for such inequalities explored in other chapters in this volume. We will then conclude by suggesting that an adequate understanding of racism is fundamental to an understanding of ethnic inequalities in health. But we will begin by discussing the ethnic/racial make-up of modern industrial societies and the extent of social disadvantage associated with ethnicity/race, using the US and UK as examples.

12.2 **Ethnic/racial composition of industrialized nations**

The non-White populations of the US and UK have quite different histories and a quite different composition. Although some non-White people settled in the UK prior to World War II (mainly in London and the ports on the west coast—Bristol, Cardiff, Liverpool, Glasgow—and primarily related to the slave trade), most of the non-White migration to Britain occurred after World War II. This was driven by the post-war economic boom and consequent need for labour—a need that could be filled from British Commonwealth countries (primarily countries in the Caribbean and the Indian sub-continent). This 'economic' migration was followed by migration of spouses and children and, sometimes, older relatives, in a climate when the legislation regulating entry into the UK became increasingly restrictive. Migration from these countries was not evenly spread over time: immigration from the Caribbean and India occurred throughout the 1950s and 1960s, peaking in the early 1960s; from Pakistan, largely in the 1970s; from Bangladesh, mainly in the late 1970s and early 1980s; and from Hong Kong, in the 1980s and 1990s. In addition, there was a notable flow of immigrants from East Africa in the late 1960s and early 1970s, made up of migrants from India to East Africa who were subsequently expelled. Over the past 10 years, migration to the UK has taken a very different form, including many refugees.

However, alongside this 'visible' migration, there has been a long history of migration to England from Ireland, which continued during the active recruitment of labour from the Caribbean and the Indian subcontinent. The history of Irish migration to England, as to the US, holds important lessons on the circumstances of economic migrants and their descendants, and how far skin colour is a demarcating factor.

The collection of data on ethnicity in the UK Census has happened only twice, for 1991 and 2001. Data from the 2001 Census of England, which included a fairly comprehensive assessment of ethnicity, are shown in Table 12.2, along with an estimate of the percentage in each group who were born in England. Table 12.2 shows that at the 2001 Census, nine per cent of the English population identified themselves as belonging to one of the non-White ethnic minority groups, with a further four per cent identifying themselves as a member of a White ethnic minority group. It also shows that less than half of the non-White ethnic minority population was born in England, though this varies across specific groups, reflecting both period of migration and patterns of fertility.

In contrast to the UK, racial categories have been used in the US Census since the first census in 1790, illustrating the centrality of race to US society (Nobles 2000;

Table 12.2 Ethnic composition of the English population

	Number	Per cent	Per cent migrant*
White British	42,747,000	87	2
White Irish	624,000	1.3	49
Other White	1,308,000	2.7	69
Black Caribbean (incl. mixed)	793,000	1.6	47
Black African (incl. mixed)	552,000	1.1	83
Other Black	95,000	0.2	60
Indian Asian	1,029,000	2.1	75
Pakistani Asian	707,000	1.4	67
Bangladeshi Asian	275,000	0.6	87
Other Asian	238,000	0.5	88
Mixed White and Asian	184,000	0.4	47
Chinese	221,000	0.5	81
Other (incl. other mixed)	336,000	0.7	88

Source: 2001 Census.

* Estimated from Health Survey for England 1999 (see Erens et al. 2001)

Williams 1997). In compliance with Article One of the US Constitution, three racial categories were utilized in the 1790 census that reflected a hierarchy of racial preference which was driven by a racist ideology: Whites, Blacks (as three fifths of a person), and 'civilized Indians' (that is those who paid taxes).

Every US Census has subsequently categorized the population by race, although the racial categories utilized have changed at almost every Census (as the ethnic categories did between the 1991 and 2001 UK Censuses). In some censuses, racial categories were used to capture various degrees of racial admixture between White and Black; for example, the 1890 census included the categories of mulatto, quadroon, and octoroon. The Thirteenth Amendment to the US Constitution abandoned the Three-Fifths Rule, but Indians continued to be divided into the categories of 'civilized Indians' and 'Indians not taxed' until all American Indians were granted US citizenship by Congress in 1924 (Anderson and Fienberg 1995).

Over time, new racial categories were added as the need arose to keep track of new immigrant groups. So, for example, Japanese was added as a new category in the 1890 Census; and Filipino, Hindu, and Korean in the 1920 Census; and Mexican in the 1930 Census. Thus, changes in racial classification have historically captured the emergence or redefinition of marginal population groups.

The American ideology of a clear racial hierarchy that reflected the 'one drop rule' (one drop of non-White blood made one non-White) was also evident in how race was assigned to all newborns for the tabulation of natality statistics prior to 1989 (National Center for Health Statistics 2003). A child would only be assigned the White race if both parents were White. If an infant's parents were of different races and one parent was White, the child would always be assigned the other parent's race. However, if either parent was Hawaiian, the child would be classified as Hawaiian. In all other cases, the child would be assigned the father's race.

Guidelines established in 1978 by the federal government's Office of Management and Budget (OMB) for the uniform assessment of race and ethnicity (Office of Management and Budget 1978), continue to shape how race is assessed in the US. These guidelines recognized four racial groups—White, Black, American Indian or Alaskan Native, and Asian or Pacific Islander (API)—and one ethnic category (Hispanic). Prior to the 2000 Census, there was considerable debate regarding how race ethnicity should be conceptualized and measured (Evinger 1995). After mulling over the suggestions, the OMB issued new guidelines in 1997 that made only a few changes. The biggest change was that persons of mixed racial ancestry were allowed to list themselves in as many racial categories as apply. Other changes included the expansion of the racial categories by one, with Native Hawaiian and Other Pacific Islander constituting a new racial category separate from Asian. Changes in terminology allow for 'Black or African American' and 'Hispanic or Latino' to be utilized. These new guidelines were used in the 2000 Census and all Federal statistical agencies were required to use them by 2003. The OMB argues that they are only minimal standards, but few agencies go beyond them and they have shaped how other organizations and researchers assess race.

In the 2000 Census, the US population was 75.1% White, 12.3% Black, 0.9% American Indian or Alaskan Native, 3.6% Asian, 0.1% Native Hawaiian and Other Pacific Islander, 12.5% Hispanic, and 2.4% belonging to two or more races (Grieco and Cassidy 2001). There is considerable heterogeneity within each of the major racial/ethnic groups. For example, the American Indian and Alaskan Native category consists of over 450 federally recognized tribes and Alaskan Native villages (Norton and Manson 1996). American Indian tribes share a common history of exploitation and oppression, but there is great diversity in tribal cultures, socio-economic circumstances, and health. In a similar vein, the Hispanic category consists of more than 25 national origin groups that share a common language, religion, and traditions, but vary in terms of the timing of their migration to the US, regional concentration, incorporation experiences, and socio-economic status and health (Sorlie *et al.* 1993; Vega and Amaro 1994).

The Asian population in the US consists of persons from some 28 Asian countries, each of which has its own distinctive history, culture, and language (Lin–Fu 1993). Although the Asians have the highest median level of income in the US, some Asian subgroups (such as the Hmong, Laotian, and Cambodian) have a lower median income and higher poverty rates than Blacks or American Indians (US Census 1993). The Pacific Islander population consists of persons from some 25 Pacific Island cultures (Lin–Fu 1993). There is also considerable cultural and ethnic diversity in both the Black and the White population. Regional variations in morbidity and mortality have been noted among Blacks (Fang *et al.* 1997), and migration status also predicts variations in health within the Black population of the US (David and Collins 1997; Fruchter *et al.* 1985).

The US Census also collects data on many White ethnic subgroups but the extent to which ethnicity predicts variations in health for the White population has not received much attention in recent health research in the US.

12.3 **Ethnic/racial disadvantage—variation and similarities across groups and countries**

There is considerable demographic and socio-economic diversity among the major racial/ethnic groups in the US. Some of this is summarized in Table 12.3, which shows that:

- Asians and Hispanics have much higher proportions of immigrants than the other groups;
- The age structure of these groups varies with American Indians, Native Hawaiians, and Hispanics having a lower median age than Whites, Asians, and Blacks;
- Whites and Asians have the lowest levels of female-headed households and Blacks have the highest;
- Whites and Asians have higher levels of educational attainment, percentage of persons in managerial and professional occupations, and lower rates of poverty than the other population groups;
- Whites have higher levels of home ownership than all other racial/ethnic groups.

Much is this is complicated by the geographical segregation of ethnic and racial minority groups, something which is a prominent theme in the US (Williams and Collins 2001). Indeed, racial residential segregation is the foundation on which Black–White disparities in socio-economic position have been built in the US (Massey

Table 12.3 Demographic and socio-economic characteristics by race and ethnicity, US, 2000

Indicator	White	Black	Am. Indian / Alaska Native	Asian	Native Hawaiian / Pacific Islander	Other race	Hispanic
% Hispanic	8.0	2.0	16.4	1.2	11.4	97.0	n/a
% foreign born	3.5	6.1	5.4	68.9	19.9	43.4	40.2
Median age	37.7	30.2	28.0	32.7	27.5	24.6	25.8
% female headed	9.2	30.8	20.9	9.1	16.1	19.3	17.8
% white collar	36.6	25.2	24.3	44.6	23.3	14.2	18.1
% high school +	85.5	72.3	70.9	80.4	78.3	46.8	52.4
% college grad.+	27.0	14.3	11.5	44.1	13.8	7.3	10.4
% poor	8.1	24.9	25.7	12.6	17.7	24.4	22.6
% own home	71.3	46.3	55.5	53.4	45.0	40.5	48.0

Source: US Census 2000.

and Denton 1993). Segregation refers to the physical separation of the races that limited the housing options of Blacks to the least desirable residential areas. In the late 19th and early 20th century, segregation emerged most aggressively in the developing industrial urban centres to ensure that Whites were protected from residential proximity to Blacks. It was imposed by legislation, supported by major economic institutions, enshrined in the housing policies of the federal government, enforced by the judicial system, and legitimized by an ideology of White supremacy that was advocated by the church and other cultural institutions (Cell 1982; Jaynes and Williams 1989).

Although the Civil Rights Act of 1968 made discrimination in the sale or rental of housing units illegal in the US, studies reveal that explicit discrimination in housing persists (Clark 1992; Fix and Struyk 1993). Moreover, in more subtle ways, Blacks are discouraged from residing in White residential areas, and Whites continue to move out of communities when the Black population increases (Shihadeh and Flynn 1996; Turner 1993). Thus, although African Americans express the highest support for residence in integrated neighbourhoods (Bobo and Zubrinsky 1996), their residential exclusion remains high and distinctive; an analysis of the 2000 Census data showed the national index of dissimilarity for the US was 0.66 (Glaeser and Vigdor 2001), meaning that 66 per cent of Black residents would have to move to achieve equal representation of their group in residential areas. Generally, a dissimilarity index value above 0.60 is thought to represent extremely high segregation (Massey and Denton 1989). So, although most immigrant groups have experienced some residential segregation in the US, no immigrant group has ever lived under the high levels of segregation that currently characterize the African American population (Massey and Denton 1993).

Such residential segregation has truncated socio-economic mobility for African Americans by determining access to education and employment opportunities, and been a central mechanism through which racial inequality has been created and reinforced (Jaynes and Williams 1989; Massey and Denton 1993). In the US, residence determines which public school students can attend, so residential segregation has led to highly segregated elementary and high schools. The funding of public education is under the control of local government, so community resources determine the quality of the neighbourhood school, and the concentration of poverty and consequent low community resources in Black neighbourhoods is a fundamental cause of racial differences in the quality of education (Orfield 1996). Although there are millions of poor Whites in the US, poor White families tend to be dispersed throughout the community with many residing in desirable residential areas (Wilson 1987). Accordingly, most poor White students go to schools where the majority of students come from middle-class backgrounds (Orfield 1996). In contrast, public schools with a high proportion of Blacks and Hispanics are dominated by poor children.

Research also reveals that institutional discrimination, based on residential segregation, severely restricts access to jobs for Blacks. In the last several decades there has been a mass movement of low-skilled, high-paid jobs from many of the urban areas where Blacks are concentrated to the suburbs (Wilson 1987, 1996). Some corporations explicitly use the racial composition of areas in their decision-making process regarding the placement of new plants and the relocation of existing ones (Cole and Deskins 1988). Negative racial stereotypes of African Americans and of the areas where they are concentrated play an important role in these decisions (Kirschenman and Neckerman 1991; Neckerman and Kirschenman 1991).

An empirical analysis of the effects of segregation on young African Americans making the transition from school to work documented that segregation is a key determinant of racial differences in socio-economic mobility (Cutler *et al.* 1997). This study found that getting rid of residential segregation would lead to the elimination of Black–White differences in earnings, high-school graduation rates, and unemployment, and would reduce racial differences in single motherhood by two thirds. Segregation also creates health-damaging conditions in the social and physical environment. High levels of segregation create distinctive ecological environments on multiple dimensions for African Americans. Sampson and Wilson (1995) reported that in the 171 largest cities in the US, there was not even one where Whites lived in comparable ecological conditions to Blacks in terms of poverty rates or rates of single parent households. These researchers came to the striking conclusion that 'the worst urban context in which Whites reside is considerably better than the average context of Black communities' (Sampson and Wilson 1995).

Although analyses of residential segregation are less developed in the UK, they also show marked differences between the geographical locations of ethnic minority and White people. Analysis of the 1991 Census (Owen 1992, 1994) has shown that the non-White ethnic minority population is largely concentrated in England, mainly in the most populous areas. Key findings are:

- More than half of the ethnic minority population lives in South East England, where less than a third of the White population lives.

- Greater London contains 44.8 per cent of the ethnic minority population and only 10.3 per cent of the White population.

- Elsewhere, the West Midlands, West Yorkshire, and Greater Manchester display the highest relative concentrations of people from ethnic minorities.

- Almost 70 per cent of ethnic minority people live in Greater London, the West Midlands, West Yorkshire, and Greater Manchester, compared with just over 25 per cent of Whites.

- There are even greater differences when smaller areas (enumeration districts) are considered: more than half of ethnic minority people live in areas where the total ethnic minority population exceeds 44 per cent, compared with the 5.5 per cent national average at the 1991 Census.

Analysis of the areas where ethnic minority people live in England show that they are much more likely to live in deprived areas (Karlsen *et al.* 2002). For example, 81 per cent of Pakistani and Bangladeshi people, 72 per cent of Caribbean people, and 49 per cent of Indian people lived in the bottom quintile of areas, using a standard area deprivation score.

As for the US, there are also marked economic inequalities by ethnic group in the UK. Some indicators of this are summarized in Table 12.4. The first part of the table shows rates of paid employment for men aged 16 to 65. For the White English group, three-quarters of men are in paid employment. Figures are lower for all of the ethnic minority groups (except for the Chinese group), with particularly low rates in the Caribbean and Pakistani groups, and even lower rates for the Bangladeshi group (with less than half in paid employment). The second part of the table shows occupational class of the head of household. The data suggest that the profiles of White English and Indian households are similar, with White minority and possibly Chinese households better off, and Caribbean, Pakistani, and particularly Bangladeshi households worse off. Four out of five Bangladeshi households are headed by someone in a manual occupation. The third and final part of Table 12.4 shows equivalized household income from all sources, split into tertiles on the basis of the general population distribution. The data suggest that on this measure, the two White groups are equivalent, with the Indian and the Caribbean group worse off, and the Pakistani and the Bangladeshi group particularly poorly off—two-thirds of the Pakistani group and almost 90 per cent of the Bangladeshi group are in the bottom tertile. In terms of the top income tertile, the Chinese group is equivalent to the two White groups, but it has substantially more households in the bottom tertile, suggesting greater inequality within the Chinese group.

Table 12.4 Ethnic differences in socio-economic indicators in England

	Caribbean (%)	Indian (%)	Pakistani (%)	Bangladeshi (%)	Chinese (%)	White minority (%)	White English (%)
Male employment rates, aged 16–65	58	69	59	46	67	72	75
Registrar General's class							
I/II	24	34	23	12	40	46	35
IIINM	19	12	10	7	16	13	14
IIIM	28	29	40	39	34	25	32
IV/V	29	26	27	42	11	16	19
Equivalized household income							
Bottom tertile	47.8	45.1	68.8	89.6	41.3	26.8	30.9
Middle tertile	28.0	31.0	19.7	5.1	22.3	30.5	35.5
Top tertile	24.1	23.9	11.5	5.3	36.4	42.7	33.6

Source: Health Survey for England 1999 (see Erens et al. 2001).

12.4 **Heterogeneity of the ethnic patterning of health**

Table 12.5, containing data on mortality rates for 1999, illustrates the patterning of mortality by racial/ethnic group and age in the US (Hoyert *et al.* 2001; Mathews *et al.* 2002). The pattern is one that is familiar (Sorlie *et al.* 1995). Rates for non-Hispanic Black people are more than twice as high as those for non-Hispanic White people until early old age, when their relative rates begin to drop. A similar pattern is found for Native Americans, though differences are smaller at younger ages, and the 'cross-over' with non-Hispanic White people at older ages is clearer. Rates for Hispanic people are generally lower than those of non-Hispanic Whites, though the differences are small at younger ages. Rates for Asian/Pacific Islanders are uniformly lower than those for non-Hispanic Whites.

The pattern reveals heterogeneity in experience across racial/ethnic groups, with some doing well in comparison with non-Hispanic Whites, others doing badly, and differences varying across the life course. Notable, perhaps, is the position of Hispanic people, given their relatively poor socio-economic position.

It has been suggested that these findings reflect one or more of a 'protective' Hispanic culture (Frisbie *et al.* 2001); health selection (Jasso *et al.* 2002); or poor data quality, with under-coverage of denominators and inaccuracies in the reporting of numerators (Rosenberg *et al.* 1999). Indeed, there are important limitations linked to the quality of these mortality data for all groups (Hahn 1992). The numerator for the officially

Table 12.5 Race/ethnic inequalities in mortality in the US, 1999

	Non-Hispanic White	Non-Hispanic Black	Hispanic origin	Asian or Pacific Islander	Native American
Infant mortality					
Infant mortality rate (per 1000 live births)	5.8	14.1	5.7	4.8	9.3
Rate ratio vs. non-Hispanic Whites	–	2.43	0.98	0.83	1.60
Younger adult mortality					
Rate (per 100,000) for ages 20–24	78.8	163.0	97.9	48.1	151.8
Rate ratio vs. non-Hispanic Whites	–	2.07	1.24	0.61	1.93
Rate (per 100,000) for ages 40–44	208.0	466.2	192.8	101.7	331.9
Rate ratio vs. non-Hispanic Whites	–	2.24	0.93	0.49	1.60
Rate (per 100,000) for ages 60–64	1225.8	2060.8	913.8	706.2	1379.3
Rate ratio vs. non-Hispanic Whites	–	1.68	0.75	0.58	1.13
Older adult mortality					
Rate (per 100,000) for ages 70–74	2997.8	4227.5	2115.3	1812.5	2785.7
Rate ratio vs. non-Hispanic Whites	–	1.41	0.71	0.60	0.93
Rate (per 100,000) for ages 80–84	7546.4	8702.5	4838.3	4979.3	4770.9
Rate ratio vs. non-Hispanic Whites	–	1.15	0.64	0.66	0.63

Sources: Hoyert *et al.* 2001; Mathews *et al.* 2002.

reported death rates in the US comes from death certificates. Funeral home directors and other officials who record racial status on the death certificate misclassify as many as 26 per cent of self-identified American Indians and 18 per cent of Asians and Pacific Islanders as belonging to a different race, with most of them being misclassified as White (Sorlie *et al.* 1992). There appears to be little misclassification of Blacks and Whites, but 10 per cent of Hispanics are also misclassified as non-Hispanic. This undercount in the numerator suppresses the death rates for these groups and slightly inflates the death rates for Whites.

Problems with the denominator can also affect the quality of mortality statistics (Notes and Comments 1994). Census data are used to calculate the denominators for mortality rates. Using a denominator that has an undercount inflates the obtained rate in exact proportion to the undercount in the denominator. Although the overall undercount for the US population is relatively small, it is much higher for Blacks than Whites, with evaluation based on demographic analysis suggesting that there is a net census undercount of 11–13 per cent for all of the 10-year age groups for Black males between the ages of 25–64 (National Center for Health Statistics 1994). Thus, all of the officially reported morbidity and mortality rates for African American males in these age groups are 11–13 per cent too high. Some evidence suggests that the undercount rate for Hispanics and Indians residing on reservations may be even higher than the undercount for the Black population (Hogan 1993).

However, generally, the heterogeneity in mortality rates parallels heterogeneity in migration, settlement, and socio-economic experiences. This does, of course, point to the need to reflect the diversity of groups in data collection efforts, but also to be aware of, and sensitive to, potential ethnic differences within groups (as described above, we cannot assume that all Pacific Islanders or all Hispanics are equivalent). For example, differences among Hispanic subgroups include median age, immigration history, geographic distribution, fertility and family patterns, health status and mortality rates, income, education levels, and occupational distribution (Sandefur *et al.* 2001).

In the UK, mortality data are not available by ethnic group. Country of birth is recorded on death certificates, but this carries three significant problems. First, and most obvious, it ignores the situation of ethnic minority people born in the UK, whose experiences might be quite different. Second, given forced migration patterns and the artificial construction of national borders after the 'fall' of the British Empire, country of birth groupings do not necessarily reflect ethnic groups (e.g. the heterogeneity of those born in South Asia or India, the large South Asian population who migrated to Britain from the Caribbean). Third, British colonial history means that a significant number of White people were born in ex-colonies and migrated back to Britain after the World War II. And, as for the US, the denominator is calculated from Census data, with evidence of significant under-counting of some ethnic groups.

Although the UK does not have mortality data by ethnicity, there has been a growth in data on ethnic differences in morbidity over the last decade. Figure 12.1, drawn from

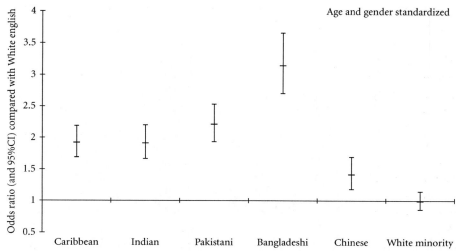

Fig. 12.1 Ethnic differences in reported fair or bad general health in England.

Source: Health Survey for England 1999; see Erens *et al*. 2001.

the 1999 Health Survey for England (Erens *et al*. 2001), shows differences in self-reported health across ethnic groups. It charts the odds ratio and 95% confidence intervals, in comparison with a White English group, for reporting health as fair or bad. Immediately obvious is the heterogeneity in experience across ethnic groups. Most notable is the wide variation for the three South Asian groups—Indian, Pakistani, and Bangladeshi—who are typically treated as one and the same ethnic group in British data (e.g. McKeigue *et al*. 1988; Gupta *et al*. 1995). Again, the diversity in health experience across ethnic minority groups in the UK is paralleled by differences in migration history, patterns of settlement in the UK, and economic experiences, as illustrated earlier.

12.5 Socio-economic patterning of health within and across ethnic groups

It is now reasonably clear that a socio-economic patterning of health is present within ethnic groups in industrialized countries. Figure 12.2 shows all-cause mortality rates over the 16-year follow-up period in the US MRFIT study, stratified by mean income in the area of residence of respondents (individual socio-economic data were not included in the study) (Davey Smith *et al*. 1998). The figure shows a very clear gradient for White and Black men, which is similar for both groups. The extent of the socio-economic inequality in health is shown by the twofold difference in mortality rates between those in the top and bottom income groups for both Black and White men. Table 12.6 shows a marker for morbidity, self-reported fair or poor health, and level of income for Black, Hispanic, and White men and women. Again, there is a clear gradient that is similar for all groups.

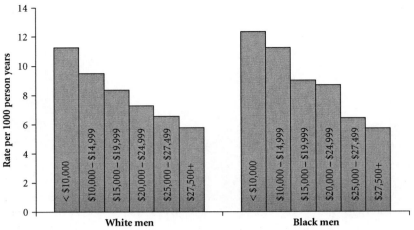

Fig. 12.2 Death rate in the US by median family income in the area of residence.

Source: MRFIT (Multiple Risk Factor Intervention Trial) data.

Table 12.6 Percentage of men and women reporting fair or poor health, by race and income, US, 1995

	Men			Women		
Household income	White	Black	Hispanic	White	Black	Hispanic
Poor	30.5	37.4	26.9	30.2	38.2	30.4
Near poor	21.3	22.6	19.2	17.9	26.1	24.3
Middle income	9.3	13.1	11.9	9.2	14.6	13.5
High income	4.2	5.0	4.8	5.8	9.2	7.0

Poor = below federal poverty level; near poor = less than twice the poverty level; middle income = more than twice poverty level but less than $50,000; high income = $50,000 or more

Source: Pamuk *et al.* 1998.

Figure 12.3 contains data from the Health Survey for England, showing rates of reporting fair or bad health by ethnicity with each of the ethnic groups stratified by income (equivalized tertiles) (Nazroo 2003). As for the US data, Fig. 12.3 shows a clear relationship between reported general health and economic position for each ethnic group. Important here is that both the US and the UK data again point to heterogeneity within broad ethnic groupings. It is misleading to consider, for example, Black Americans to be uniformly disadvantaged in terms of their health; those in better socio-economic positions have better health. There is nothing inevitable, or inherent, in the link between being Black American, Bangladeshi, etc. and a greater risk of mortality and morbidity.

However, the figures also raise the possibility that socio-economic effects do not explain ethnic inequalities in health. For example, Fig. 12.3 shows that for the top and

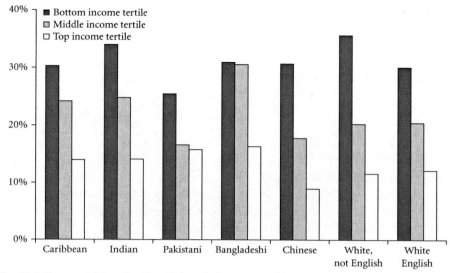

Fig. 12.3 Reported fair or bad health by ethnic group and income tertile in England.

middle-income groups, those in the Bangladeshi group were more likely than those in the White English group to report fair or bad health, and the same is true for differences between Black and White men for many of the income bands in Fig. 12.2 and is particularly obvious for Black and White women and the top and middle-income - groups of Hispanic women in Table 12.6. Although this might suggest that socio-economic factors do not contribute to ethnic inequalities in health, it is important to recognize that the process of standardizing for socio-economic position when making comparisons across groups, particularly ethnic groups, is not as straightforward as it might at first seem.

As Kaufman *et al.* (1997, 1998) point out, the process of standardization is effectively an attempt to deal with the non-random nature of samples used in cross-sectional population studies—controlling for all relevant 'extraneous' explanatory factors introduces the *appearance* of randomization. But, attempting to introduce randomization into cross-sectional studies by adding 'controls' has a number of problems, summarised by Kaufman *et al.* in the following way:

> When considering socioeconomic exposures and making comparisons between racial/ethnic groups . . . the material, behavioral, and psychological circumstances of diverse socioeconomic and racial/ethnic groups are distinct on so many dimensions that no realistic adjustment can plausibly simulate randomization. (Kaufman *et al.* 1998, p. 147)

Evidence from the British Fourth National Survey of Ethnic Minorities illustrates this point clearly. The first part of Table 12.7 shows the mean equivalized household income for individuals within particular classes by ethnic group. Each ethnic group

Table 12.7 Ethnic variations in income within occupational classes in the UK

Mean income by Registrar General's class pounds[1]	White	Indian or African Asian	Pakistani or Bangladeshi	Caribbean
I/II	250	210	125	210
IIINM	185	135	95	145
IIIM	160	120	70	145
IV/V	130	110	65	120

[1] Based on bands of equivalized household income. The mean point of each band is used to make this calculation, which is rounded to the nearest 5.

shows the expected income gradient by occupational class. However, when comparisons are drawn across ethnic groups, the table shows that, within each occupational class, Caribbean and Indian or African Asian people appear to have similar locations, while White people were better off than them, and Pakistani or Bangladeshi people worse off than them. Indeed, comparing the White and Pakistani or Bangladeshi groups shows that, within each occupational class band, those in the Pakistani or Bangladeshi group had on average half the White income, and class I or II Pakistani or Bangladeshi people had an equivalent average income to class IV or V White people. This suggests that using a measure such as Registrar General's class to adjust for socio-economic status is far from adequate for comparisons across ethnic groups, even if this indicator does reflect socio-economic differences within ethnic groups.

Similar findings have been reported in the US (Lillie–Blanton and Laveist 1994; Williams et al. 1994). For example, there are racial differences in the quality of education, income returns for a given level of education or occupational status, wealth or assets associated with a given level of income, the purchasing power of income, the stability of employment, and the health risks associated with occupational status (Williams and Collins 1995). Similarly, Oliver and Shapiro (1995) report that, within occupational groups, White people have higher incomes than Black people; among those below the poverty line, Black people are more likely to remain in this situation than White people; and, within income strata, Black people have considerably lower wealth levels than White people and are less likely to be home owners. The parallels with Table 12.1, which showed data on infant mortality by mother's education status in the US, are striking.

The overall conclusion, then, is that using single or crude indicators of socio-economic position is of little use for 'controlling out' the impact of socio-economic position when attempting to reveal the extent of a 'non-socio-economic' ethnic/race effect. Within any given level of a particular socio-economic indicator, the social circumstances of ethnic minority people in the UK and the US are less favourable than those of White people. This leads to two related problems with approaches that attempt to adjust for socio-economic effects when making comparisons across ethnic groups. The first is that if socio-economic position is simply regarded as a confounding factor that needs to be controlled out to reveal the 'true' relationship between ethnicity and health, data will be presented and interpreted once controls have been applied. This will result in the impact of socio-economic factors becoming obscured and their explanatory role in determining the health of ethnic minority people will be lost. The second is that the presentation of 'standardized' data allows the problems with such data, outlined by Kaufman *et al.* (1997, 1998) and Nazroo (1997*a*, 1998) and illustrated by Table 12.7, to be ignored, leaving both the author and reader to assume that all that is left is an 'ethnic/race' effect, be that cultural or genetic.

Nevertheless, if these cautions are considered, there are some benefits in attempting to control for socio-economic effects. In particular, if controlling for socio-economic effects alters the pattern of ethnic inequalities in health, despite the limitations of the indicators used, we can conclude that at least some of the differences we have uncovered are a result of a socio-economic effect.

These conclusions are supported by Fig. 12.4, which uses data from the 1999 Health Survey for England to show changes in the odds of reporting fair or bad health for ethnic minority groups compared with White English people, before and after the data had been standardized for a variety of socio-economic factors. Comparing the adjusted and unadjusted figures shows a clear and large reduction in odds ratios for most ethnic groups (to give an accurate visual impression of the size of the change in odds, the natural logarithm of the odds ratio compared with White English people is used). Exceptions are the White minority (predominantly Irish) and Indian groups. This

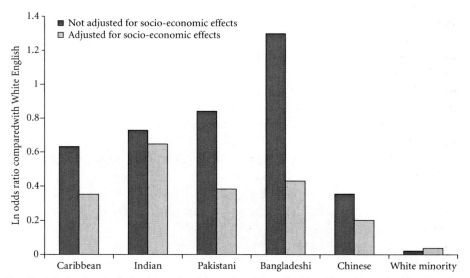

Fig. 12.4 Reduction in (Ln) odds ratio of reporting fair or bad health compared with white English after adjusting for socio-economic effects.

Source: Health Survey for England 1999; see Erens *et al.* 2001.

impression is strengthened if the process is repeated across outcomes as has been shown using data from the British Fourth National Survey (Nazroo 2001, 2003).

Returning to US data, Davey Smith *et al.* (1998) show that standardizing for mean household income in area of residence reduces the relative risk for Black compared with White men for all-cause mortality from 1.47 to 1.19. Conversely, adjusting the Black–White mortality differential for a number of medical risk factors (diastolic blood pressure, serum cholesterol, cigarette smoking, existing diabetes, and prior hospitalization for coronary heart disease) only decreased the relative risk from 1.47 to 1.40 (Davey Smith *et al.* 1998). This demonstrates that socio-economic position—as indexed by income of area of residence—is a considerably more important determinant of Black–White differentials in mortality than biological markers of risk and behavioural factors, such as cigarette smoking or diet (to the extent to which the diet influences serum cholesterol and blood pressure).

So, these data suggest that differences in socio-economic position make a key contribution to ethnic inequalities in health, particularly if we take seriously Kaufman *et al.*'s (1997, 1998) and Nazroo's (1997a, 1998) cautions on the difficulties with making effective adjustments for socio-economic position. It is also worth emphasizing that the analyses shown here simply reflect current socio-economic position: data on the life course and on other forms of social disadvantage were not included and are almost universally not available in existing studies of ethnic inequalities in health. We turn to these issues next.

12.6 Age and the life course

There is growing evidence that socio-economic conditions across the life course can influence current health (Kuh and Ben–Shlomo 1997; see also Chapters 3 and 4 in this volume). This could occur in two ways. First, an early 'exposure', perhaps prenatal (Barker 1991) or in early childhood, might set an adverse biological process in train. For example, low birth weight, which is strongly influenced by adverse material circumstances acting over the lifetime of the mother, is associated with high rates of diabetes, coronary heart disease, respiratory disease, and hypertension in adult life. Similarly, short stature, influenced by nutrition in early life, is related to an increased risk of respiratory and cardiovascular mortality (Kuh and Ben–Shlomo 1997). Second, the impact of socio-economic disadvantage on health might accumulate across the life course—a process that has been referred to as 'weathering' with respect to the health of Black women in the US (Geronimus 1992).

Figure 12.5 uses data from the 1999 Health Survey for England to explore how, in England, the ethnic patterning of reported fair or bad health varies by age group. It suggests relatively small absolute differences at a younger age, with large differences beginning to emerge in the mid 20s and becoming very prominent by the mid 30s. In relative terms, though, the ethnic inequalities in health are prominent at a young age,

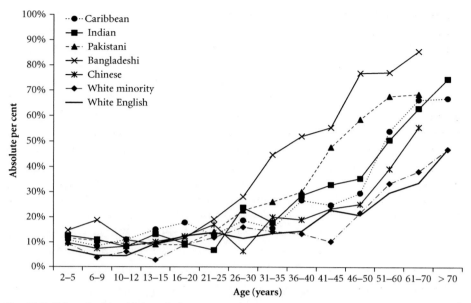

Fig. 12.5 Fair or bad health by ethnic group and age.

Source: Health Survey for England 1999; see Erens *et al.* 2001.

as well as from late 20s onwards, but are more or less absent in teenage years and the early 20s. As described earlier (see Table 12.5), variations in ethnic inequalities in health across the life course are also apparent in US data, but these seem to show a narrowing of differences at older ages and much discussion of possible 'cross-over' effects for Black–White differences (Kestenbaum 1992; Nam 1995), which may be an artefact resulting from poor data quality.

The interpretation of such patterns is not straightforward, but does point to the need for sophisticated approaches to the explanation of the complex patterning of ethnic inequality. In particular, we need to place ethnic inequalities in health within a wide social context. For example, the pattern shown in Fig. 12.5 could reflect a number of co-existing explanations:

- The growth in absolute differences in risk of fair or bad health with increasing age could reflect the accumulation of risk across the life course (weathering).

- The presence of large relative differences in risk of fair or bad health in early and middle to late life could reflect the impact of early life and prenatal differences in risk.

- In the British context, the growth of absolute differences in risk over age could reflect differences between first and second generation migrants, as older people are migrants and younger people second generation. Cross-sectional differences across age groups reported in US data could also reflect cohort effects.

The final point above reminds us of the need to be aware of a number of potential effects related to migration. First, selection into a migrant group will be related to both health and economic capital. Second, the childhood experiences of migrants will be very different from those of the second generation. So, insofar as these lead to long-term adverse health outcomes or to an accumulation of social and health disadvantage, differences in health across generations might be expected. Third, the experience of migration itself will occur alongside social and economic upheavals, which might have a direct impact on health. Fourth, return migration might have a significant impact on the pattern found in the data, with selection into a return migrant group also being related to both health and economic capital. And fifth, the contemporary social and economic experiences of a migrant and non-migrant generation might be quite different, with the non-migrant generation more likely to do well economically (Nazroo 2004) and to have less traditional ethnic identities (Nazroo and Karlsen 2003). On the other hand, experiences of racism appear to be fairly universal across generations and there is growing evidence that these contribute to ethnic inequalities in health.

12.7 Impact of experiences of racial harassment and discrimination on health—the significance of social status?

Experiences of and awareness of racism appears to be central to the lives of ethnic minority people. Eighty per cent of Black respondents in a US study reported experiencing racial discrimination at some time in their lives (Krieger and Sidney 1996). Qualitative investigations of experiences of racial harassment and discrimination in Britain have found that, for many people, experiences of interpersonal racism are a part of everyday life, that the way they lead their lives is constrained by fear of racial harassment, and that being made to feel different is routine and expected (Virdee 1995; Chahal and Julienne 1999).

Experiences of racial harassment and discrimination were investigated quantitatively, in some depth, in the British Fourth National Survey (Virdee 1997). This suggested that more than one in eight ethnic minority people had experienced some form of racial harassment in the past year. Although most of these incidents involved racial insults, many of the respondents reported repeated victimization and as many as a quarter of all of the ethnic minority respondents reported being fearful of racial harassment. This National Survey also showed that, among ethnic minority respondents, there was a widespread belief that employers discriminated against ethnic minority applicants for jobs and widespread experience of such discrimination (Modood 1997). Indeed, when White respondents to the survey were asked about their own racial prejudice, 26 per cent admitted to being prejudiced against South Asian people, 20 per cent to being prejudiced against Caribbean people, and 8 per cent to being prejudiced against Chinese people.

In the few studies that have been conducted, experiences of racial harassment and discrimination appear to be related to health. Laboratory studies reveal that experiences

Table 12.8 Racial harassment, racial discrimination, and risk of fair or poor health (British Fourth National Survey)

	All ethnic minority groups	
	Odds ratio*	95% confidence intervals
Experience of racial harassment		
No attack	1.00	–
Verbal abuse	1.54	1.07–2.21
Physical attack	2.07	1.14–3.76
Perception of discrimination		
Fewer than half of employers discriminate	1.00	–
Most employers discriminate	1.39	1.10–1.76
Occupational class		
Non-manual	1.00	–
Manual	1.44	1.07–1.94
No full-time worker in the household	2.42	1.82–3.22

* Adjusted for gender and age

of discrimination are stressful and produce acute physiological effects (Harrell *et al.* 2003; Clark *et al.* 1999). Population-based studies from the US and elsewhere have shown a relationship between self-reported experiences of racial harassment and a range of health outcomes including hypertension, psychological distress, psychiatric disorders, poorer self-rated health, and days spent unwell in bed (Krieger 2000; Williams and Neighbors 2001; Williams *et al.* 2003). In Britain, analyses of the Fourth National Survey of Ethnic Minorities also suggested a relationship between experiences of racial harassment, perceptions of racial discrimination, and a range of health outcomes across ethnic groups (Karlsen and Nazroo 2002*a,b*). Table 12.8, drawn from these analyses, shows that reporting experiences of racial harassment and perceiving employers to discriminate against ethnic minority people are independently related to likelihood of reporting fair or poor health, and that this relationship is independent of socio-economic effects.

Elsewhere, it has also been shown that fear of racism *per se* also increases risk of reporting fair or poor health by about 60 per cent after adjustments for age, gender, and class (Karlsen and Nazroo 2004). It may be that these findings represent three dimensions of social and economic inequality operating simultaneously: economic disadvantage (as measured by occupational class); a sense of being a member of a devalued, low-status group (British employers discriminate, fear of racism); and the personal insult and stress of being a victim or potential victim of racial harassment.

12.8 Social support, networks, and participation—the significance of ethnic communities?

There is a paradox in the research on African American health that highlights the importance of attending to the cultural strengths and health-enhancing resources that may exist within disadvantaged ethnic populations. African Americans tend to have higher levels of ill health than Whites for most indicators of physical health. At the same time, Blacks tend to have comparable or better mental health than Whites (as measured by rates of clinical depression and other commonly occurring psychiatric disorders). The Epidemiologic Catchment Area Study (ECA), the largest study of psychiatric disorders ever conducted in the US, found very few differences between Blacks and Whites in the rates of both current and lifetime psychiatric disorders (Robins and Regier 1991). Especially striking was the absence of a racial difference in drug use history and the prevalence of alcohol and drug abuse dependence. Similarly, the National Comorbidity Survey (NCS), the first study to use a national probability sample to assess psychiatric disorders in the US, found that Blacks did not have higher rates of disorder than Whites for any of the major classes of disorders (Kessler *et al.* 1994). Instead, lower rates of disorders for Blacks than Whites are especially pronounced for the affective disorders (depression) and the substance abuse disorders (alcohol and drug abuse). Consistent with these mental health data, Blacks have markedly lower rates of suicide than Whites.

Two social institutions—the family and the church—stand out as crucial for the Black population. Strong family ties and an extended family system are important resources that may reduce some of the negative effects of stress on the health of Black Americans. Historically, the Black church was the most important social institution in the Black community. These churches have traditionally been centres of spiritual, social, and political life and may affect mental health in multiple ways. First, African American churches are involved in providing a broad range of social and human services to the African American community (Lincoln and Mamiya 1990; Williams *et al.* 1999). Second, at least some Black churches serve as a conduit to the formal mental health system (Chang *et al.* 1994), and the African American clergy are actively involved in directly providing mental health services to the community (Neighbors *et al.* 1998). Third, congregation-based friendship networks in Black churches function as a type of extended family and provide supportive social relationships to individuals (Taylor and Chatters 1988). Fourth, participation in private and public religious rituals may buffer the negative effects of stress on mental health (Griffith *et al.* 1980, 1984; Gilkes 1980).

In the UK, there is emerging evidence that the establishment of ethnic minority communities in particular geographical areas may carry benefits, despite the high levels of deprivation in these areas. For example, in contrast to the high deprivation scores for areas where ethnic minority people live, described earlier, ethnic minority people perceive the amenities in the areas where they live more positively than White people do (Karlsen *et al.* 2002). This finding appears to reflect the investment that ethnic minority people have made to establish commercial (such as shops) and civic (such as schools, places of worship, community centres) facilities for their communities, and, importantly, this is related to the quality of life of ethnic minority people (Bajekal *et al.* 2004; Grewal *et al.* 2004).

At the same time, recognition of the existence of such resources should not be used to romanticize them as if they were a panacea for a broad range of adverse living conditions. For example, while networks of mutual aid and support may facilitate survival, they are also likely to provide both stress and support. Similarly, even if religious coping is able to shield Blacks from some of the negative psychological consequences of stress, it appears to be unable to cushion the cumulative effects of exposure to chronic stress on a broad range of physical ailments. Importantly, the evidence on residential segregation and health outcomes is mixed, perhaps reflecting the positives and negatives that go with such segregation (Halpern 1993; Halpern and Nazroo 2000; Karlsen *et al.* 2002; Williams and Collins 2001).

12.9 **Conclusion**

In both the US and the UK, there remain ongoing problems with the data available to explore ethnic inequalities in health. Data often do not contain sufficiently detailed information on the ethnicity of respondents to reflect heterogeneity across ethnic groups and heterogeneity within broadly defined ethnic groups. Socio-economic data are either not collected at all, or collected at very crude levels that are plainly inadequate for drawing comparisons across ethnic groups. Those that are collected invariably reflect current position, rather than risks across the life course. And they do not include other dimensions of social inequality, such as experiences of racial harassment and discrimination and geographically based inequalities.

Nevertheless, a large body of convincing evidence now supports the possibility that ethnic inequalities in health are largely a consequence of socio-economic differentials. This applies across a range of ethnic minority groups and a range of outcomes. In addition, there is a growing body of evidence suggesting that experiences of racial harassment and discrimination, and perceptions of living in a discriminatory society, contribute to ethnic inequalities in health. These findings, however, need to be placed within a wider explanatory framework. Here there are two, not mutually exclusive, routes that can be followed.

These findings could be investigated in terms of how they relate to the individual embodiment of social risks. How do such markers of social inequality relate to psychological and biological markers of stress, and how does this translate into disease outcomes? Here the emphasis is on the causal pathways linking 'exposures' to social and economic inequality to disease outcomes. Importantly, the processes involved might vary across ethnic groups, given differences in social context and possible genetic variations across ethnic groups. So, for example, from an epidemiological perspective, it might be fruitful to explore how social inequality translates to hypertension-related diseases for Black American people in the US and Black Caribbean people in the UK, while it translates into cardiovascular disease for Pakistani and Bangladeshi people in the UK.

However, such an approach avoids more fundamental explanations for the health, economic, and social inequalities related to ethnicity. Here, it is important to consider the centrality of racism to any attempt to explain ethnic inequalities in health. Not only are personal experiences of racism and harassment likely to impact on health, but racism as a social force will play a central role in structuring the social and economic disadvantage faced by ethnic minority groups. The socio-economic differences between ethnic groups should not be considered as somehow autonomous (which is a danger of an approach which attempts to examine the extent to which socio-economic differentials 'explain' ethnic differentials in health). As Oliver and Shapiro (1995) demonstrate, the socio-economic disadvantage of Black people in the US is the outcome of a long history of institutional racism and discrimination that has produced the levels of disadvantage which are currently observed. Similarly, while the post-war migration of ethnic minority people into Britain was driven by a shortage of labour, this process, and the socio-economic disadvantage faced by ethnic minority migrants in the UK, was, and continues to be, structured by racism that has its roots in colonial history (Gilroy 1987; Miles 1982).

The concern, then, is that while the tight focus on the pathways that lead from social and economic disadvantage to poor health should contribute greatly to our understanding of aetiology, it may not contribute to our understanding of social inequality. This focus produces an exclusive concern with inequalities *in health* as an adverse outcome, and how the complex pathways leading to this outcome (which might vary across ethnic groups and across disease outcomes) can be understood and broken. The root cause, wider social inequalities, becomes obscured from view. The policy implications of this are clear—the more difficult and dramatic interventions to address social inequalities can continue to be avoided and health promotion can focus on improving our understanding of pathways and designing interventions along them. Inequalities in health become a problem requiring technical interventions tailored to individual diseases and individual circumstances; they become a problem for individuals rather than a reflection of social malaise. Williams *et al.*'s comments in this regard are worth citing:

> There is a temptation to focus on identified risk factors as the focal point for intervention efforts. In contrast, we indicate that the macrosocial factors and racism are the basic causes of racial differences in health. The risk factors and resources are the surface causes, the current intervening mechanisms. These may change, but as long as the basic causes remain operative, the modification of surface causes alone will only lead to the emergence of new intervening mechanisms to maintain the same outcome. (Williams *et al.* 1994, p. 36)

However, understanding the operation of macrosocial factors indicated by Williams *et al.* (1994) and appropriate policy interventions is by no means straightforward. Certainly, there is a need to recognize the overriding importance of national and historical context on the 'making' of ethnic groups; how this is related to economic processes and inequities in this; and how this influences the lives of ethnic minority and migrant populations. Here, comparisons across industrialized nations may particularly help us to understand the underlying social and economic processes.

References

Anderson, M. and Feinberg, S.E. (1995) Black, white, and shades of gray (and brown and yellow). *Chance*, **8(1)**, 15–18.

Bajekal, M., Blane, D., Grewal, I., Karlsen, S., and Nazroo, J. (2004) Ethnic differences in influences on quality of life at older ages: a quantitative analysis. *Ageing and Society*, **24(5)**, 709–28.

Barker, D. (1991) The foetal and infant origins of inequalities in health in Britain. *Journal of Public Health Medicine*, **13**, 64–8.

Bhopal, R. (1997) Is research into ethnicity and health racist, unsound, or important science? *British Medical Journal*, **314**, 1751–6.

Bobo, L. and Zubrinsky, C.M. (1996) Attitudes on residential integration: perceived status differences, mere in-group preference, or racial prejudice? *Social Forces*, **74(3)**, 883–909.

Cell, J. (1982) *The highest stage of white supremacy: the origin of segregation in South Africa and the American South*. New York: Cambridge University Press.

Chahal, K. and Julienne, L. (1999) *We can't all be white!: racist victimisation in the UK*. London: YPS.

Chang, P., Williams, D.R., Griffith, E., and Young, J.L. (1994) Church–agency relationships in the Black community. *Nonprofit and Voluntary Sector Quarterly*, **23(2)**, 91–105.

Clark, R., Anderson, N.B., Clark, V.R., and Williams, D.R. (1999) Racism as a stressor for African Americans: a biopsychosocial model. *American Psychologist*, **54(10)**, 805–16.

Clark, W.A.V. (1992) Residential preferences and residential choices in a multiethnic context. *Demography*, **29**, 451–66.

Cole, R.E. and Deskins Jr., D.R. (1988) Racial factors in site location and employment patterns of Japanese auto firms in America. *California Management Review*, **31(1)**, 9–22.

Cutler, D.M., Glaeser, E.L., and Vigdor, J.L. (1997) Are ghettos good or bad? *Quarterly Journal of Economics*, **112**, 827–72.

Davey Smith, G., Neaton, J.D., Wentworth, D., Stamler, R., and Stamler, J. (1998) Mortality differences between black and white men in the USA: contribution of income and other risk factors among men screened for the MRFIT. *Lancet*, **351**, 934–9.

David, R.J. and Collins Jr., J.W. (1997) Differing birth weight among infants of US-born Blacks, African-born Blacks, and US-born Whites. *New England Journal of Medicine*, **337(17)**, 1209–14.

Department of Health and Human Services (1985) *Report of the Secretary on Black and Minority Health*. Washington, DC: US Department of Health.

Erens, B., Primatesta, P., and Prior, G. (2001) *Health Survey for England 1999: the health of minority ethnic groups*. London: The Stationery Office.

Evinger, S. (1995) How shall we measure our nation's diversity? *Chance*, **8(1)**, 7–14.

Fang, J., Madhavan, S., and Alderman, M.H. (1997) Nativity, race, and mortality: influence of region of birth on mortality of US-born residents of New York City. *Human Biology*, **69(4)**, 533–44.

Fix, M. and Struyk, R.J. (1993) *Clear and convincing evidence: measurement of discrimination in America*. Washington, DC: Urban Institute Press.

Frisbie, W.P., Cho, Y., and Hummer, R. (2001) Immigration and health of Asian and Pacific Islander adults in the United States. *American Journal of Epidemiology*, **153**, 372–80.

Fruchter, R.G., Wright, C., Habenstreit, B., Remy, J.C., Boyce, J.G., and Imperato, P.J. (1985) Screening for cervical and breast cancer among Caribbean immigrants. *Journal of Community Health*, **10(3)**, 121–35.

Geronimus, A.T. (1992) The weathering hypothesis and the health of African-American women and infants: evidence and speculations. *Ethnicity and Disease*, 2, 207–21.

Gilkes, C. (1980) The Black Church as a therapeutic community: suggested areas for research into the Black religious experience. *Journal of Interdenominational Theological Center* 8, 29–44.

Gilroy, P. (1987) *There ain't no black in the Union Jack: the cultural politics of race and nation.* London: Hutchinson.

Glaeser, E.L. and Vigdor, J.L. (2001) *Racial segregation in the 2000 Census: promising news*, Survey series. Washington, DC: The Brookings Institution.

Grewal, I., Nazroo, J., Bajekal, M., Blane, D., and Lewis, J. (2004) Influences on quality of life: a qualitative investigation of ethnic differences among older people in England. *Journal of Ethnic and Migration Studies*, 30(4), 737–61.

Grieco, E.M. and Cassidy, R.C. (2000) *Overview of race and Hispanic origin*. United States Census 2000, US Department of Commerce, Economics, and Statistics Administration.

Griffith, E.E.H., English, T., and Mayfield, V. (1980) Possession, prayer and testimony: therapeutic aspects of the Wednesday night meeting in a Black church. *Psychiatry*, 43, 120–8.

Griffith, E.E.H., Young, J., and Smith, D. (1984) An analysis of the therapeutic elements in a Black church service. *Hospital and Community Psychiatry*, 35, 464–9.

Gupta, S., de Belder, A., and O'Hughes, L. (1995) Avoiding premature coronary deaths in Asians in Britain: spend now on prevention or pay later for treatment. *British Medical Journal*, 311, 1035–6.

Hahn, R.A. (1992) The state of federal health statistics on racial and ethnic groups. *Journal of the American Medical Association* 267(2), 268–71.

Halpern, D. (1993) Minorities and mental health. *Social Science and Medicine*, 36, 597–607.

Halpern, D. and Nazroo, J. (2000) The ethnic density effect: results from a national community survey of England and Wales. *International Journal of Social Psychiatry*, 46(1), 34–46.

Harding, S. and Maxwell, R. (1997) Differences in the mortality of migrants. In: *Health inequalities: decennial supplement Series DS no. 15* (ed. F. Drever and M. Whitehead). London: The Stationery Office.

Harrell, J., Hall, S., and Taliaferro, J. (2003) Physiological responses to racism and discrimination: an assessment of the evidence. *American Journal of Public Health*, 93(2), 243–8.

Hogan, H. (1993) The 1990 post-enumeration survey: operations and results. *Journal of the American Statistical Association*, 88, 1047–57.

Hoyert, D.L., Arias, E., Smith, B.L., Murphy, S.L., and Kochanek, K.D (2001) *Deaths: final data for 1999*. National Vital Statistics Reports, 49(8). National Center for Health Statistics.

Jasso, G., Massey, D.S., Rosenzweig, M.R., and Smith, J.P. (2002) *Immigrant health—selectivity and acculturation*. Paper presented at the National Academy of Science Conference on Racial and Ethnic Disparities in Aging Health, March 2002.

Jaynes, G.D. and Williams, R.M. (1989) *A common destiny: Blacks and American society*. Washington, DC: National Academy Press.

Karlsen, S. and Nazroo, J.Y. (2002a) The relationship between racial discrimination, social class and health among ethnic minority groups. *American Journal of Public Health*, 92, 624–31.

Karlsen, S. and Nazroo, J.Y. (2002b) Agency and structure: the impact of ethnic identity and racism on the health of ethnic minority people. *Sociology of Health and Illness*, 24, 1–20.

Karlsen, S. and Nazroo, J.Y. (2004) Fear of racism and health. *Journal of Epidemiology and Community Health*, 58, 1017–18.

Karlsen, S., Nazroo, J.Y., and Stephenson, R. (2002) Ethnicity, environment and health: putting ethnic inequalities in health in their place. *Social Science and Medicine*, 55(9), 1647–61.

Kaufman, J.S., Cooper, R.S., and McGee, D.L. (1997) Socioeconomic status and health in Blacks and whites: the problem of residual confounding and the resiliency of race. *Epidemiology*, **8(6)**, 621–8.

Kaufman, J.S., Long, A.E., Liao, Y., Cooper, R.S., and McGee, D.L. (1998) The relation between income and mortality in U.S. Blacks and Whites. *Epidemiology*, **9(2)**, 147–55.

Kessler, R.C., McGonagle, K.A., Zhao, S., Nelson, C.B., Hughes, M., Eshleman, S., *et al.* (1994) Lifetime and 12-month prevalence of DSM-III-R psychiatric disorders in the United States. *Archives of General Psychiatry*, **51**, 8–19.

Kestenbaum, B. (1992) A description of the extreme age population based on improved Medicare enrollment data. *Demography*, **29**, 565–80.

Kirschenman, J. and Neckerman, K.M. (1991) 'We'd Love to Hire Them, but . . .': the meaning of race for employers. In: *The urban underclass* (ed. C. Jencks and P.E. Peterson), pp. 203–32. Washington, DC: The Brookings Institution.

Krieger, N. (2000) Discrimination and Health. In: *Social epidemiology* (ed. L. Berkman and I. Kawachi), pp. 36–75. Oxford: Oxford University Press.

Krieger, N. and Sidney, S. (1996) Racial discrimination and blood pressure: the CARDIA study of young Black and White adults. *American Journal of Public Health*, **86(10)**, 1370–8.

Krieger, N., Rowley, D.L., Herman, A.A., Avery, B., and Philips, M.T. (1993) Racism, sexism, and social class: implications for studies of health, disease, and well-being. *American Journal of Preventive Medicine*, **9 (suppl)**, 82–122.

Kuh, D. and Ben–Shlomo, Y. (1997) *A life course approach to chronic disease epidemiology*. Oxford: Oxford University Press.

Lillie–Blanton, M. and Laveist, T. (1996) Race/ethnicity, the social environment, and health. *Social Science and Medicine*, **43(1)**, pp. 83–91.

Lincoln, C.E. and Mamiya, L.H. (1990) *The Black Church in the African American experience*. Durham, North Carolina: Duke University Press.

Lin–Fu, J.S. (1993) Asian and Pacific Islander Americans: an overview of demographic characteristics and health care issues. *Asian and Pacific Islander Journal of Health*, **1**, 20–36.

Marmot, M.G., Adelstein, A.M., Bulusu, L., and OPCS (1984) *Immigrant mortality in England and Wales 1970–78: causes of death by country of birth*. London: HMSO.

Massey, D.S. and Denton, N.A. (1989) Hypersegregation in U.S. metropolitan areas: Black and Hispanic segregation along five dimensions. *Demography*, **26**, 373–92.

Massey, D.S. and Denton, N.A. (1993) *American apartheid: segregation and the making of the underclass*. Cambridge, Massachusetts: Harvard University Press.

Mathews, T.J., MacDorman, M.F., and Menacker, F. (2002) *Infant mortality statistics from the 1999 period linked birth/infant death data set*, National Vital Statistics Reports, 50(4). National Center for Health Statistics.

McKeigue, P., Marmot, M. Syndercombe Court, Y., Cottier, D., Rahman, S., and Riermersma, R. (1988) Diabetes, hyperinsulinaemia, and coronary risk factors in Bangladeshis in East London. *British Heart Journal*, **60**, 390–6.

McLennan, W. and Madden, R. (1999) *The health and welfare of Australia's aboriginal and Torres Strait Islander peoples*. Commonwealth of Australia: Australian Bureau of Statistics.

Miles, R. (1982) *Racism and migrant labour*. Routledge and Kegan Paul.

Modood, T. (1997) Employment. In: *Ethnic minorities in Britain: diversity and disadvantage* (ed. T. Modood, R. Berthoud, J. Lakey, *et al.*). London: Policy Studies Institute.

Nam, C.B. (1995) Another look at mortality crossovers. *Social Biology*, **42**, 133–42.

National Center for Health Statistics (1994) *Vital Statistics of the United States, 1990, Vol. II, Mortality, Part A*. Washington, DC: Public Health Service.

National Center for Health Statistics (2003) *Health, United States*. Hyattsville, Maryland: National Center for Health Statistics.

Navarro, V. (1990) Race or class versus race and class: mortality differentials in the United States. *Lancet*, **336**, 1238–40.

Nazroo, J.Y. (1997*a*) *The health of Britain's ethnic minorities: findings from a national survey*, London: Policy Studies Institute.

Nazroo, J.Y. (1997*b*) *Ethnicity and mental health: findings from a national community survey*. London: Policy Studies Institute.

Nazroo, J.Y. (1998) Genetic, cultural or socio-economic vulnerability? Explaining ethnic inequalities in health. *Sociology of Health and Illness*, **20(5)**, 710–30.

Nazroo, J.Y. (2001) *Ethnicity, class and health*. London: Policy Studies Institute.

Nazroo, J. (2003) The structuring of ethnic inequalities in health: economic position, racial discrimination and racism. *American Journal of Public Health*, **93(2)**, 277–84.

Nazroo, J. (2004) Ethnic disparities in aging health: what can we learn from the United Kingdom? In: *Critical perspectives on racial and ethnic differentials in health in late life* (ed. N. Anderson, R. Bulatao, and B. Cohen), pp. 677–702. Washington, DC: National Academies Press.

Nazroo, J.Y. and Karlsen, S. (2003) Patterns of identity among ethnic minority people: diversity and commonality. *Ethnic and Racial Studies*, **26(5)**, 902–30.

Neckerman, K.M. and Kirschenman, J. (1991) Hiring strategies, racial bias, and inner-city workers. *Social Problems*, **38**, 433–47.

Neighbors, H.W., Musick, M.A., and Williams, D.R. (1998) The African American minister as a source of help for serious personal crises: bridge or barrier to mental health care? *Health Education and Behavior*, **25(6)**, 759–77.

Nobles, M. (2000) History counts: a comparative analysis of racial/color categorization in US and Brazilian censuses. *American Journal of Public Health*, **50(11)**, 1738–45.

Norton, I.M. and Manson, S.P. (1996) Research in American Indian and Alaskan Native communities: navigating the cultural universe of values and process. *Journal of Consulting and Clinical Psychology*, **65(5)**, 856–60.

Notes and Comments (1994) Census undercount and the quality of health data for racial and ethnic populations. *Ethnicity and Disease*, **4(1)**, 98–100.

Office of Management and Budget (1978) *U.S. Directive No. 15: Race and Ethnic Standards for Federal Statistics and Administrative Reporting*. Washington, DC: Office of Federal Statistical Policy and Standards, U.S. Department of Commerce.

Oliver, M.L. and Shapiro, T.M. (1995) *Black wealth/white wealth: a new perspective on racial inequality*. New York: Routledge.

Orfield, G. (1996) The growth of segregation: African Americans, Latinos, and unequal education. In: *Dismantling desegregation: the quiet reversal of Brown V. Board of Education* (ed. G, Orfield and S.E. Eaton), pp. 53–71. New York: The New Press.

Owen, D. (1992). *Ethnic minorities in Great Britain: settlement patterns, national ethnic minority data archive 1991. Census statistical paper no.1*. University of Warwick: Centre for Research in Ethnic Relations.

Owen, D. (1994). Spatial variations in ethnic minority groups populations in Great Britain. *Population Trends*, **78**, 23–33.

Pamuk, E., Makuc, D., Heck, K., Reuben, C., and Lochner, K. (1998) *Socioeconomic status and health chartbook. Health, United States, 1998*. Hyattsville, Maryland: National Center for Health Statistics.

Pan American Health Organization (June 2001) *Equity in health: from an ethnic perspective.* Washington, DC: Pan American Health Organization.

Polednak, A.P. (1989) *Racial and ethnic differences in disease.* New York: Oxford University Press.

Robins, L.N. and Regier, D.A. (1991) *Psychiatric disorders in America: the epidemiologic catchment area study.* New York: Free Press.

Rogers, R. (1992) Living and dying in the USA: sociodemographic determinants of death among blacks and whites. *Demography,* **29(2),** 287–303.

Rogot, E., Sorlie, P.D., Johnson, N.J., and Schmitt, C. (1993) *A mortality study of 1.3 million persons by demographic, social and economic factors: 1979–1985. Follow-up, US National Longitudinal Mortality Study.* Washington: NIH.

Rosenberg, H.M., Maurer, J.D., Sorlie, P.D., Johnson, N.J., MacDorman, M.F., Hoyert, D.L., et al. (1999) Quality of death rates by race and Hispanic origin: a summary of current research. *Vital Health Statistics,* **2(128).** National Center for Health Statistics

Rudat, K. (1994) *Black and minority ethnic groups in England: health and lifestyles.* London: Health Education Authority.

Sampson, R.J. and Wilson, W.J. (1995) Toward a theory of race, crime, and urban inequality. In: *Crime and inequality* (ed. J. Hagan and R.D. Peterson) pp. 37–54. Stanford, CA: Stanford University Press.

Sandefur, G.D., Martin, M.A., Eggerling–Boeck, J., Mannon, S., and Meier, A. (2001) An overview of racial and ethnic demographic trends. In: *America becoming: racial trends and their consequences* (ed. N.J. Smelser, W.J. Wilson, and F. Mitchell). Washington, DC: National Academy Press.

Sheldon, T.A. and Parker, H. (1992) Race and ethnicity in health research. *Journal of Public Health Medicine,* **14(2),** 104–10.

Shihadeh, E.S. and Flynn, N. (1996) Segregation and crime: the effect of Black social isolation on the rates of Black urban violence. *Social Forces,* **74(4),** 1325–52.

Sidiropoulos, E., Jeffery, A., Mackay, S., Forgey, H., Chipps, C., and Corrigan, T. (1997) *South Africa Survey 1996/97.* Johannesburg: South African Institute of Race Relations.

Smaje, C. (1996) The ethnic patterning of health: new directions for theory and research. *Sociology of Health and Illness,* **18(2),** 139–71.

Soni Raleigh, V. and Balarajan, R. (1992) Suicide and self-burning among Indians and West Indians in England and Wales. *British Journal of Psychiatry,* **161,** 365–8.

Sorlie, P.D., Backlund, E., Johnson, N.J., and Rogot, E. (1993) Mortality by Hispanic status in the United States. *Journal of the American Medical Association,* **270,** 2464–8.

Sorlie, P.D., Backlund, E., and Keller, J. (1995) U.S. mortality by economic, demographic and social characteristics: the Natioanl Longitudinal Mortality Study. *American Journal of Public Health,* **85,** 949–56.

Sorlie P., Rogot, E., Anderson, R., Johnson, N.J., and Backlund, E. (1992) Black–white mortality differences by family income. *Lancet,* **340,** 346–50.

Stewart, J.A, Dundas, R., Howard, R.A., Rudd, A.G., and Woolfe, C.D.A. (1999) Ethnic differences in incidence of stroke: prospective study with stroke register. *British Medical Journal,* **318,** 967–71.

Taylor, R.J. and Chatters, L.M. (1988) Church members as a source of informal social support. *Review of Religious Research,* **30,** 193–203.

Turner, M.A. (1993) Limits on neighborhood choice: evidence of racial and ethnic steering in urban housing markets. In: *Clear and convincing evidence: measurement of discrimination in America,* (ed. M. Fix and R.J. Struyk), pp. 117–52. Washington, DC: The Urban Institute Press.

Vega, W.A. and Amaro, H. (1994) Latino outlook: good health, uncertain prognosis. *Annual Review of Public Health,* **15,** 39–67.

Virdee, S. (1995) *Racial violence and harassment*. London: Policy Studies Institute.

Virdee, S. (1997) Racial harassment. In: *Ethnic minorities in Britain: diversity and disadvantage* (ed. T. Modood, R. Berthoud, J. Lakey, *et al.*). London: Policy Studies Institute.

Wild, S. and McKeigue, P. (1997) Cross sectional analysis of mortality by country of birth in England and Wales. *British Medical Journal*, **314**, 705–10.

Williams, D.R. (1997) Race and health: basic questions, emerging directions. *Annals of Epidemiology*, **7(5)**, 322–33.

Williams, D.R. (1999) Race, SES, and health: the added effects of racism and discrimination. *Annals of the New York Academy of Sciences*, **896**, 173–88.

Williams, D.R. (2001) Racial variations in adult health status: patterns, paradoxes and prospects. In: *America becoming: racial trends and their consequences* (ed. N.J. Smelser, W.J. Wilson, and F. Mitchell), Washington, DC: National Academy Press.

Williams, D.R. and Collins, C. (1995) U.S. socioeconomic and racial differences in health. *Annual Review of Sociology*, **21**, 349–86.

Williams, D.R. and Collins, C. (2001) Racial residential segregation: a fundamental cause of racial disparities in health. *Public Health Reports*, **116**, 404–16.

Williams, D.R. and Neighbors, H.W. (2001) Racism, discrimination and hypertension: evidence and needed research. *Ethnicity & Disease*, **11**, 800–16.

Williams, D.R., Griffith, E.E.H., Young, J., Collins, C., and Dodson, J. (1999) Structure and provision of services in New Haven Black churches. *Cultural Diversity and Ethnic Minority Psychology*, **5(2)**, 118–33.

Williams, D.R., Lavizzo–Mourey, R., and Warren, R.C. (1994) The concept of race and health status in America. *Public Health Reports*, **109(1)**, 26–41.

Williams, D.R., Neighbors, H.W., and Jackson, J.S. (2003) Racial/ethnic discrimination and health: findings from community studies. *American Journal of Public Health*, **93(2)**, 200–8.

Wilson, W.J. (1987) *The truly disadvantaged*. Chicago: University of Chicago Press.

Wilson, W.J. (1996) *When work disappears: the world of the new urban poor*. New York: Alfred A. Knopf.

Chapter 13

Social determinants of health in older age

Anne McMunn, Elizabeth Breeze, Alissa Goodman, James Nazroo, and Zoe Oldfield

13.1 Introduction

This chapter focuses on the social determinants of health (both physical and mental) and disability among older people. Rapid increase in life expectancy, coupled with declining fertility rates during the last century, has meant that older people make up a growing proportion of the population. For example, by 2020, the over-50s will constitute nearly 40% of the British population, and by 2040, almost 30% will be aged 60 or over (Government Actuaries Department 2002). Over the first part of the twentieth century, increases in life expectancy were concentrated among children and younger adults as improvements in nutrition and public health reduced the incidence of infectious illnesses. From about the 1970s, life expectancy began to increase more for those aged 55 and older, perhaps because of improvements in medical care or perhaps as a result of living in healthier conditions during early life (Marmot and Nazroo 2001).

This phenomenon of an 'ageing population' has led to policy concerns about the potential impact of changing dependency ratios and increasing disability trends on health and social services. For example, by 2031, in the UK, there will be 2.5 persons of working age for every person of pensionable age, compared to 3.4 in 2002. However, in addition to changes in the age structure of the population, the dynamics of ageing appear also to be changing. For example, the compression of morbidity hypothesis (Fries 1980, 1989; Fries and Grapo 1981) predicts that levels of morbidity are falling more rapidly than mortality in the US, resulting in an older, but healthier population. There is some cross-sectional data to support this hypothesis (Bebbington 1991; Manton *et al.* 1997; Singer and Manton 1998; Spillman 2004; Waidmann and Manton 1998); although, without longitudinal data, it is impossible to do more than speculate on changing patterns of disability and the causal forces that might underlie cross-sectional shifts.

In the US, the concept of 'successful ageing' (Rowe and Kahn 1998) has emerged as a response to the traditional stereotypes of ageing as associated with inevitable sickness and decline. Rowe and Kahn define successful ageing as the absence of disease or disability, the maintenance of cognitive and physical function, and engagement with life (meaning engagement both with other people and in productive labour). Their main emphasis is that successful ageing is within the control of individuals through lifestyle choices and health behaviour. In the UK, the theory of the 'third age' (Laslett 1989) portrays later life as potentially a period of self-fulfilment in which individuals are freed from the responsibilities of paid work and childcare to plan their lives and to pursue those plans.

However, the ideas of successful ageing and the third age are predicated on access to wealth and health in older age, without acknowledgment of economic or health inequalities among older people (Bury 1995). The experience of healthy, active ageing is by no means uniform, nor random. For example, for the period 1997–1999, life expectancy for men in a social class I occupation at age 65 (at 17.5 years) was 30% longer than for men in a social class V occupation (Donkin *et al.* 2002).

In addition to inequalities in life expectancy, it is possible that the hypothesized compression in morbidity is occurring for some population groups but not for others. Melzer and colleagues (2000) have shown marked differences by occupational class in expected life free of disability for both men and women in the 65–69 age group. The UK government has espoused greater independence among older people at least since 1998 (Department of Health 1998). A crucial policy question, therefore, is which sections of the older population will live healthy active lives and which will be dependent on formal and informal sources of support in order to undertake activities of daily living. To answer this, we need to understand how inequalities in health are distributed in the older population and what the underlying processes are.

This chapter first reviews research on social and economic inequalities in health in older ages, concluding that much of the work on inequalities in older age has focused on documenting differences rather than testing theories as to what the generative mechanisms may be. The chapter then discusses several of the specific social determinants that may contribute to these inequalities, either as aspects of socio-economic position or as mediators on the pathway between socio-economic position and health. While secular changes in longevity and a potential simultaneous compression of morbidity are related to the topic of social determinants of health among older people, the factors that underlie these secular changes are not a focus of this chapter.

13.2 Inequalities in health at older ages: evidence from Europe and North America

The large body of empirical and theoretical work on health inequalities has been characterized by an 'employment bias' (Dahl and Birkelund 1997) as, since the 1980 Black Report (Townsend and Davidson 1982), this debate has primarily focused on the working age population (Feinstein 1993; Fox 1989; Whitehead 1987). Research into the relationships between socio-economic position and health in older age began a decade or two after studies of health inequalities in the working age population (Arber and Ginn 1993; Dahl and Birkelund 1997). The results of studies of health inequalities in older age have been somewhat less consistent than findings for working age individuals, particularly in studies using occupational class as a measure of social position. Studies in the US have tended to examine education and/or income inequalities, while British studies have preferred to focus mainly on occupational class. This section reviews studies of inequalities in health in older age, many of which suggest continuing socio-economic inequalities in health and functioning in older age, although with reductions in the size of this difference with increasing age.

13.2.1 Education

The most consistent relationship among studies in the US is that educational attainment is inversely related to physical disability in older age in both cross-sectional (Berkman and Gurland 1998; Longino *et al.* 1989; Ross and Wu 1996; Smith and Kington 1997) and longitudinal (Guralnik and Simonsick 1993; Harris *et al.* 1989; Hubert *et al.* 1993; Liao *et al.* 1999; Maddox and Clark 1992; Maddox *et al.* 1994; Palmore *et al.* 1985; Strawbridge *et al.* 1996) studies, after adjusting for functioning at baseline and, in some cases, other socio-economic indicators. This finding is further supported by evidence from cross-sectional studies in Finland (Rautio *et al.* 2001; Sakari–Rantala *et al.* 1995) and Italy (Amaducci *et al.* 1998), as well as a two-year follow-up study in Spain (Beland and Zunzunegui 1999). Indeed, only one longitudinal study, conducted in Spain (Beland and Zunzunegui 1999), showed that the relationship between education and functional decline over the subsequent two years among those aged 65 and over was explained by health status at baseline.

Longitudinal studies examining the relationship between education and successful ageing in North America have been contradictory. For example, Roos and Havens (1991) found that neither occupation, education, nor income at baseline predicted successful ageing (defined as not being in an institution, not reporting dependency on an ADL, rating their health as excellent to fair, and having good mental health) after 12 years of follow-up among men and women in the Manitoba Longitudinal Study of Ageing. Conversely, in the Honolulu Heart Program, both education and previous occupation were associated with successful ageing (defined as absence of life-threatening illness and maintenance of physical and mental functioning) among those aged 45–68 at baseline after 15 and 25 years of follow-up respectively (Reed *et al.* 1998). This was after adjusting for baseline smoking, biological measures, and number of years spent in Japan. Of course, the differences in the results of these two studies may be due to their differing definitions of successful ageing.

In addition, a few cross-sectional studies in Europe and Canada have shown relationships between health outcomes other than physical functioning are also associated with educational attainment among older people, such as self-reported health (Cairney 2000; Cairney and Arnold 1996; Reijneveld and Gunning–Schepers 1995;

Veenstra 2000) (although one study showed that this relationship declined with older-age cohorts in relative terms), cognition in older age (Rautio *et al.* 2001; Steel *et al.* 2003), as well as certain dimensions of the SF-20 (Kempen *et al.* 1999) or SF-36 (Regidor *et al.* 1999).

13.2.2 Occupational class

Cross-sectional studies in Britain and mainland Europe have documented relationships between occupational class and self-reported health (Arber and Ginn 1993; Damian *et al.* 1999; Falaschetti *et al.* 2002; McMunn *et al.* 2003; Rakhonen and Takala 1998; Thorslund and Lundberg 1994; Victor 1989, 1991), reported physical disability (Arber and Ginn 1993; Blaxter 1990; Hirani and Malbut 2002; Parker *et al.* 1994; Rakhonen and Takala 1998; Steel *et al.* 2003), limiting longstanding illness (McMunn *et al.* 2003; Rakhonen and Takala 1998; Victor 1989, 1991); and, in one case, physical functioning based on performance measures (Parker *et al.* 1994) in older age.

Swain (1993) studied class inequalities in health among older people longitudinally, following-up men and women from the Health and Lifestyles Study (HALS) seven years after their first interview. Among those who had been 60 or over at baseline, being in a manual class household carried a disadvantage in reporting poor health seven years later regardless of health at baseline. Several European cross-sectional studies have also documented a relationship between class and cardiovascular disease in older people (Brown *et al.* 1957; McMunn *et al.* 2003; Thorslund and Lundberg 1994). However, not all studies have found relationships between class and health. Taylor and Ford (1983) examined social class differences in a host of self-reported outcomes in a sample of over 600 men and women in Aberdeen aged 60 and over and found that gender and age accounted for class differences in reported chronic conditions, acute symptoms, and self-reported poor health. They did not find class differences in reported difficulties in functioning, self-esteem, or morale. In a national sample of Italians aged 65 to 84, farmers were more likely than other workers to report limitation on adjusted for disability life years (ADLs), but there were no differences between those who had been manual or non-manual workers (Amaducci *et al.* 1998). Also, some studies have documented gender differences in the class–health relationship. In Norway, men aged 65 or over, whose main job was manual, were more likely than non-manual workers to have poor mental health; while the study found no association between class of main occupation and mental health for women aged 65 and older (Dahl and Birkelund 1997).

In the case of occupational class, several studies have also found that these relationships decline with age, with respect to both self-reported health (Damian *et al.* 1999) and physical disability (Blaxter 1990; Steel *et al.* 2003), in both absolute and relative terms. This association may decline in older age groups due to a survivor effect related to selective mortality. Additionally, the declining association between class and health with age raises questions about the use of occupation-based measures of social position in older age, something that has long been identified as a methodological problem for studying inequalities in health among women (for example, see Kreiger *et al.* 1999; Macran *et al.* 1994; Martikainen 1995) due to lower levels of female labour force participation and persistent occupational downgrading after childbearing (Dex 1987). Most studies of older people have dealt with this issue by using the last or main occupational class of individuals, or the head of household or spouse in the case of married women.

As an illustration of the problem of using occupation-based measures of socio-economic position after working age, analysis of the first Whitehall study of British civil servants (of men aged 40–69 when first studied) showed that the power of occupational grade to predict mortality declined quite dramatically after retirement, while the predictive power of car access declined much less after retirement (Marmot and Shipley 1996). This suggests that different aspects of socio-economic position are important for pre-retirement mortality (both the specific effects of position in the occupational hierarchy and more general socio-economic factors) than are important for post-retirement mortality, where, perhaps, the specific effects of work diminish but other influences related to socio-economic position remain important. However, further work on the first Whitehall cohort has shown that occupational grade strongly predicted functioning in older age (Breeze *et al.* 2001).

13.2.3 Income and wealth

Many studies in the US have examined relationships between material circumstances, particularly income, and health or functioning in older age. When material circumstances have been considered in Britain, studies have tended to focus on housing tenure rather than income, with a few exceptions. Looking at respondents aged 65 and over in the General Household Survey (GHS), Arber and Ginn (1993) found that current household income was inversely associated with both self-reported poor health and functioning after adjusting for other socio-economic factors. Living in rented rather than owned accommodation or being without a car in the household were each accompanied by greater risk of poor health. Poor functioning was associated with being in rented accommodation for women and with lacking a car for men.

One longitudinal study of material circumstances and health among older people in Britain was conducted using the British Household Panel Survey (BHPS) (Salas 2002). Among those who were aged 60 and over at baseline in 1991, income predicted self-reported health four years later among men and car ownership predicted self-reported health four years later for women, after adjusting for other socio-economic factors. Tenure did not predict self-reported health four years later after adjustments. Analysis of the Longitudinal Study showed that tenure and access to a car in late middle and early old age predicted limiting longstanding illness 20 years later (Breeze *et al.* 1999). In other European countries, lower income has generally been shown to accompany worse health outcomes in older age (Beland and Zunzunegui 1999; Dahl and Birkelund

1997; Martelin 1994; Rautio *et al.* 2001), although one Finnish study showed that income was not significantly associated with mobility after adjusting for other indicators of health status and living arrangements (Sakari–Rantala *et al.* 1995).

In North America, several cross-sectional studies have found household income to be positively associated with functioning (as well as self-reported health in two studies and life satisfaction in one study) in older respondents, after adjusting for numerous factors (Berkman and Gurlund 1998; Cairney 2000; Forbes *et al.* 1991; Newacheck *et al.* 1980; Smith and Kington 1997; Usui *et al.* 1985; Veenstra 2000). In addition, many American longitudinal studies have shown relationships between income and later-life functioning (Guralnik and Kaplan 1989; Guralnik and Simonsick 1993; Strawbridge *et al.* 1996), although results from some studies have been mixed. For example, Palmore and colleagues (1985) found that low individual income was associated with a decline in mental functioning, but not in physical functioning, over a 10-year period, among those in their early 70s or older at baseline. In the Alameda County study, among those aged 50 to 89 at baseline, lower income predicted incident mobility problems, but not incident self-care problems, over 10 years of follow-up, adjusting for gender, age, social isolation, smoking, weight, and depression at baseline (Kaplan 1992). In a 10-year follow-up of those aged 50 to 77 in the 1971 US National Health and Nutrition Examination Survey (NHANES), lower family income predicted onset of disability (adjusting for education), but only for men (Hubert *et al.* 1993).

Other studies have found no relationship between poverty and functioning. For example, in the Longitudinal Study of Ageing (Rogers *et al.* 1992), poverty was not associated with disability at baseline or onset of disability over two years in those aged 70 and over at baseline. In the Longitudinal Retirement History Study, in which five interviews were conducted over 10 years, poverty did not consistently predict onset of functional impairment over the subsequent two years, but impairment did consistently predict onset of poverty among those who were employed and aged 58 to 63 years (and unmarried in the case of women) at baseline, suggesting reverse causation in the relationship between material circumstances and functioning (Maddox *et al.* 1994).

Although many American studies have focused on income inequalities in health (as well as health effects on income), far fewer have focused on wealth. As with the use of occupational class as a measure of social position, income is problematic as a measure of economic position among retirees whose earnings are low, but whose wealth, and therefore consumption, may be high. For older individuals, accumulated wealth is generally a more useful indicator of lifetime economic status, as well as of economic resources to draw on, than income. Robert and House (1996) found that liquid financial assets and tenure were better predictors of functional health among those aged 65 to 84, and assets were a better predictor of number of chronic illnesses among those aged 75 to 84, than education or income (own or spouses), although wealth was not a better predictor of self-reported health than education or income among older people.

In the UK, studies of wealth inequalities in health have been rare, not least because of a lack of available data. The English Longitudinal Study of Ageing (ELSA) (Marmot *et al.* 2003)—a panel study of a representative sample of people aged 50 and over in England—is the first study in the UK to include detailed measures of wealth, income, and health. Results from ELSA show a strong wealth gradient in the likelihood of reporting poor health among those aged 50 and over, with median wealth for those reporting good health around three times that of those reporting fair or poor health which persists at all ages (Banks *et al.* 2003). Again, these relationships are cross-sectional and only when future waves of ELSA are available can the investigation of causal directions begin. However, other studies have shown that, even when controlling for individuals' initial health state, their position in the wealth distribution is an important determinant of their subsequent mortality (Attanasio and Emmerson 2003).

As well as providing a comprehensive measure of wealth amongst the elderly, the emergence of ELSA has meant that direct comparisons of the relationship between material circumstances and health in older age can be made between England and the US using the Health and Retirement Study (HRS), which formed the basis for much of ELSA. Figure 13.1 shows unpublished analysis using the first wave of ELSA (2002) and the 2000 wave of HRS. The figure shows the percentage of individuals aged 60–74 years who report excellent or very good health, by financial wealth decile. As well as showing a clear, positive relationship between good health and financial wealth, it also reveals that the gradients in self-reported health in the two countries are very similar despite their markedly different health care and welfare systems.

In summary, a large number of studies reviewed here suggest continuing socio-economic inequalities in health and functioning into older ages, although in relative terms they may be smaller than at younger ages. This evidence documents structural

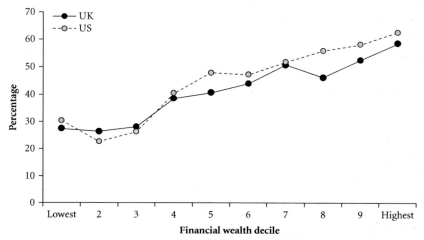

Fig. 13.1 Percentage of individuals aged 60–74 reporting excellent or very good health, by financial wealth decile.

inequalities based on occupational class, education, and income, but does little to elucidate the mechanisms behind these inequalities. They may signify structural constraints in more specific social determinants of health, such as material circumstances, social integration, or control over the environment. This chapter now turns to some of the specific social determinants of health that may underlie health inequalities generally, and discusses how they may apply to inequalities among older people specifically.

13.3 A life-course perspective on health in older age

13.3.1 Early vs. adult determinants of health in older age

In the context of thinking about social determinants of health in older age, one question that comes to mind is the relative importance of current circumstances as compared with circumstances earlier in life. For example, if social and environmental stress affect health through biological pathways (see Chapter 2), when in the life course, and for what durations, is this stress most influential? Research on the British birth cohorts and the Whitehall II study have led to the development of at least three models of relationships between early life influences and health in older adults.

- Life-course hypotheses emphasize the accumulation of advantage and disadvantage across the entire life course (Brunner *et al.* 1999; Kuh *et al.* 1997; Power and Hertzman 1997).

- A second model describes a latency effect whereby exposures early in life, including in utero, have later effects on health (Barker 1994, 1995; Marmot and Wadsworth 1997).

- A third model suggests that there is no direct effect of social circumstances from earlier life on health in later life, but that such circumstances determine the social and economic position that a person reaches in later life, and it is the factors attendant on socio-economic position in later life acting concurrently that affect health (Marmot *et al.* 2001).

These models of pathways between circumstances in early life and health in older age (discussed in Chapter 3), each of which may be accurate and inter-relate, suggest the need for long-term detailed longitudinal studies of individuals. In particular, for policy purposes, it is important to know whether there are modifiable factors in later life that still influence health inequalities in old age. The British birth cohort studies are likely to provide valuable information on the relative importance of early vs. later life influences on morbidity and mortality in older age. Analysis of the 1946 cohort has shown childhood social class to be an independent predictor of adult obesity at age 53 (Hardy *et al.* 2000; Langenberg *et al.* 2003). Alternatively, analysis of women in the same cohort has shown that neither childhood social class, nor education was associated with self-reported health at age 54, but adult social class was (McMunn 2004).

However, men and women born in 1946 (the oldest of the British birth cohorts) are only just beginning to reach the age groups with which we are concerned. In the main, we must currently look to other data sources to address questions regarding the influence of social determinants across the life course on health in older age. In investigating Barker's in utero programming hypothesis, Koupilova and colleagues (1997) found a clear inverse relationship between birth weight and hypertension at age 70 in men above median height, but not in those below median height. Evidence from the West of Scotland Collaborative Study (reviewed in Chapter 4), for which 21 years of follow-up mortality data are available on about 5500 male employees aged 35–64 at baseline from a representative range of workplaces, supported a cumulative life-course model (Davey Smith et al. 1997). Respondents were categorized according to the number of times, between zero and three, they were assigned a manual class occupation, based on father's occupation, social class of first occupation, and occupational class during later adulthood. All-cause mortality, systolic and diastolic blood pressure, serum choles-terol, height, body mass index, lung function, as well as symptomatic angina and chronic bronchitis, were all related in a graded, stepwise fashion to this measure of cumulative lifetime social class. Adjustment for a range of behavioural and physiological risk factors only modestly attenuated this relationship with respect to mortality.

Further analysis of the West of Scotland Collaborative Study showed that various phases of the life course varied in their importance for different diseases and causes of death (Davey Smith et al. 1998). Deaths due to cancer (apart from stomach), coronary heart disease, and respiratory disease, as well as behavioural and physiological risk factors, were shown to be related to adult, and not to childhood, social class. Conversely, stroke and stomach cancer mortality, as well as body mass index (BMI), were associated most strongly with childhood socio-economic circumstances (consistent with the findings from the 1946 cohort).

In the US, the National Longitudinal Survey of Labour Market Experience of Mature Men (NLS) (reviewed in Chapter 4)—a panel study of about 5000 men aged 45–59 in 1966, followed up to 1983—found that controlling for education largely eliminated the association seen between father's occupation and later mortality risk (Mare 1990). Also, further analysis suggested that the influence of education on later mortality worked through the wealth associated with occupational position in adulthood that was made possible by educational attainment, suggesting that the influence of early circumstances was transmitted mainly through later experiences. A Norwegian study found that economic hardship in childhood was a predictor of serious illness in old age for men after adjusting for own adult social class (Dahl and Birkelund 1997). Also, the Level of Living Survey in Sweden followed over 500 men and women from 1968 to 1991 and found that education predicted self-reported physical functioning among those aged 76 and over at follow-up (Parker et al. 1994). Education also predicted outcomes on physical performance tests for men, but not for women.

Taken together, these studies show education to be a potentially important determinant of health status in later life, probably in the establishment of subsequent social and economic trajectories, but also potentially through the promotion of healthy behaviours and by increasing options (as well as awareness of options) for dealing with ill health and stress. It is clear that there have been dramatic increases in educational attainment in the UK over the past half century. Analysis of the British birth cohorts has shown that successive cohorts of Britons have faced, on average, better opportunities for education than their own parents, particularly their mothers. For example, 16% of the 1946 cohort obtained a diploma, degree, or higher educational qualification compared with 26% of the 1958 cohort and 36% of the 1970 cohort (Makepeace *et al.* 2003). Initially, these secular increases in educational attainment included dramatic gender divisions in education. However, women's educational attainment in the UK grew dramatically over the 1970s, and particularly in the 1980s, so that by the end of the 1980s they had caught up with men, reducing gender differences in human capital (Corti *et al.* 1995; Crompton 1993; Dale and Egerton 1995; Joshi *et al.* 1999). As the British birth cohorts age, it will be interesting to see whether secular increases and decreasing gender divisions in educational attainment will leave a small but clearly disadvantaged low-attainment group, with decreasing gender differences in levels of morbidity or functional impairment in older age, or whether the mechanisms driving these inequalities will vary by cohort. Recent work examining changes in educational attainment between the 1958 and 1970 cohorts (Machin and Vignoles 2004) suggests that increases in educational participation between these two cohorts were disproportionately concentrated among those from more advantaged backgrounds in terms of income and class, therefore increasing rather than decreasing inequality.

13.3.2 Retirement as a key transition period in older age

In addition to education, retirement stands out as a key period of transition when thinking about social determinants of health in older age. The nature of retirement is increasingly blurred as pathways to retirement and the age at which retirement occurs become more diverse. Many OECD countries have been experiencing a trend towards earlier labour market exits among older, particularly male workers. This trend is striking to the extent that, for the majority of men, the 'statutory' retirement age is no longer relevant for many retirement decisions. For instance, cross-sectional analysis of the first wave of ELSA has shown that the majority of people up to five years younger than the state pension age are not in paid work and rates of labour force participation are lowest at both ends of the wealth spectrum; high rates for inactivity are found for both the wealthiest individuals and for those in the lowest wealth groups (Banks and Casanova 2003).

The nature of one's labour market exit appears to be linked with subsequent health outcomes. In Sweden, those who became unemployed were more likely to have a subsequent hospitalization, after adjusting for previous hospitalization and health at work (Hyde *et al.* 2004*b*). Conversely, among Whitehall II participants, the better subsequent health of those who took voluntary redundancy or voluntary early retirement was explained by pre-retirement health in the case of the former and occupational grade in the case of the latter (Hyde *et al.* 2004*a*). Nationally representative, longitudinal data on the health, wealth, and lifestyles of older people in England will make a major contribution to understanding how important the timing and nature of labour market exit is for subsequent health.

13.3.3 Social determinants and health in older age: the question of direction

A life-course perspective is also integral to the question of the direction of relationships. Causal links may operate in both ways, with those in better health in early life more able to participate and gain a higher level of education, occupation, and income. One way of trying to ascertain the direction of relationships is to adjust statistically for pre-existing health conditions when examining the relationship between socio-economic position and later health in longitudinal data. Camacho and colleagues (1993) showed that socio-economic effects on functioning persisted after adjustment for health problems in the previous two decades. Similarly, Swain (1993) showed that, among men and women who were aged 60 or over in the 1984/5 HALS, those in manual class households were more likely to report fair or poor health seven years later than their counterparts in non-manual households after stratifying for self-reported health at baseline. Sundquist and Johansson (1997) showed that education differentials in mortality rates persisted after adjusting for baseline self-reported health and marital status in a large population-based follow-up study in Sweden, while Rogers and colleagues (1992) showed that education was associated with onset of disability over two years of follow-up. Melzer and colleagues (2001) showed that educational differences in disability arise largely in the time of incidence rather than in duration or mortality rates once disabled. However, the only study to look specifically at transitions in socio-economic status in older age and subsequent functioning or health (Maddox *et al.* 1994) found that these relationships worked both ways. Also, endogenous health effects for older people have been found in the US. Using data from the HRS and AHEAD studies, Smith (1999) has shown that new episodes of poor health do lead to lower wealth accumulation.

Certainly, an understanding of changes in socioeconomic circumstances in older years and how these changes relate to changes in health is a crucial element of understanding the social determinants of health in older age.

13.4 Risk factors in the post-retirement social environment

The first part of this chapter reviewed studies investigating class differences in health in older age and noted that neither the meaning of social position nor which aspects of social position may be important for health, were as well addressed. Towards the end of the twentieth century, authors in both the UK and the US highlighted the necessity of using measures of socio-economic position that are directly derived from theory

(Bartley *et al.* 1999; Krieger *et al.* 1997; Sacker *et al.* 2001). There are several social and economic constructs that may be captured by a measure of social class such as material circumstances, working conditions, and social status or prestige (Bartley *et al.* 1999; Krieger *et al.* 1997; Sacker *et al.* 2001).

13.4.1 Control

In relation to working conditions, several studies have identified psychosocial factors such as control at work to be an important factor in social inequalities in health (see Chapter 6; Hallqvist *et al.* 1998; Hemingway and Marmot 1998; Karesek *et al.* 1981; Marmot *et al.* 1991). If control at work is important for those who are employed, an important question for the study of inequalities in health in older age is whether control over life in general has relevance for those who do not work, including the retired. Evidence from the Whitehall II study on control at home showed its greater relevance for women, but did not provide evidence for retired individuals (Chandola *et al.* 2004). To address this question, the first wave of ELSA included demand and control questions related to both the work and home environments. Results from ELSA showed that only 9% of men and women had low control at home, compared with about a fifth of both men and women who had low control at work (McMunn *et al.* 2003). There were no discernable age or gender patterns in low control at home.

13.4.2 Perceived social status

In addition to control, the Whitehall II studies (Singh–Manoux *et al.* 2003) and ELSA, as well as studies in the US (Adler *et al.* 2000; Ostrove *et al.* 2000), have identified perceived social status, as captured by 'ladder position'[1], to be an important explanatory factor in inequalities in health, over and above other measures of social position. Preliminary analysis of ELSA data shown in Fig. 13.2 reveals that the likelihood of reporting good health increased with perceived social status even after adjusting for total non-pension wealth (Banks *et al.* 2003). Results were similar for reported functional limitations (using ADLs), and adjusting further for age. Whether the importance of perceived social status differs for people pre- and post-retirement is an empirical question that ELSA will allow us to address, although current analysis shows that mean ladder position did decline with age among ELSA respondents (Banks *et al.* 2003).

---

[1] 'The ladder' is a self-anchoring pictorial scale in the form of a 10-rung ladder, used to measure perceived social status. Respondents were asked: 'Think of this ladder as representing where people stand in our society. At the top of the ladder are the people who are the best off—those who have the most money, most education, and best jobs. At the bottom are the people who are the worst off—who have the least money, least education, and the worst jobs or no jobs. The higher up you are on this ladder, the closer you are to the people at the very top, and the lower you are, the closer you are to the people at the very bottom. Please mark a cross on the rung on the ladder where you would place yourself.'

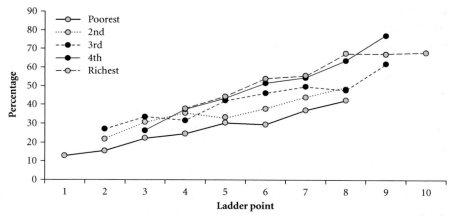

Fig. 13.2 Percentage of ELSA respondents aged 50+ reporting excellent/very good/good health, by perceived social position within wealth quintile.

13.4.3 Social support

Chapter 8 reviews the considerable evidence showing the beneficial health effects of social relations. With respect to health in older age, social support is a determinant of the morbidity and declines in functioning that become more prevalent with age, and also acts as a buffer for important life events that are more likely to occur in older age, such as the death of a partner or the onset of a chronic illness.

In terms of the direct effects of social support on health, studies have shown that blood pressure response to a challenge differs according to whether someone believes that they can call on someone for support or not, and social engagement has been shown to have a direct effect in maintaining cognitive function in older age (Berkman and Glass 2000). In addition to its protective effect in preventing illness, Chapter 8 reviews many studies showing social support to be helpful in coping with the stress of a chronic illness (Berkman *et al.* 1992; Cameron 1996; Fitzpatrick *et al.* 1991; Frasure–Smith and Prince 1985; Kiecolt–Glaser and Glaser 1995; Lesperance *et al.* 1996; Ruberman *et al.* 1984; Williams *et al.* 1992). As well as moderating the effect of illness onset, social support may mediate the relationship between economic position and health. For instance, those in poor health who are married may be less dependent on formal health care, have less need to spend their resources on outside care, and, therefore, have more ability to protect their economic position.

Equally, class may act to constrain or foster social relationships. For example, one study found higher income and education to be associated with larger social networks, more contact with network members, and more voluntary associations (Fischer 1982). Also, both a Canadian study and Whitehall II have found that higher levels of perceived social support were associated with higher social position (Stansfeld *et al.* 1998; Turner and Marino 1994). Of course, the form and quality of support are important. For instance, close relationships can have negative, as well as positive, aspects (see Chapter 8).

The ELSA study has added considerably to our knowledge of social support among older people in England (Janevic *et al.* 2003). Adult offsprings appear to play a central role in the social networks of older people, with more than half of older people seeing their children at least once a week. Also, while isolation may be a problem for women in their 70s and 80s, as they are more likely to live on their own, there is also some evidence that the quality of social relationships improves with age, as reflected by measures of positive and negative social support reported by older people in ELSA. However, it is not possible to determine whether this represents an age or a cohort effect in cross-sectional analysis. There also appear to be important gender differences in the social worlds of older people, with older women more disadvantaged than older men in terms of perceived social capital and access to local amenities, but more advantaged in terms of social networks. In the ELSA sample, women had more face-to-face, phone, and written contact with others than their male counterparts.

13.4.4 **Caring**

Aside from the care of one's own children, the majority of individuals who assume caring roles are likely to do so in midlife and older age (Hirst 2002). Being a carer has been shown to have a particularly strong influence on one's ability to participate in paid employment, as well as on mental and physical health and participation in social activities. Stress associated with providing care, particularly when the care recipient is cognitively impaired, may result in high levels of psychological distress (Schulz *et al.* 1995), negative effects on immune, neuroendocrine, and cardiovascular functioning (Vitaliano *et al.* 1997), and increased mortality (Schulz and Beach 1999). The effects of caring on the self-reported health of ELSA respondents depended on the recipient of care and the age of the carer. Prior to age 75, the higher the number of hours spent caring for a spouse or partner, the more likely the respondent was to report fair or poor health. This pattern did not hold universally across different care recipients, however (Hyde and Janevic 2003). Also, with the exception of women aged 60 to 75 looking after grandchildren or parents, carers in ELSA were much more likely than non-carers to be economically inactive (Hyde and Janevic 2003).

Despite the enormous increases in women's labour force participation over the last several decades, a substantial gender division in responsibility for household labour continues with respect to the role of carer, such that women are more likely to assume a caring role (Martin and Campbell 1995). In addition, there appear to be qualitative gender differences in the nature of care giving, with women providing more hands-on and personal care than men, and also exhibiting more psychological distress as carers (Martin and Campbell 1995)—though these gender differences are less apparent in spouse carers. In ELSA, overall, men and women were about equally likely to provide care to a spouse, with women more likely before age 70 and men more likely after age

70. However, women are more likely to care for children, grandchildren, parents, or in-laws (Hyde and Janevic 2003). Gender imbalances in caring responsibilities might be a factor in explaining gender differences in both labour force participation and social participation.

13.5 Material risk factors and health in older age

The exact relationship between material circumstances and health has long been debated. Lack of resources may lead to poor health outcomes through a number of pathways, some related directly to the ability to afford health-promoting goods (e.g. high-quality health care or nutritious food, high- quality housing, good neighbourhoods); others relating to the sense of security or control that access to economic resources may bring. Of course, a further longstanding empirical puzzle has been to understand the importance of this direction of causation (from material resources to health) compared to the causation the other way (from health to material resources) in explaining the inequalities in health described in the first section of this chapter. A further, related issue revolves around understanding how far these causal mechanisms overlap with ones associated with other markers of socio-economic status discussed in this chapter, such as occupational status and education.

While the relative importance of material circumstances and other socio-economic constructs have yet to be disentangled, the material circumstances associated with older age may also be changing. Old age is traditionally portrayed as a time of economic decline, as well as physical and mental decline. Is this stereotype an accurate picture of the current economic circumstances of the elderly, and to what extent are these circumstances changing? Although income typically drops around retirement (Banks *et al.* 1998), pensioner incomes have risen over time, as successive cohorts retire with higher lifetime incomes and access to income from occupational pensions. Pensioner poverty has also fallen in recent years, largely due to increases in the generosity of means-tested benefits (Goodman *et al.* 2003). However, behind these age trends are large inequalities in the distribution of income, with a large proportion of the pensioner population dependent on means-tested benefits, whilst the number of 50–64 year-old men claiming invalidity or incapacity benefits has almost doubled since 1980 and the number of women aged 50–59 claiming the benefits has risen by a factor of over four (Banks *et al.* 2002). For older people on low incomes, poverty tends to be persistent, rather than temporary, as relatively few will have recourse to the labour market to add to their incomes (Department for Work and Pensions 2004).

Though these patterns in income are informative, for the older population, it can be argued that wealth is a better gauge of material resources than income, particularly since earnings tend to be low, and only small proportions of total wealth are typically annuitized. Compared with income, wealth gives a better measure of access to resources which can be drawn from to finance consumption, and since it also provides

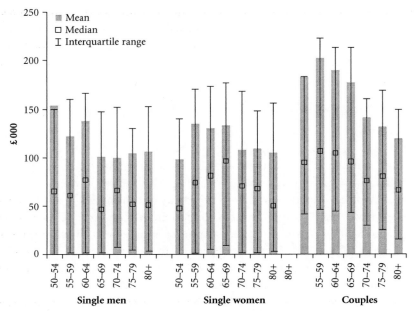

Fig. 13.3 Mean, median, and interquartile range of total (non-pension) wealth among ELSA respondents, 2002.

information on the accumulated sum of past saving and borrowing, it can provide a good measure of lifetime living standards. Until recently, we had relatively little information on patterns of wealth holding among the older population. Evidence from ELSA has so far been very revealing about levels of non-pension wealth and on holdings of private pensions; much future work will revolve around calculating levels of private and state pension wealth amongst survey members.

Using ELSA data, Fig. 13.3 shows that in cross-section, older individuals generally have lower non-pension wealth (housing, financial assets, and physical assets) than younger individuals (Banks *et al.* 2003), although this should not be interpreted as wealth drawn down over time due to differences that may exist across cohorts. The interquartile range shown in Fig. 13.3 reveals that inequalities in wealth amongst the older population are very pronounced. For example, amongst single men aged 55–59, mean total (non-pension) wealth is around £122,000, but around a quarter of these men have more than £160,000 and a quarter have almost zero wealth. Across the whole ELSA sample, despite average financial wealth being over £40,000, half the population aged 50 and over had less than £12,000 and a quarter had less than £1500 in financial assets outside of a pension, indicating the degree to which average wealth is driven by a small number of very wealthy individuals. In addition, a considerable number of individuals (particularly single people) report having very little non-pension wealth (Banks *et al.* 2003).

Though it is harder to measure the value of pension wealth held by individuals, it is helpful to think about pension wealth as arising from two sources—private pension wealth, and entitlement to state pension payments. Whilst access to occupational pensions has been growing over time, and a large proportion of individuals in their 50s and 60s have contributed to a private pension at some point in time, evidence from ELSA shows that the main forms of wealth—housing, pensions, and financial assets—were positively correlated, so that those without housing or financial wealth also had the lowest likelihood of holding a private pension.

13.6 **Health behaviour and health in older age**

According to Rowe and Kahn (1998), healthy behaviour is the route to successful ageing. How one ages is not genetically determined, but is determined by the lifestyle choices of individuals. However, health behaviour is known to be influenced by social position, culture (Elstad 1998), and financial constraints (Stitt *et al.* 1995)—at least in middle age. Relationships between social position and health behaviours in older age are less clear.

People at high risk may die before reaching old age and habits may change, either with age or with cohort changes in acceptability, such as cohort differences in smoking. For instance, the prevalence of smoking typically declines with age (Boreham *et al.* 1999; McMunn *et al.* 2003), partly due to the selective mortality of heavy smokers (Peto *et al.* 1994). In addition, cultural forces have influenced both the uptake and the cessation of smoking in different countries and social groups (Schooling and Kuh 2002). Historically, women's smoking started in the 1920s in the US and the UK (Husten and Malarcher 2000; Todd 1959); somewhat later elsewhere in northern Europe; and later still in southern Europe—for example, in the mid 1960s in parts of Spain (Borras *et al.* 2000) and Italy (La Vecchia *et al.* 1995). Women's smoking peaked about 40 years later, so rates are declining in northern Europe and the US but not (yet) in southern Europe (Graham 1996; Husten and Malarcher 2000). Men's smoking started earlier, reached higher levels, and peaked earlier. The decline in smoking has been less marked in women than in men, so prevalence rates for men and women are converging (Husten and Malarcher 2000; Rayner and Petersen 2000).

There also appear to be socio-economic differences in smoking, physical activity, and alcohol consumption in older age (McMunn *et al.* 2003). In ELSA, those in routine or manual class households were particularly likely to be current smokers, although the relationship between class and smoking decreased dramatically with age (McMunn *et al.* 2003). Looking at leisure-time activity (excluding job-related physical activity), people in routine or manual class households were least likely to have the highest levels of physical activity, and women were more likely than men to be sedentary (McMunn *et al.* 2003). Also, people in routine or manual occupational class households were most likely to abstain from drinking alcohol or to only drink alcohol on special occasions.

Conversely, people from professional or managerial households were more likely to drink moderately, in line with the pattern now thought to be protective against chronic illness (McMunn *et al.* 2003). Cairney (2000) found relationships similar to those seen in ELSA: among those aged 55 and over, both low levels of income and education were associated with smoking, being a non-drinker, and being sedentary. In Spain, Lasheras and colleagues (2001) found that women with low levels of education were most likely to smoke, while Amaducci and colleagues (1998) found the converse in Italy.

In older age, health behaviours are also known to be associated with health outcomes. For example, a systematic review of risk factors for functional decline identified smoking, low levels of physical activity, and no alcohol consumption as among the most important factors (Stuck *et al.* 1999). Several studies have shown associations between smoking in older age and cardiovascular and cancer mortality (Benfante *et al.*1991; Davis *et al.* 1994; LaCroix *et al.* 1993; Paffenbarger *et al.* 1993), although there are exceptions (Barrett–Connor *et al.* 1984; Branch 1985; Branch and Jette 1984; Korten *et al.* 1999). Physical activity has been shown to have protective effects against several chronic physical and mental illnesses (Pate *et al.* 1995). In the EPESE study, moderately active walking was protective against mortality among those aged 65 and over (Simonsick *et al.* 1993).

As there is some evidence to indicate that health behaviour is associated with health and social position in older age, this is likely to provide one set of pathways through which social determinants influence health in older age. However, very few British studies of health inequalities in older age have taken health behaviours into account (some exceptions are Breeze *et al.* 2004 and Shahtahmasebi *et al.* 1992), while a few North American and European studies (Amaducci *et al.* 1998; Cairney 2000; Cairney and Arnold 1996; Damian *et al.* 1999; House *et al.* 1990; Parker *et al.* 1996) have included both socio-economic and behavioural factors.

13.7 **Policy in relation to health inequalities in old age—the British example**

The British government has recognized the challenges of catering for an ageing population. At the turn of the century, people aged 65 and over used almost two-thirds of general and acute hospital beds and £10.5 billion was spent on long-term care (Department of Health 2000). Survival after stopping paid work can be several decades, not only through longevity but also because about a quarter of men and a third of women are not economically active at ages 50–64/59. Funding old age is thus a major challenge. An ageing population was a prime factor in anticipated increased calls on the health service, which was addressed in a report commissioned from Sir Derek Wanless (Wanless 2002). The Government also places high priority on dealing with health inequalities (HM Treasury 2002). As in many countries, their existence among older people was recognized long after their existence at working ages. The Acheson report (1998) was the first to consider older people in any depth.

The evidence cited above shows that, despite state provision for health care alongside an extensive social security system, health differences between socio-economic groups, genders, and ethnic groups remain. The Cross-Cutting Review (HM Treasury 2002) strategy and the subsequent programme for action (Department of Health 2003) were broadranging, in recognition of the multi-faceted nature of inequalities. While there were specific mentions of older people, the strategy was not clear as to the extent to which gender or socio-economic differences were to be explicitly addressed within the age group.

Policies specifically aimed at helping the poorest older people include the Minimum Income Guarantee, introduced in 1999 and replaced by Pension Credit in 2003, and the Fuel Poverty scheme. The Warm Front scheme was designed to protect vulnerable people against health risks of cold homes but has not necessarily helped those who need it most (National Audit Office 2004). Means testing and complexity of benefits tend to inhibit take-up (McConaghy *et al.* 2003) such that intentions to reduce inequalities in resources are, at best, partially realized. The Single Assessment Process, as announced in the National Service Framework (Department of Health 2001), was designed to facilitate co-ordination of different kinds of health and social service support and to improve efficiency in dealing with people's needs. Although, potentially, this process could be of great benefit to those who are least able to control and command the resources they need, this will only be achieved with considerable commitment from the various services involved, and it is too early to judge its value in the context of health inequalities.

Generally, the policies to tackle health inequalities place considerable responsibility on local health and administrative authorities to take up the baton. At local level, the London Borough of Camden's Quality of Life Strategy is an example of an initiative to improve the involvement and independence of older people, with outreach to the isolated and the minority ethnic groups as priorities (Camden Council 2002).

Wanless (2002) described a 'full engagement' scenario in which members of the public are active in securing improved health and quick to respond to health care initiatives. If this vision were realized, there would be a substantial increase in life expectancy, a marked shift to healthier lifestyles, and a 10% reduction in ill health among the elderly by 2022. His recommendations include providing information (Wanless 2004), but information is of little use unless people can and will use it. The National Audit Office (2002) noted that, even after a massive publicity campaign, many low-income pensioners were not well versed about the Minimum Income Guarantee. Wanless' assumptions about people's ability to take greater responsibility for their health have been called heroic (Hunter 2003). However, attempts at 'full engagement' could increase health inequalities if there is differential ability to become engaged.

Resource limitations at the national level may constrain the reduction of health inequalities. If an ageing population pushes governments into increasing the expected age of retirement and relying more on private savings, this could cause a further relative deterioration in health and economic prospects of those who retire before the age of 60 years for health reasons or because they cannot find work. The British Government encourages private saving but will provide a safety net for those who cannot save for retirement (Department of Social Security 1998). However, it is not so straightforward to save sufficient to provide an income for old age. A study of people in their 50s, in the lower half of the income distribution, found that they were unable to predict well the income they would have in retirement and they anticipated only being able to afford small contributions to domiciliary care costs (Deeming and Keen 2002). Despite a Minimum Income Guarantee, 40% of the pensioners in this study were exhausting their income every week. In Britain, the Pensions Commission (2004) recognizes that there are no easy options and that there are major barriers to sufficient voluntary saving. A problem for the health and social services is to find resources to do preventive work alongside management of existing disease, disability, and care needs.

13.8 Conclusion

Changing sociodemographics in wealthier countries, such as increasing longevity, decreasing fertility, the ageing of the baby boom generation, as well as increasingly early labour market exit, have made older age a central policy and research topic. The concepts of successful ageing in the US and the third age in the UK have suggested a shift in perceptions of older age from a period of sickness, poverty, and decline, to one of active self-fulfilment, a period free from the constraints of employment and childcare.

Whilst the bulk of research on inequalities in health has concentrated on the working age adult population, initial studies of socio-economic inequalities in health in older age suggest that the rosy picture of healthy, active ageing presented by recent theories are by no means universal. An increasing body of evidence shows that health inequalities continue in older age, regardless of which measure of socio-economic circumstances is used. There is some evidence to suggest that health inequalities diminish somewhat in the oldest age groups, but this evidence is based on studies using occupational class, which is unlikely to be the best measure of socio-economic circumstances for people who are no longer in the labour market. This decline in a social gradient in health with age may also be the result of selective mortality.

This chapter has highlighted a number of areas in need of further research, and research questions for which longitudinal, cross-national data are starting to become available. For example, pathways into retirement are becoming increasingly diverse. Longitudinal data will allow us to examine whether and how these changes will impact health outcomes in older age, as well as the extent of endogenous health effects on the timing and nature of labour market exit. In addition, the ageing of the British birth cohorts will allow researchers to better address questions regarding the relative importance of socio-economic circumstances in earlier and later life on health outcomes in older age. Currently available evidence suggests that socio-economic circumstances in early life are more important than adult socio-economic circumstances for certain diseases in older age, but not for others.

In addition to the need for further longitudinal focus in studies of health inequalities in older age, further studies of risk factors in the social environment of older people would prove useful. Studies have shown control and subjective social status to be important components of socio-economic inequalities in health among people of working age. Studies are needed to investigate how sources of control and perceived status might change in the post-retirement environment. We know from existing evidence that social support continues to play an important role as an independent influence on health and as a mediator of life events in older age. It is also well known that a number of older people assume a caring role, and that caring influences health as well as participation in paid employment and other social activities.

As well as risk factors in the social environment, material circumstances are likely to be an important determinant of health in older age. Existing evidence regarding relationships between material circumstances and health mainly focuses on income inequalities among people of working age. Wealth is likely to be a more useful measure of material circumstances in older age, and detailed data on wealth among older people in England are only just beginning to become available.

Finally, besides social and economic risk factors, the concept of successful ageing emphasizes the importance of healthy behaviour, yet the majority of studies of health inequalities in older age have not taken health behaviour into account. Clearly, our understanding of the social determinants of health in older age is in its infancy. Fortunately, data sources are becoming available that will help provide answers to these and many other relevant questions in this field.

This chapter reports on health inequalities in old age but it does not provide a message of pessimism about the consequences of an ageing population. To quote the National Service Framework: 'people living longer is something to celebrate' (Department of Health 2001, p. 2). Although there is much work to be done in reducing health inequalities, the high percentages of older people reporting excellent or very good health (McMunn et al. 2003), and the existence of differentials, show us that many problems associated with old age are not inevitable products of age per se. Undoubtedly, social care costs are a concern but could be reduced if health improves. Sensitivity analyses (Sutherland 1999) revealed major absolute and relative differences in overall long-term care costs 25 years ahead, depending on longevity, disability prevalence, care costs, informal care provision. Health care costs are more influenced by nearness to death than chronological age (Seshamani and Gray 2004), and the lower birth rate should reduce the dependency costs of bringing up children. Moreover, the resources of older people themselves should not be underestimated. For example, long-term residents can contribute knowledge of the neighbourhood to planners, older people can be peer leaders in physical activity and other programmes, and they are major providers of child care.

Acknowledgement

The authors are grateful to the ESRC, whose funding of the project 'Inequalities in health in an ageing population: patterns, causes and consequences' (RES–000–23–0590) supported work on this chapter.

References

Acheson, D. (1998) *Independent inquiry into inequalities in health: report*. London: The Stationery Office.

Adler, N.E., Epel, E.S., Castellazzo, G., and Ickovics, J.R. (2000) Relationship of subjective and objective social status with psychological and physiological functioning: preliminary data in healthy white women. *Health Psychol.* **19**:586–592.

Amaducci, L., Maggi, S., Langlois, J., Minicuci, N., Baldereschi, M., Di Carlo, A., *et al.* (1998) Education and the risk of physical disability and mortality among men and women aged 65 to 84: the Italian Longitudinal Study on Aging. *J. Gerontol. A. Biol. Sci. Med. Sci.* **53**:M484–M490.

Arber, S. and Ginn, J. (1993) Gender inequalities in health in later life. *Soc. Sci. Med.* **36**:33–46.

Attanasio, O. and Emmerson, C., (2003) Mortality, health status and wealth. *J. Eur. Econ. Assoc.* **1**:821–50.

Banks, J. and Casanova, M. (2003) Work and retirement. In: *Health, wealth and lifestyles of the older population in England: the 2002 English Longitudinal Study of Ageing* (ed. M. Marmot, J. Banks, R. Blundell, *et al.*). London: Institute for Fiscal Studies.

Banks, J., Blundell, R., Disney, R., and Emmerson, C. (2002) *Retirement, pensions and the adequacy of savings: a guide to the debate*. London: Institute for Fiscal Studies briefing note no. 29.

Banks, J., Blundell, R., and Tanner, S. (1998) Is there a retirement-savings puzzle? *Am. Econ. Rev.* **88**:769–88.

Banks, J., Karlsen, S., and Oldfield, Z. (2003) Socio-economic position. In: *Health, wealth and lifestyles of the older population in England: the 2002 English Longitudinal Study of Ageing* (ed. M. Marmot, J. Banks, R. Blundell, *et al.*). London: Institute for Fiscal Studies.

Barker, D.J.P. (1994) *Mothers, babies and disease in later life*. London: British Medical Journal Publishing.

Barker, D.J. (1995) Fetal origins of coronary heart disease. *BMJ* **311**:171–4.

Barrett–Connor, E., Suarez, L., Khaw, K., Criqui, M.H., and Wingard, D.L. (1984) Ischemic heart disease risk factors after age 50. *J. Chronic Dis.* **37**:903–8.

Bartley, M., Sacker, A., Firth, D., and Fitzpatrick, R. (1999) Understanding social variation in cardiovascular risk factors in women and men: the advantage of theoretically based measures. *Soc. Sci. Med.* **49**:831–45.

Bebbington, A. (1991) The expectation of life without disability in England and Wales. *Pop. Trends* **66**:26–9.

Beland, F. and Zunzunegui, M.V. (1999) Predictors of functional status in older people living at home. *Age Ageing* **28**:153–9.

Benfante, R., Reed, D., and Frank, J. (1991) Does cigarette smoking have an independent effect on coronary heart disease incidence in the elderly? *Am. J. Public Health* **81**:897–9.

Berkman, C.S. and Gurland, B.J. (1998) The relationship among income, other socioeconomic indicators, and functional level in older persons. *J. Aging Health* **10**:81–98.

Berkman, L.F. and Glass, T.A. (2000) Social integration, social networks, social support and health. In: *Social epidemiology* (ed. L.F. Berkman and I. Kawachi), pp. 137–73. Oxford: Oxford University Press.

Berkman, L.F., Leo–Summers, S., and Horwitz, R.I. (1992) Emotional support and survival after myocardial infarction: a prospective, population-based study of the elderly. *Ann. Int. Med.* **117**:1003–9.

Blaxter, M. (1990) *Health and lifestyles.* London: Tavistock/Routledge.

Boreham, R., Erens, B., Falaschetti, E., Hirani, V., and Primatesta, P. (1999) Risk factors for cardiovascular disease. In: *Health survey for England 1998: cardiovascular disease* (ed. B. Erens and P. Primatesta). London: The Stationery Office.

Borras, J.M., Fernandez, E., Schiaffino, A., Borrell, C., and La Vecchia, C. (2000) Pattern of smoking initiation in Catalonia, Spain, from 1948–1992. *Am. J. Public Health* **90**:1459–62.

Branch, L.G. (1985) Health practices and incident disability among the elderly. *Am. J. Public Health* **75**:1436–9.

Branch, L.G. and Jette, A.M. (1984) Personal health practices and mortality among the elderly. *Am. J. Public Health* **74**:1126–9.

Breeze, E., Fletcher, A.E., Leon, D.A., Marmot, M.G., Clarke, R.J., and Shipley, M.J. (2001) Do socioeconomic disadvantages persist into old age? Self-reported morbidity in a 29-year follow-up of the Whitehall study. *Am. J. Public Health* **91**:277–83.

Breeze, E., Jones, D.A., Wilkinson, P., Latif, A.M., Bulpitt, C.J., and Fletcher, A.E. (2004) Association of quality of life in old age in Britain with socioeconomic position: baseline data from a randomized controlled trial. *J. Epidemiol. Community Health* **58**:667–73.

Breeze, E., Sloggett, A., and Fletcher, A.E. (1999) Socioeconomic status and transitions in status in old age in relation to limiting long-term illness measured at the 1991 Census: results from the UK Longitudinal Study. *Eur. J. Public Health* **9**:265–70.

Brown, R.G., Davidson, L.A.G., McKeown, T., and Whitfield, A.G.W. (1957) Coronary-artery disease. Influences affecting its incidence in males in the seventh decade. *Lancet* (1957): 1073–7.

Brunner, E.J., Shipley, M.J., Blane, D., Davey Smith, G., and Marmot, M.G. (1999) When does cardiovascular risk start? Past and present socioeconomic circumstances and risk factors in adulthood. *J. Epidemiol. Community Health* **53**:757–64.

Bury, M. (1995) Ageing, gender and sociological theory. In: *Connecting Gender and Ageing* (ed. S. Arber and J. Ginn). Buckingham: Open University Press.

Cairney, J. (2000) Socio-economic status and self-rated health among older Canadians. *Can. J. Aging* **19**:456–78.

Cairney, J. and Arnold, R. (1996) Social class, health and aging: socioeconomic determinants of self-reported morbidity among the noninstitutionalized elderly in Canada. *Can. J. Public Health* **87**:199–203.

Camacho, T., Strawbridge, W.J., Cohen, R.D., and Kaplan, G.A. (1993) Functional ability in the oldest old. Cumulative impact of risk factors from the previous two decades. *J. Aging Health* **5**:439–54.

Camden Council (2002) *The quality of life strategy for Camden's older citizens.* Camden Council.

Cameron, O. (1996) Depression increases post-MI mortality: how? *Psychosom. Med.* **58**:111–12.

Chandola, T., Kuper, H., Singh-Manoux, A., Bartley, M., and Marmot, M. (2004) The effect of control at home on CHD events in the Whitehall II study: gender differences in psychosocial domestic pathways to social inequalities in CHD. *Soc. Sci. Med.* **58**:1501–9.

Corti, L., Laurie, H., and Dex, S. (1995) *Highly qualified women.* Employment Department Research Series No. 50.

Crompton, R. (1993) *Class and stratification.* Cambridge: Polity.

Dahl, E. and Birkelund, G.E. (1997) Health inequalities in later life in a social democratic welfare state. *Soc. Sci. Med.* **44**:871–81.

Dale, A. and Egerton, M. (1995) *Highly educated women: evidence from the National Child Development Study*. Report to the Employment Department.

Damian, J., Ruigomez, A., Pastor, V., and Martin–Moreno, J.M. (1999) Determinants of self assessed health among Spanish older people living in at home. *J. Epidemiol. Community Health* 53:412–16.

Davey Smith, G., Hart, C.L., Blane, D., Gillis, C., and Hawthorne, V.M. (1997) Lifetime socioeconomic position and mortality: prospective observational study. *BMJ* 314:547–52.

Davey Smith, G., Hart, C., Blane, D., and Hole, D. (1998) Adverse socioeconomic conditions in childhood can cause specific adult mortality: prospective observational study. *BMJ* 316:1631–5.

Davis, M.A., Neuhaus, J.M., Moritz, D.J., Lein, D., Barclay, J.D., and Murphy, S.P. (1994) Health behaviors and survivial among middle-aged and older men and women in the NHANES I Epidemiologic Follow-up Study. *Prev. Med.* 23:369–76.

Deeming, C. and Keen, J. (2002) Paying for old age: can people on lower incomes afford domiciliary care costs? *Soc. Pol. Admin.* 36:465–81.

Department of Health (1998) *Modernising social services. Promoting independence; improving protection; raising standards*. Cm 4169. London: The Stationery Office.

Department of Health (2000) *The NHS plan: the Government's response to the Royal Commission on Long- Term Care*. CM4818-II. London: The Stationery Office.

Department of Health (2001) *The National Service Framework for older people*. London: Department of Health.

Department of Health (2003) *Tackling health inequalities. A programme for action*. London: Department of Health.

Department of Social Security (1998) *A new contract for welfare: partnership in pensions*. London: Department of Social Security.

Department for Work and Pensions. Households Below Average Income 1994/95 *2002/02*. Leeds: Corporate Document Services, 2004.

Dex, Shirley. Women's Occupational Mobility: A Lifetime Perspective. London: Macmillan, 1987.

Donkin, Angela, Peter Goldblatt, and Kevin Lynch. "Inequalities in life expectancy by social class, 1972–1999." *Health Statistics Quarterly*, 15 (2002): 5–15.

Elstad, J.I. (1998) The psycho-social perspective on social inequalities in health. In: *The sociology of health inequalities* (ed. M. Bartley, D. Blane, and G. Davey Smith), pp. 39–58. Oxford: Blackwell Publishers.

Falaschetti, E., Malbut, K., and Primatesta, P. (2002) The general health of older people and their use of health services. In: *Health survey for England 2000* (ed. G. Prior and P. Primatesta). London: The Stationery Office.

Feinstein, J.S. (1993) The relationship between socioeconomic status and health—a review of the literature. *Milbank Quart.* 71:279–322.

Fischer, C.S. (1982) *To dwell among friends*. Chicago: University of Chicago Press.

Fitzpatrick, R., Newman, S., Archer, R., and Shipley, M. (1991) Social support, disability and depression: a longitudinal study of rheumatoid arthritis. *Soc. Sci. Med.* 33:605–11.

Forbes, W.F., Hayward, L.M., and Agwani, N. (1991) Factors associated with the prevalence of various self-reported impairments among older people residing in the community. *Can. J. Public Health* 82:240–4.

Fox, J. (ed.) (1989) *Health inequalities in European countries*. Aldershot: Gower.

Frasure–Smith, N. and Prince, R. (1985) The ischemic heart disease life stress monitoring program: impact and mortality. *Psychosom. Med.* 47:431–45.

Fries, J.F. (1980) Aging, natural death, and the compression of morbidity. *New Eng. J. Med.* 303:130–5.

Fries, J.F. (1989) The compression of morbidity: near or far? *Milbank Quart.* **67**:208–32.

Fries, J.F. and Grapo, L.M. (1981) *Vitality and aging.* San Francisco: Freeman.

Goodman, A., Myck, M., and Shephard, A. (2003) *Sharing in the nation's prosperity? Pensioner poverty in Britain.* Commentary no. 93. London: Institute for Fiscal Studies.

Government Actuaries Department (2002) *Population projections: population of Great Britain in five-year age bands* (*http://www.gad.gov.uk/Population/2002/gb*).

Graham, H. (1996) Smoking prevalence among women in the European Community 1950–90. *Soc. Sci. Med.* **43**:243–54.

Guralnik, J.M. and Kaplan, G.A. (1989) Predictors of healthy aging: prospective evidence from the Alameda County study. *Am. J. Public Health* **79**:703–8.

Guralnik, J.M. and Simonsick, E.M. (1993) Physical disability in older Americans. *J. Gerontol.* **48**: 3–10.

Hallqvist, J., Diderichsen, F., Theorell, T., Reuterwall, C., Ahlbon, A., and the SHEEP study (1998) Is the effect of job strain on myocardial infarction due to interaction between high psychological demands and low decision latitude. Results from the Stockholm Heart Epidemiology Program (SHEEP). *Soc. Sci. Med.* **46**:1405–15.

Hardy, R., Wadsworth, M., and Kuh, D. (2000) The influence of childhood weight and socioeconomic status on change in adult body mass index in a British national birth cohort. *Intern. J. Obesity* **24**:725–34.

Harris, T., Kovar, M.G., Suzman, R., Kleinman, J.C., and Feldman, J.J. (1989) Longitudinal study of physical ability in the oldest-old. *Am. J. Public Health* **79**:698–702.

Hemingway, H. and Marmot, M. (1998) Psychosocial factors in the primary and secondary prevention of coronary heart disease: a systematic review. In: *Evidence based cardiology* (ed. S. Yusuf, J. Cairns, J. Camm, *et al.*), pp. 269–85. London: BMJ Publishing Group.

Hirani, V. and Malbut, K. (2002) Disability among older people. In: *Health survey for England 2000* (ed. G. Prior and P. Primatesta). London: The Stationery Office.

Hirst, M. (2002) Transitions to informal care in Great Britain during the 1990s. *J. Epidemiol. Community Health* **56**:579–87.

HM Treasury, Department of Health (2002) *Tackling health inequalities: 2002 crosscutting review.* London: The Stationery Office.

House, J.S., Kessler, R.C., and Herzog, A.R. (1990) Age, socioeconomic status, and health. *Milbank Quart.* **68**:383–411.

Hubert, H.B., Bloch, D.A., and Fries, J.F. (1993) Risk factors for physical disability in an aging cohort: the NHANES I epidemiologic follow-up study. *J. Rheumatol.* **20**:480–8.

Hunter, D. (2003) The Wanless Report and public health. *BMJ* **327**:573–4.

Husten, R.F. and Malarcher, A.M. (2000) Cigarette smoking: trends, determinants, and health effects. In: *Women and health* (ed. M.B. Goldman and M.C. Hatch). San Diego, CA: Academic Press.

Hyde, M. and Janevic, M. (2003) Social activity. In: *Health, wealth and lifestyles of the older population in England: the 2002 English Longitudinal Study of Ageing* (ed. M. Marmot, J. Banks, R. Blundell, *et al.*) London: Institute for Fiscal Studies.

Hyde, M., Ferrie, J., Higgs, P., Mein, G., and Nazroo, J. (2004*a*) The effects of pre-retirement factors and retirement route on circumstances in retirement: findings from the Whitehall II study. *Ageing Soc.* **24**:279–96.

Hyde, M., Hagberg, J., Oxenstierna, G., Theorell, T., and Westerlund, H. (2004*b*) Bridges, pathways and valleys: labour market position and risk of hospitalization in a Swedish sample aged 55–63. *Scand. J. Public Health* **32**:1–6.

Janevic, M., Gjonca, E., and Hyde, M. (2003) Physical and social environment. In: *Health, wealth and lifestyles of the older population in England: the 2002 English Longitudinal Study of Ageing* (ed. M. Marmot, J. Banks, R. Blundell, *et al.*) London: Institute for Fiscal Studies.

Joshi, H., Paci, P., and Waldvogel, J. (1999) The wages of motherhood: better or worse? *Cambridge J. Econ.* 23:543–64.

Kaplan, G.A. (1992) Maintenance of functioning in the elderly. *Ann. Epidemiol.* 2:823–34.

Karasek, R., Baker, D., Marxer, F., Ahlbom, A., and Theorell, T. (1981) Job decision latitude, job demands and cardiovascular disease: a prospective study of Swedish men. *Am. J. Public. Health* 71:694–705.

Kempen, G.I., Brilman, E.I., Ranchor, A.V., and Ormel, J. (1999) Morbidity and quality of life and the moderating effects of level of education in the elderly. *Soc. Sci. Med.* 49:143–9.

Kiecolt–Glaser, J. and Glaser, R. (1995) Psychoneuroimmunology and health consequences: data and shared mechanisms. *Psychosom. Med.* 57:269–74.

Korton, A.E., Jorm, A.F., Jiao, Z., Letenneur, L., Jacomb, P.A., Henderson, A.S., *et al.* (1999) Health, cognitive, and psychosocial factors as predictors of mortality in an elderly community sample. *J. Epidemiol. Community Health* 53:83–8.

Koupilova, I., Leon, D.A., Lithell, H.O., and Berglund, L. (1997) Size at birth and hypertension in longitudinally followed 50–70-year-old men. *Blood Press.* 6:223–8.

Krieger, N., Chen, J.T., and Selby, J.V. (1999) Comparing individual-based and household-based measures of social class to assess class inequalities in women's health: a methodological study of 684 US women. *J. Epidemiol. Community Health* 53:612–23.

Krieger, N., Williams, D.R., and Moss, N.E. (1997) Measuring social class in US public health research: concepts, methodologies, and guidelines. *Ann. Rev. Public Health* 18:341–78.

Kuh, D., Power, C., Blane, D., and Bartley, M. (1997) Social pathways between childhood and adult health. In: *A lifecourse approach to chronic disease epidemiology* (ed. D. Kuh and Y. Ben–Shlomo), pp. 169–98. New York: Oxford University Press.

LaCroix, A.Z., Guralnik, J.M., Berkman, L.F., Wallace, R.B., and Satterfield, S. (1993) Maintaining mobility in late life. II. Smoking, alcohol consumption, physical activity, and body mass index. *Am. J. Epidemiol.* 137:858–69.

Langenberg, C., Hardy, R., Kuh, D., Brunner, E., and Wadsworth, M. (2003) Central and total obesity in middle aged men and women in relation to lifetime socioeconomic status: evidence from a national birth cohort. *J. Epidemiol. Community Health* 57:816–22.

Lasheras, C., Patterson, A.M., Casado, C., and Fernandez, S. (2001) Effects of education on the quality of life, diet, and cardiovascular risk factors in an elderly Spanish community population. *Exp. Aging Res.* 27:257–70.

Laslett, P. (1989) *A fresh map of life*. London: Weidenfield and Nicholson.

La Vecchia, C., Decarli, A., and Pagano, R. (1995) Patterns of smoking initiation in Italian males and females from 1955 to 1985. *Prev. Med.* 24: 293–6.

Lesperance, F., Frasure–Smith, N., and Talajic, M. (1996) Major depression before and after myocardial infarction: its nature and consequences. *Psychosom. Med.* 58:99–110.

Liao, Y., McGee, D.L., Kaufman, J.S., Cao, G., and Cooper, R.S. (1999) Socioeconomic status and morbidity in the last years of life. *Am. J. Public Health* 89:569–72.

Longino Jr., C.F., *et al.* (1989) Class, aging and health. In: *Aging and health: perspectives on gender, race, ethnicity, and class* (ed. K.S. Markides). London: Sage.

Machin, S. and Vignoles, A. (2004) Education inequality: the widening socio-economic gap. *Fiscal Studies* 25:107–28.

Macran, S., Clarke, L., Sloggett, A., and Bethune, A. (1994) Women's socio-economic status and self-assessed health: identifying some disadvantaged groups. *Sociol. Health Illn.* **16**:182–208.

Maddox, G.L. and Clark. D.O. (1992) Trajectories of functional impairment in later life. *J. Health Soc. Behav.* **33**: 114–25.

Maddox, G.L., Clark, D.O., and Steinhauser, K. (1994) Dynamics of functional impairment in late adulthood. *Soc. Sci. Med.* **38**:925–36.

Makepeace, G., Dolton, P., Woods, L., Joshi, H., and Galinda–Rueda, F. (2003) From school to the labour market. In: *Changing Britain, changing lives* (ed. E. Ferri, J. Bynner, and M. Wadsworth). London: Institute of Education.

Manton, K.G., Corder, L., and Stallard, E. (1997) Chronic disability trends in elderly United States populations: 1928–1994. *Pro. Nat. Acad. Sci. Med. Sci.* **94**:2593–8.

Mare, R.D. (1990) Socioeconomic careers and differential mortality among older men in the United States. In: *Measurement and analysis of mortality: new approaches* (ed. J. Vallin, S. D'Souza, and A. Palloni), pp. 362–87. Oxford: Clarendon Press.

Marmot, M.G. and Nazroo, J.Y. (2001) Social inequalities in health in an ageing population. *Eur. Rev.* **9**:445–60.

Marmot, M.G. and Shipley, M. (1996) Do socioeconomic differences in mortality persist after retirement? 25-year follow-up of civil servants from the Whitehall Study. *BMJ* **313**:117–80.

Marmot, M.G. and Wadsworth, M.E.J. (ed.) Fetal and early childhood environment: long-term health implications. *Br. Med. Bull.* **53(1)**.

Marmot, M., Banks, J., Blundell, R., Lessof, C., and Nazroo, J. (eds) (2003) *Health, wealth and lifestyles of the older population in England: the 2002 English Longitudinal Study of Ageing.* London: Institute for Fiscal Studies.

Marmot, M.G., Davey Smith, G., Stansfeld, S.A., *et al.* (1991) Health inequalities among British civil servants: the Whitehall II study. *Lancet* **337**:1387–93.

Marmot, M., Shipley, M., Brunner, E., and Hemingway, H. (2001) Relative contribution of early life and adult socioeconomic factors to adult morbidity in the Whitehall II study. *J. Epidemiol. Community Health* **55**:301–7.

Martelin, T. (1994) Mortality by indicators of socioeconomic status among the Finnish elderly. *Soc. Sci. Med.* **38**:1257–78.

Martikainen, P. (1995) Socioeconomic mortality differentials in men and women according to own and spouse's characteristics in Finland. *Sociol. Health Illn.* **17**:353–75.

Martin Matthews, A. and Campbell, L.D. (1995) Gender roles, employment and informal care. In: *Connecting gender and ageing: a sociological approach* (ed. S. Arber and J. Ginn). Buckingham: Open University Press.

McConaghy, M., Hill, C., Kane, C., Lader, D., Costigan, P., and Thornby, M. (2003) *Entitled but not claiming? Pensioners, the Minimum Income Guarantee, and Pension Credit.* Leeds: Corporate Document Services, Department of Work and Pensions.

McMunn, A.M. (2004) *Social roles and women's health: need satisfaction or normative satisfaction?* Unpublished Ph.D thesis, University College London.

McMunn, A., Hyde, M., Janevic, M., and Kumari, M. (2003) Health. In: *Health, wealth and lifestyles of the older population in England: the 2002 English Longitudinal Study of Ageing* (ed. M. Marmot, J. Banks, R. Blundell, *et al.*). London: Institute for Fiscal Studies.

Melzer, D., Izmirlian, G., Leveille, S.G., and Guralnik, J.M. (2001) Educational differences in the prevalence of mobility disability in old age: the dynamics of incidence, mortality, and recovery. *J. Gerontol. B Psychol. Sci. Soc. Sci.* **56**:S294–301.

Melzer, D., McWilliams, B., Brayne, C., Johnson, T., and Bond, J. (2000) Socioeconomic status and the expectation of disability in old age: estimates for England. *J. Epidemio. Community Health* **54**:286–92.

National Audit Office (2002) *Tackling pensioner poverty: encouraging take-up of entitlements. Report by the Comptroller and Auditor General.* HC37. London: The Stationery Office,.

National Audit Office (2004) *Warm front helping to combat fuel poverty.* HC 769. London: The Stationery Office.

Newacheck, P.W., Butler, L.H., Harper, A.K., Piontkowski, D.L., and Franks, P.E. (1980) Income and illness. *Med. Care* **18**:1165–76.

Ostrove, J.M., Adler, N.E., Kuppermann, M., and Washington, A.E. (2000) Objective and subjective assessments of socioeconomic status and their relationship to self-rated health in an ethnically diverse sample of pregnant women. *Health Psychol.* **19**:613–18.

Paffenbarger Jr., R.S., Hyde, R.T., Wing, A.L., Lee, I.M., Jung, D.L., and Kampert, J.B. (1993) The association of changes in physical-activity level and other lifestyle characteristics with mortality among men. *N. Eng. J. Med.* **328**:538–45.

Palmore, E.B., Nowlin, J.B., and Wang, H.S. (1985) Predictors of function among the old-old: a 10-year follow-up. *J. Gerontol.* **40**:244–50.

Parker, M.G., Thorslund, M., and Lundberg, O. (1994) Physical function and social class among Swedish oldest old. *J. Gerontol.* **49**:S196–S201.

Parker, M.G., Thorslund, M., Lundberg, O., and Kareholt, I. (1996) Predictors of physical function among the oldest old: a comparison of three outcome variables in a 24-year follow-up. *J. Aging Health* **8**:444–60.

Pate, R.R., Pratt, M., Blair, S.N., Haskell, W.L., Macera, C.A., Bouchard, C., et al. (1995) Physical activity and public health. A recommendation from the Centers for Disease Control and Prevention and the American College of Sports Medicine. *JAMA* **273**: 402–7.

Pensions Commission (2004) *Pensions, challenges and choices. First report.* London: The Stationery Office.

Peto, R., Lopez, A.D., Boreham, J., et al. (1994) *Mortality from smoking in developed countries 1950–2000.* Oxford: Oxford University Press.

Power, C. and Hertzman, C. (1997) Social and biological pathways linking early life and adult disease. *Br. Med. Bull.* **53**:210–21.

Rakhonen, O. and Takala, P. (1998) Social class differences in health and functional disability among older men and women. *Int. J. Health Serv.* **28**:511–24.

Rautio, N., Heikkinen, E., and Heikkinin, R–L. (2001) The association of socio-economic factors with physical and mental capacity in elderly men and women. *Arch. Gerontol. Geriatr.* **33**: 163–78.

Rayner, M. and Petersen, S. (2000) *European cardiovascular disease statistics.* London: British Health Foundation.

Reed, D.M., Foley, D.J., White, L.R., Heimovitz, H., Burchfiel, C.M., and Masaki, K. (1998) Predictors of healthy aging in men with high life expectancies. *Am. J. Public Health* **88**: 1463–8.

Regidor, E., G. Barrio, A. Domingo, C. Rodriguez, and J. Alonso. "Association between education level and health related quality of life in Spanish adults." *J. Epidemiol. Community Health,* 53 (1999): 75–82.

Reijneveld, S.A. and Gunning–Schepers, L.J. (1995) Age, health and the measurement of the socio-economic status of individuals. *Eur. J. Public Health* **5**:187–92.

Robert, S. and House, J.S. (1996) SES differentials in health by age and alternative indicators of SES. *J. Aging Health* **8**:359–88.

Rogers, R.G., Rogers, A., and Belanger, A. (1992) Disability-free life among elderly in the United States. *J. Aging Health* **4**:19–42.

Roos, N.P. and Havens, B. (1991) Predictors of successful aging: a twelve-year study of Manitoba elderly. *Am. J. Public Health* **81**:63–8.

Ross, C.R. and Wu, C.L. (1996) Education, age, and the cumulative advantage in health. *J. Health Soc. Behav.* **37**:104–20.

Rowe, J.W. and Kahn, R.L. (1998) *Successful aging.* New York: Dell.

Ruberman, W., Weinblatt, E., Goldberg, J.D., and Chaudhary, B.S. (1984) Psychosocial influences on mortality after myocardial infarction. *N. Engl. J. Med.* **311**:552–9.

Sacker, A., Bartley, M., Firth, D., and Fitzpatrick, R. (2001) Dimensions of social inequality in the health of women in England: occupational, material and behavioural pathways. *Soc. Sci. Med.* **52**:763–81.

Sakari–Rantala, R., Heikkinen, E., and Ruoppila, I. (1995) Difficulties in mobility among elderly people and their association with socioeconomic factors, dwelling environment and use of services. *Aging (Milano)* **7**:433–40.

Salas, C. (2002) On the empirical association between poor health and low socioeconomic status at old age. *Health Econ.* **11**:207–20.

Schooling, M. and Kuh, D. (2002) A life course perspective on women's health behaviours. In: *A Life course approach to women's health* (ed, D. Kuh and R. Hardy). Oxford: Oxford University Press.

Schulz, R. and Beach, S.R. (1999) Caregiving as a risk factor for mortality: the Caregiver Health Effects Study. *JAMA* **282**:2215–9.

Schulz, R., O'Brien, A.T., Bookwala, J., and Fleissner, K. (1995) Psychiatric and physical morbidity effects of dementia caregiving: prevalence, correlates and causes. *Gerontologist* **35**:771–91.

Seshamani, M. and Gray, A. (2004) Time to death and health expenditure: an improved model for the impact of demographic change on health care costs. *Age Ageing* **33**:556–61.

Shahtahmasebi, S., Davies, R., and Wenger, G.C. (1992) A longitudinal analysis of factors related to survival in old age. *Gerontologist* **32**:404–13.

Simonsick, E.M., Lafferty, M.E., Phillips, C.L., Mendes de Leon, C.F., Kasl, S.V., Seeman, T.E., *et al.* (1993) Risk due to inactivity in physically capable older adults. *Am. J. Public Health* **83**: 1443–50.

Singer, B.H. and Manton, K.G. (1998) The effects of health changes on projections of health service needs for the elderly population of the United States. *Pro. Nat. Acad. Sci.* **95**:15618–22.

Singh–Manoux, A., Adler, N.E., and Marmot, M.G. (2003) Subjective social status: its determinants and its associations with measures of ill-health in the Whitehall II study. *Soc. Sci. Med.* **56**: 1321–33.

Smith, J.P. (1999) Healthy bodies and thick wallets: the dual relation between health and economic status. *J. Econ. Perspectives* **13**:145–66.

Smith, J.P. and Kington, R. (1997) Demographic and economic correlates of health in old age. *Demography* **34**:159–70.

Spillman, B.C. (2004) Changes in elderly disability rates and the implications for health care utilization and cost. *Milbank Quart.* **82**:157–94.

Stansfeld, S.A., Head, J., and Marmot, M.G. (1998) Explaining social class differences in depression and well being. *Soc. Psych. Psych. Epidemiol.* **33**:1–9.

Steel, N., Huppert, F.A., McWilliams, B., and Melzer, D. (2003) Physical and cognitive function. In: *Health, wealth and lifestyles of the older population in England: the 2002 English Longitudinal Study of Ageing* (ed. M. Marmot, J. Banks, R. Blundell, *et al.*). London: Institute for Fiscal Studies.

Stitt, S., O'Connell, C., and Grant, D. (1995) Old, poor and malnourished. *Nutr. Health* **10**:135–54.

Strawbridge, W.J., Cohen, R.D., Shema, S.J., and Kaplan, G.A. (1996) Successful aging: predictors and associated activities. *Am. J. Epidemiol.* **144**:135–41.

Stuck, A.E., Walthert, J.M., Nikolaus, T., Bula, C.J., Hohmann, C., and Beck, J.C. (1999) Risk factors for functional status decline in community-living elderly people: a systematic literature review. *Soc. Sci. Med.* **48**:445–69.

Sundquist, J. and Johansson, S.E. (1997) Self reported poor health and low educational level predictors for motality: a population-based follow-up study of 39,156 people in Sweden. *J. Epidemiol. Community Health* **51**:35–40.

Sutherland, S. (1999) *With respect to old age: long-term care—rights and responsibilities. Report of the Royal Commission on Long-term Care.* CM 4192-I. London: The Stationery Office.

Swain, V.J. (1993) Changes in self-reported health. In: *The Health and Lifestyle Survey: seven years on* (ed. B.D. Cox, F.A. Huppert, and M.J. Whichelow), pp. 49–72. Aldershot: Dartmouth.

Taylor, R. and Ford, G. (1983) Inequalities in old age: an examination of age, sex and class differences in a sample of community elderly. *Ageing Society* **3**:183–208.

Thorslund, M. and Lundberg, O. (1994) Health inequalities among the oldest old. *J. Aging Health* **6**: 51–69.

Todd, G.F. (1959) *Statistics of smoking.* London: Tobacco Manufacturers Standing Committee.

Townsend, P. and Davidson, N. (1982) *Inequalities in health. The Black Report.* Harmondsworth: Penguin Books.

Turner, R.J. and Marino, F. (1994) Social support and social structure: a descriptive epidemiology of a central stress mediator. *J. Health Soc. Behav.* **35**:193–212.

Usui, W.M., Keil, T.J., and Durig, K.R. (1985) Socioeconomic comparisons and life satisfaction of elderly adults. *J. Gerontol.* **40**:110–14.

Veenstra, G. (2000) Social capital, SES and health: an individual-level analysis. *Soc. Sci. Med.* **50**:619–29.

Victor, C.R. (1989) Inequalities in health in later life. *Age Ageing* **18**:387–91.

Victor, C.R. (1991) Continuity of change: inequalities in health in later life. *Ageing Soc.* **11**:23–9.

Vitaliano, P.P., Schulz, R., Kiecolt–Glaser, J., and Grant, I. (1997) Research on physiological and physical concomitants of caregiving: where do we go from here? *Ann. Behav. Med.* **19**:117–23.

Waidmann, T.A. and Manton, K.G. (1998) *International evidence on disability trends among the elderly (abstract).* US Department of Health and Human Services.

Wanless, D. (2002) *Securing our future health: taking a long term view. Final report.* London: HM Treasury.

Wanless, D. (2004) *Securing good health for the whole population. Final report.* London: The Stationery Office.

Whitehead, M. (1987) *The health divide: inequalities in health in the 1980s.* London: The Health Education Council.

Williams, R.B., Barefoot, J.C., Califf, R.M., *et al.* Prognostic importance of social and economic resources among medically treated patients with angiographically documented coronary artery disease. *JAMA* **267**:520–4.

Chapter 14

Neighbourhoods, housing, and health

Mai Stafford and Mark McCarthy

14.1 Introduction

Differences in rates of mortality and morbidity across countries were presented in Chapter 1. At a more local level, does place of residence influence health? The UK has official targets to 'narrow the gap between deprived neighbourhoods and the rest of the country, so that within 10 to 20 years, no-one should be seriously disadvantaged by where they live' (Cabinet Office 2001, p. 8). But what is the evidence that neighbourhood and housing quality are related to health? Is the neighbourhood and housing environment important for both physical health and mental health? Which particular features of the neighbourhood might be important for health? Is there any evidence linking changing neighbourhood or housing environment to health improvement? Dealing firstly with neighbourhood influences on health and then moving on to review the housing and health literature, this chapter summarizes findings from several recent studies, highlights limitations of this literature, and points to possible ways that researchers and policy makers may move the field forward.

14.2 Neighbourhood environment and residents' health

Mortality and disease rates vary across neighbourhoods in the UK and in other developed countries (Humphreys and Carr–Hill, 1991; Duncan et al,1995; Wiggins et al. 1998; Krieger 1992; Diez–Roux et al. 1997; Martikainen et al. 2003). Figure 14.1 illustrates the variation in limiting long-term illness for women across the country, with the highest rates of limiting illness clustering in parts of the north, north–west, and Wales. The differences between neighbourhoods may be widening (Shaw et al. 1998). It is clear that health in certain areas is worse than in other areas. What is less clear is whether differences can be explained simply by the association between individual risk factors and health combined with the clustering of individuals with similar risk profiles into the same areas (a compositional effect), or whether they are due to additional effects of area of residence over and above individual risk factors (a contextual effect).

Several designs have been used to study the association between neighbourhood environment and health: ecological studies which relate population characteristics to

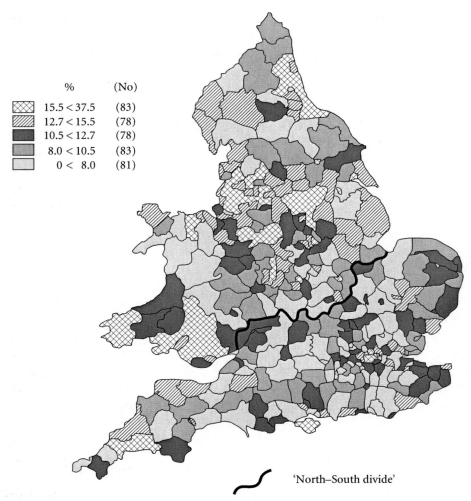

Fig. 14.1 Percentage of women in England and Wales aged 36–65 with limiting long-term illness, by county district.

Source: ONS Longitudinal Study, Wiggins *et al.* 2002, with permission from Elsevier.

population health (Bobak and Leon 1999); individual quantitative or in-depth studies which relate perceptions of the local environment to health (Pevalin 2004; Cattell 2001); and multilevel studies which combine neighbourhood level data with individual health (Duncan *et al.* 1995). Only the latter types of studies can be used to tease out contextual and compositional explanations for neighbourhood differences in health. Multilevel analysis allows the investigation of the health of individuals living not just in the same type of area (for example, deprived or affluent area) but for individuals living in the same area, sharing the same physical space, the same transport, retail and health services, and the same neighbours. In this chapter, we focus mainly on evidence from multilevel studies of the neighbourhood environment and health.

One of the challenges to studying neighbourhoods is deciding how the neighbourhood should be operationalized. Administrative boundaries, such as census wards in the UK or census tracts in the US, are often used in quantitative studies, for practical rather than theoretical reasons. Arguably, census wards and census tracts cover a fairly small geographical area that most residents could walk round and where they share the same shops, churches, pubs, and so on and are a reasonable approximation to geographical community. Campbell and McLean's work (2002) suggests that many people do express some identification with the census ward they live in, indicating a degree of overlap between geographically and psychologically defined communities. Nevertheless, the field will be advanced if more sophisticated ways of defining neighbourhoods can be found.

Economic, social-relational, service, and physical aspects of the neighbourhood may be important for health (Macintyre *et al.* 1993). Examples of studies relating to each of these characteristics in turn are provided below.

14.2.1 **Neighbourhood economic characteristics and health**

Economic factors such as concentrated deprivation, de-industrialization, and unemployment rate have received the most attention in the empirical literature, partly because data capturing economic factors are the most readily available. In the UK, indices of multiple deprivation, for example, are typically captured by census measures of the proportion of men who are unemployed, the proportion of residents who are in occupations in social class IV or V, the proportion of households which are overcrowded, the proportion of households without access to a car, and the proportion of households that are not owner-occupied (Carstairs and Morris 1991; Townsend 1979). Area-based deprivation indices have been reviewed elsewhere (Gordon 2003) and are also covered in Chapter 10.

Studies have shown associations between residence in a multiply-deprived area and infant and child health (Morgan and Chinn 1983; O'Campo *et al.* 1997; Roberts 1997), health-related behaviours (Duncan *et al.* 1993, 1999; Yen and Kaplan 1998), perceived general and mental health (Humphreys and Carr–Hill 1991; Duncan *et al.* 1995; Shouls *et al.* 1996; Wiggins *et al.* 1998; Sloggett and Joshi 1998), coronary heart disease (Diez–Roux *et al.* 1997, 2001), violence and murder (Sampson *et al.* 1997; Cubbin *et al.* 2000; Shaw *et al.* 2005), and all-cause mortality (Fox *et al.* 1984; Haan *et al.* 1987; Jones *et al.* 2000; Bosma *et al.* 2001; Martikainen *et al.* 2003). Most studies have found these associations to be graded, with steadily increasing deprivation being associated with incremental increases in the risk of morbidity and mortality. For example, Fig. 14.2 shows an increasing likelihood of smoking as deprivation in the local area increases. Residents in the most deprived areas are about 1.8 times as likely to smoke as those in the least deprived areas, after allowing for their personal socio-economic characteristics.

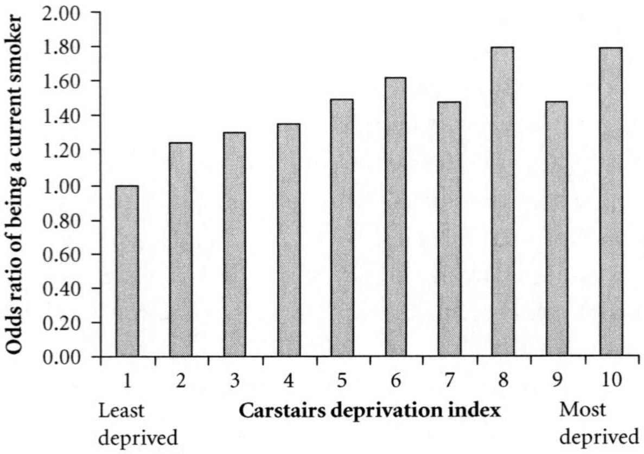

Fig. 14.2 Smoking increases by decile of Carstairs deprivation index; adjusted for age, social class, and economic activity.

Source: Health Survey for England 1994–99, men only.

A recent review of multilevel studies concluded that the majority found significant associations between neighbourhood deprivation and health, though these were generally modest in comparison with the size of associations between individual characteristics and health (Pickett and Pearl 2001).

14.2.2 Neighbourhood social environment and health

Social-relational factors include social capital, social cohesion, and social control. The definition and measurement of these constructs has been much debated and there is no universal agreement as yet. (See the extensive discussion in the *International Journal of Epidemiology* (2004), volume 33, for example.) Taking Putnam's widely quoted approach, social capital can be defined as 'features of social organisations, such as networks, norms, and trust, that facilitate action and co-operation for mutual benefit' (Putnam 1993). This can be applied to neighbourhoods (although it can equally apply to workplaces, special interest groups, professions, and so on). Social interactions between people resident in a given neighbourhood may produce externalities which have the potential to influence the health and well-being of people who do not take part in those social interactions but who live in the same locality. At the neighbourhood level, this has been operationalized in many ways, for example, as proportion of residents who report that they trust others, proportion of residents involved in local associations, and proportion of residents who report that their neighbours can be relied on. A typical design is to ask one set of respondents about their perceptions of their local social environment, aggregate these responses up to neighbourhood level, and link aggregate scores to a different database which includes data on individual health. In this way, perceptions of the social environment are obtained externally from perceptions of health.

The neighbourhood social environment may also be observed directly. This approach was taken in the Public Health and Development in Chicago Neighborhoods Study, where public incivilities were recorded by independent, trained observers (Sampson 1999). In multilevel studies adjusting for residential composition, neighbourhood

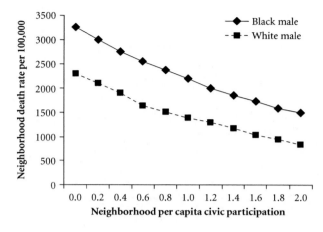

Fig. 14.3 Death rate for 45–64 year-olds is associated with civic participation; adjusted for neighbourhood deprivation.

Source: Lochner *et al.* 2003, with permission from Elsevier.

indicators of social capital have been related to birth weight (Buka *et al.* 2003), health-related behaviours (Weitzman and Kawachi 2000), perceived general and mental health (Cutrona *et al.* 2000; Wen *et al.* 2003; Stafford *et al.* 2004), and homicide and all-cause mortality (Sampson *et al.* 1997; Lochner *et al.* 2003). The inverse relationship between civic participation (measured in the Public Health and Development in Chicago Neighborhoods Study) and mortality (Lochner *et al.* 2003) is shown in Fig. 14.3. Mohan and colleagues (2004) created novel synthetic estimates of various neighbourhood level indicators of altruistic activities and informal sociability and related these to mortality. Volunteering and social activity showed significant associations with mortality over and above individual age, sex, and socio-economic characteristics.

Analysis of longitudinal individual-level data from the British Household Panel Survey showed that perceived attachment to the neighbourhood did not predict subsequent onset of common mental illness (Pevalin 2004). The lack of longitudinal association suggests that, if neighbourhood attachment is causally related to mental health, the effect is fairly immediate and does not have a long lag time.

Although the US General Social Survey is an important source of information, capturing social capital at the state level (Kawachi *et al.* 1997), it has not been used for neighbourhood-level research and studies based on this survey are not reviewed here, although Chapter 8 covers some of this literature. Studies capturing social processes within the neighbourhood and child and adolescent development have been reviewed by Sampson and colleagues (2002). The literature relating neighbourhood social-relational factors to health outcomes, especially in the UK, lags behind current evidence linking socio-economic features of the neighbourhood to health.

14.2.3 **Neighbourhood amenities and health**

The service environment covers publicly and privately provided facilities and amenities, such as health services, transport, and retail outlets. Multilevel studies of the service environment are few and far between. Cummins and colleagues (2005*a*) collected information on transport, health, retail, and financial services from a wide range of routine and non-routine sources including central government departments, local authorities, voluntary and public sector agencies, and commercial and industrial organizations. A positive association between perceived health and health service provision and access to financial services was found for women and a positive association between perceived health and access to large foodstores was found for men (Stafford *et al.* 2005). It seems unlikely that these associations represent direct pathways linking service environment to health, and it is possible that financial services and foodstores are markers of other features of the neighbourhood. For example, the presence of a new supermarket in an area might be an indicator of inner-city or suburban location, or local purchasing power. Data from the Alameda County study suggest that the presence of a high number of commercial stores (pharmacies, beauty salons/barbers, launderettes/dry cleaners, and supermarkets) was associated with increased risk of death (Yen and Kaplan 1999).

A scale measuring ease of access to four different services (corner shop, large supermarket, post office, and general practitioner) was created using Health Survey for England 2000 participants' self-reports. Responses were aggregated up to neighbourhood level. Ease of access was not associated with perceived general or mental health, smoking, or obesity over and above individual socio-economic factors (Boreham *et al.* 2002). However, a social class gradient in ease of access was found, so it is possible that access to services mediates some of the social inequality in other health outcomes.

Participants in the Alameda County study were asked about potential neighbourhood problems (Balfour and Kaplan 2002). Those reporting inadequate lighting at night or limited access to transportation were more likely to experience loss of physical function over the previous year compared to those reporting no problems with lighting or transportation (Fig. 14.4). Lower extremity functioning was especially affected. The authors speculate that neighbourhood problems might curtail the level of activity outside the home, thereby increasing the risk of functional decline.

Participants in the General Household Survey 2000 were also asked about facilities in their local area. Items included social and leisure facilities, facilities for young children, facilities for teenagers, health services, schools and colleges, and the police service and incorporated perceptions of both the quality and quantity of these facilities. Men who perceived their area to have poor local facilities were more likely to rate their health as less than good compared with men who perceived their area to have better facilities. No such association was seen for women (Ginn and Arber 2004).

It is apparent that the simple summation of the number of services and amenities which are located in an area does not capture adequately the everyday experience of residents and their contact with these facilities. The quality of these facilities is likely to be just as important and, if access to these facilities is easy, it may not matter that they are not located within one's immediate neighbourhood. Additionally, the potential

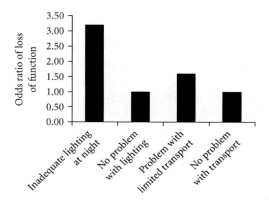

Fig. 14.4 Loss of physical function is associated with neighbourhood amenities in older adults; adjusted for age, sex, and baseline function.

Source: Balfour and Kaplan 2002.

importance of a balance of land use (for commercial and residential purposes) for local social interactions and for health has been highlighted elsewhere (Sampson *et al.* 2002).

14.2.4 **Neighbourhood physical environment and health**

In developed countries, physical aspects of the neighbourhood which may be salient for health include pollution levels, presence of industrial and waste disposal sites, degree of urbanization, green spaces, and other aspects of urban design. Many physical aspects, such as climate and water hardness, vary over relatively large areas and are not relevant for neighbourhood studies. Multilevel studies suggest that a run-down built environment is associated with poorer perceived general health, accounting for individual socio-economic characteristics (Cummins *et al.*, 2005*b*). Housing stock characterized by predominantly deck access and predominantly recent (post-1969) construction are associated with poor mental health over and above individual factors (Weich *et al.* 2002). The presence of attractive walkable spaces has recently received attention and has been shown to predict survival amongst older people (Takano *et al.* 2002) and physical activity in the general adult population (see review by Humpel *et al.* 2002). Physical environmental factors, personal attitudes, and peer support appear to be equally important in encouraging walking (Giles–Corti and Donovan 2003). Total particulate concentration and sulphur dioxide levels are positively associated with all-cause mortality after accounting for individual characteristics (Finkelstein *et al.* 2003). Ecological designs have been employed in most other studies of the physical environment and provide further evidence that air pollution, proximity to main roads, and cold climate are associated with worse health (Schwartz 1994; Maheswaran and Elliott 2003; Blane *et al.* 2000; Mitchell *et al.* 2002).

14.2.5 **Co-varying pathogenic features of the neighbourhood**

The evidence covering economic, social-relational, service, and physical features of the neighbourhood may be reviewed separately, but the reality is that these are likely to co-vary. More economically deprived areas are likely to have different physical and social-relational characteristics from more affluent areas. Neighbourhood deprivation shows a large inverse correlation with social cohesion (Stafford *et al.* 2004) and work in the US suggests that the preservation of informal social control and social cohesion is highly dependent upon neighbourhood affluence (Wen *et al.* 2003). Physical aspects of the built environment are associated with neighbouring (Skjaeveland and Garling 1997) and other aspects of social interaction (Leyden 2003). For example, semi-private space (buffers between the house and public space), living at street level compared with higher levels, and spaciousness are associated with greater neighbouring. The presence of suitable meeting places facilitates social interaction (Cattell and Herring 2002; Witten *et al.* 2001). Poor quality housing is more common in areas of the UK with a harsher climate, as illustrated in Fig. 14.5 (Blane *et al.* 2000).

Some of these environmental characteristics may only be associated with health in the presence of other risk factors. For example, over and above individual risk factors, harsh climate is associated with poorer lung function and higher blood pressure for those who live in poor quality housing stock, but this association is less apparent for people living in better quality housing (Blane *et al.* 2000; Mitchell *et al.* 2002). In another example, ecological analysis showed that male lung cancer rates were positively correlated with air pollution in neighbourhoods of high economic deprivation only (Dayal *et al.* 1984). It is probably beyond the scope of any single study to measure accurately all these features of the neighbourhood, so we must piece together evidence from various sources.

The study of neighbourhood environment and health is further complicated by the possibility that certain sections of the population will be more exposed to or more vulnerable to local features than others. In other words, there are likely to be statistical interactions between individual characteristics, features of the neighbourhood environment, and health. Associations between neighbourhood environment and health may vary by sex, social position, employment status, and race (Sloggett and Joshi 1998; Yen and Kaplan 1999; Jones *et al.* 2000; Diez–Roux *et al.* 2001; Stafford and Marmot 2003). We could speculate that retired people, children, and parents with young children might also be more exposed and dependent on locally provided facilities.

14.3 **Intervention studies**

One further study design has not yet been mentioned. Intervention studies of the link between neighbourhood and health address the problem of selection bias in neighbourhood research. An important example is the Moving to Opportunity (MTO) program which started in five US cities in 1994 (US Department of Housing and Urban Development 2003). Eligible participants (families with very low income with children who lived in social housing) were randomly assigned to one of three groups:

1 an experimental group receiving housing subsidies to move into low-poverty areas, plus assistance in finding suitable accommodation;

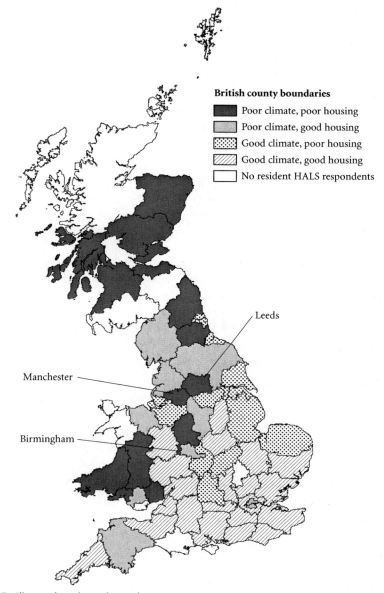

British county boundaries

■ Poor climate, poor housing

▓ Poor climate, good housing

▒ Good climate, poor housing

▨ Good climate, good housing

□ No resident HALS respondents

Leeds

Manchester

Birmingham

Fig. 14.5 Climate–housing mismatch.

Source: Blane *et al*. 2000, with permission from the BMJ Publishing Group.

2   a group receiving housing subsidies which were not limited geographically;

3   a control group.

At baseline, health status was not included in the survey of participants, so the MTO program has not yet been able to look at change in health status by randomization group. However, recent findings indicate that adults in the experimental group had less psychological distress at follow-up than the other two groups (Leventhal and Brooks–Gunn 2003). No differences in general health, smoking, alcohol consumption, or blood pressure were demonstrated. Findings for children's health were less clear, although boys and younger children in the experimental group appeared to show less distress/anxiety problems compared with controls. This, and other controlled studies of social housing interventions, are reviewed in Anderson *et al.* (2003).

An intervention designed to improve the social and physical fabric of selected 'distressed' neighbourhoods in Israel was evaluated by comparing before and after measures in an experimental versus a control group of neighbourhoods, matched on socio-economic characteristics (Carmon and Baron 1994). Despite some success in improving housing conditions, social services, and resident involvement in the experimental areas, the intervention was not successful in raising the socio-economic characteristics in comparison with control areas. The authors conclude that improved services can reduce inequalities in living conditions but a degree of residential turnover is required in order to raise an area's socio-economic profile. They suggest that gentrification is one way of achieving this population change, but new residential construction (without displacement of the original inhabitants) is another.

14.3.1 Neighbourhood-based initiatives

Several area-based initiatives have been introduced in recent years. Examples include Health Action Zones, Employment Action Zones, and the Deprived Urban Post Office scheme to prevent post office closure (which may help retain other local shops and businesses). More general schemes such as the Neighbourhood Renewal Fund (which aims to boost and co-ordinate spending in the 88 most deprived local authorities) and the New Deal for Communities (which provides funding and encourages partnership working in deprived areas) also take an area-based approach. What most of these initiatives have in common is that the target population is defined geographically; typically, areas which score highly on indices of multiple deprivation are selected. Some of these then use the allocated resources to aim to improve local economic, social, or service conditions. For example, the key aim of the Neighbourhood Renewal program is 'to deliver economic prosperity, safe communities, high quality schools, decent housing, improved physical environment and better health to the poorest parts of the country' (Cabinet Office 2001).

Some initiatives use the allocation to target specific groups of people within the catchment area. The area-based approach of the latter group of initiatives could perhaps be considered more of a (blunt) tool for identifying individuals with greatest need rather than a strategy to improve local living conditions. However, the former group of initiatives could provide a valuable opportunity to assess the extent to which features of the neighbourhood can be changed through a multi-agency approach and to identify any corresponding improvements in the health of the resident population.

Some of these initiatives are being evaluated with respect to health outcomes, although assessment of the health impact has not been built into the program, so valuable information may be lost. Admittedly, the potential for health gains following neighbourhood regeneration may be limited (Curtis *et al.* 2002). For example, schemes may tackle some of the neighbourhood-level barriers to healthy living, but many more may not be addressed by any given initiative.

Having reviewed the wide range of contextual factors that may be important for health, it is clear that complex and wide-ranging, long-term interventions will be required. Disruption and change in itself may additionally have a negative impact on health, at least in the short term.

14.4 **Evidence for causation?**

A whole host of pathways linking neighbourhood environment to various health outcomes through behavioural, biological, and psychosocial mediators can be hypothesized. A limitation of much of the existing research linking neighbourhoods to health outcomes is that these pathways are not described and tested explicitly. In large part, this comes from the fact that many of these studies use secondary analysis of existing data, but it is time to move on from describing associations between summary indices of deprivation and health towards explicit testing of possible causal pathways.

Using Bradford–Hill's criteria for helping to establish causality, we can assess the current state of knowledge relating neighbourhood environment to health.

Consistency

Studies based in several developed countries, using different geographical units, investigating many different outcomes, have demonstrated statistically significant associations between neighbourhood environment and health. The breadth of the literature is perhaps greatest for economic aspects of the neighbourhood. There is still a need to develop, test, and repeat models linking different aspects of the local economic, social, and physical environment to specific health outcomes.

Strength of association

Whilst the majority of published studies have demonstrated statistically significant associations between neighbourhood environment and health, these associations are generally reckoned to be smaller in magnitude than the associations between individual socio-economic and demographic characteristics and health (Pickett and Pearl 2001). Nevertheless, if a large number of residents is exposed to even a small environmental risk, the public health implications may be considerable.

Dose–response relationship

On the whole, graded relationships between features of the neighbourhood and risk of adverse health have been found.

Temporal sequence

These findings are largely based on cross-sectional data, so reverse causation cannot be excluded. This is perhaps more clearly the case for social-relational aspects of the neighbourhood; indeed, a person's health has been found to predict future social participation (Pevalin and Rose 2003). Relating change in neighbourhood characteristics to change in health is difficult for several reasons. Collecting primary data over a time period during which neighbourhoods could reasonably be expected to change would be costly. Routine administrative data collected over several years can be used but administrative neighbourhood boundaries usually change over time and this must be dealt with analytically. In- and out-migration must also be taken into account.

Biological plausibility

The majority of studies have used secondary analysis of existing data sources. Using best available data has limited the extent to which we have been able to test biologically plausible pathways. In more recent years, there has been an increase in purpose-built studies, so the capacity to test biological plausibility should be increasing.

Specificity

It is very difficult to isolate the effects of neighbourhood characteristics. Places can influence people and people can influence places (Macintyre and Ellaway 2003). The separation of variation in health into that which is between individuals and that which is between neighbourhoods is a statistical tool used for the multilevel analysis of person and place. This approach has been useful in highlighting the influence of the residential context on health. The separation is, however, an artificial one. To ask the question 'do people, regardless of how they differ on individual characteristics, have different health status according to where they live?' (which is what is done when area-level and individual- level variables are included together in a multilevel model), is to ignore the reality of residential segregation and the limited option for mobility experienced by some sections of the population. Previous housing policy and market forces have resulted in residential segregation, with poorer individuals being obliged to live in cheaper, less salutary areas. Personal socio-economic disadvantage therefore increases the risk of being exposed to residential socio-economic disadvantage.

A further complication is that effects which are attributed to the area may be due to unmeasured individual differences. In addition, area of residence in the formative years can influence educational attainment, income, and occupation (Jencks and Mayer 1990). This means that attempts to separate out the effect of area of residence from individual risk factors are somewhat hypothetical. Spatial dependencies also need to be considered in a more sophisticated way (Sampson *et al.* 1999). Presently, studies tend to consider each neighbourhood in isolation from contiguous areas. Existing data (and until recently, statistical software) are limited in their ability to model feedback over time and this spatial complexity. The limits of multilevel modelling techniques are discussed by Subramanian and colleagues (2003).

14.5 **Housing quality and health**

Housing is frequently described as a determinant of health. For example, the 2004 Report by the UK Sustainable Development Commission says:

> Everyone should share in the benefits of increased prosperity and a clean and safe environment. We have to improve access to services, tackle social exclusion, and reduce the harm to health done by poverty, poor housing, unemployment, and pollution. (Department for Environment, Food, and Rural Affairs 2004, p. 15)

Here, housing is considered as an independent social characteristic, akin to income and employment. But housing can also be used as a proxy for personal capital appreciation and socio-economic status—for example, comparing tenure of households in rented property with house-owners. Yet tenure is not a strong discriminant for housing characteristics: newer housing, whether public sector or private, is usually built to higher standards than older housing. Tenants of private landowners generally have poorer housing but (in England at least) are a minority of households.

Housing is linked with neighbourhoods both by being the place where 'compositional factors' (people, households) reside, and also by being the physical environment for people's lives. On the other hand, neighbourhoods have an independent dimension in the links people share across households (social relationships) and also in the mix of services and environmental factors of the urban or rural setting. Two examples of epidemiological approaches to assessing the contribution of housing to health are ecological methods and direct investigations. This chapter illustrates findings from ecological and direct studies and also points to some results from intervention evaluations, which may help demonstrate the relative benefit of policy implementation. It is not intended as a full review of housing quality on health, but see, for example, Thomson *et al.* (2001).

14.5.1 **Ecological studies—temperature and health**

Many countries in western Europe show excess mortality each year in winter time and, in some years, also in the summer time. This does not simply reflect temperature, since countries in Eastern Europe, with more pronounced minima and maxima, do not show these mortality differences. The winter and summer deaths are mostly certified for common diseases, including circulatory and respiratory diseases, rather than hypothermia or hyperthermia. The mechanism, therefore, is an exacerbation of existing liability, and the majority of excess deaths are in older people whose deaths are 'brought forward'.

Shelter in any country, from thick-walled ice igloos to black cloth berber tents, seeks to control heat loss or gain and protect the inhabitants. Houses in the west of Europe have windows that can be opened or closed at any time of the year in response to the varied temperatures of Atlantic weather systems, whereas thick-walled houses in Eastern European countries have windows that are sealed in winter. Houses in western countries have colder rooms in winter, and less well-developed heating systems, and have inadequate ventilation for hot summers. These housing differences may contribute to temperature effects on health. But housing is not the only, or necessarily primary, issue. People in western European countries dress and protect themselves less well when outside in the winter, while the southern European 'siesta' limits people going out in the summer heat. The excess mortality occurs at higher average temperature thresholds in warmer countries, suggesting adaptation—but whether it is the buildings that are adapted, or the humans themselves (and their habits), is not clear.

Some evidence comes from epidemiological studies. In England, an intervention to provide better heating and insulation for poor housing, 'Warm Front', has been evaluated in a prospective before-and-after design. The intervention itself raised room temperatures on average by one to two degrees, and there was a measurable improvement in self-perceived health and reduction in use of GP services, suggesting a benefit from improved house heating (Wilkinson, personal communication). In the US, a retrospective case-control study of deaths in the 1995 Chicago heat wave showed that people at increased risk were already ill, confined to bed, unable to care for themselves, and without air conditioning. (Semmenza et al. 1995). A recent ecological study in the US has also suggested that air conditioning has contributed to falling summer excess mortality over the past 20 years (Janssen et al. 2002).

14.5.2 Direct studies—housing characteristics

A different approach to housing and health has been to consider specific design characteristics and their associated health risks. Work in the UK has addressed both regulations for new buildings and assessment of existing housing. In 1990, the UK government adopted housing fitness standards—the house should be structurally stable, free from serious disrepair and significant damp, and have adequate lighting, heating, and ventilation, adequate piped clean water, satisfactory bathroom and toilet, and satisfactory kitchen and effective waste system. The English Housing Condition Survey of 14,000 houses in 1995 estimated, by these criteria, that 1.8 million houses failed to meet one or more of the standards and were 'unfit'. The 1997 Labour government committed itself to making all these houses fit by 2010, and the 2002 English Housing Condition survey indicated that the 1995 figure had indeed been reduced by one third. In 2003, the government identified reduction of 'unfit' housing as part of the Action Plan for reducing health inequalities in England. Households in unfit housing are more likely to be socio-economically disadvantaged, but the government did not make a prediction on how far their health would be improved by improved housing.

Also in the 1990s, in a partnership between the ministry and universities, a new assessment system was developed, widening the assessment criteria to include fire safety, air quality (especially radon), energy efficiency, and internal arrangement (especially risk of falls). The new Housing Health and Safety Rating System assesses hazards from epidemiological studies and data on falls drawn from the Home Accident Surveillance System (a sample of hospital emergency departments) (Office of the

Deputy Prime Minister 2004). It assesses risk in relation to a 'vulnerable person'—for example, for an elderly person if the staircase lighting is poor, or the danger of low windows for a child. Both the most likely outcome (for example, spraining a wrist in a fall downstairs) and the spread of risks (for example, from bruising to breaking a hip) are considered for each hazard. The rating system will be used by local authorities for monitoring the state of local housing and in making decisions on allocation of grants for housing improvements. However, there is as yet no provision for assessing whether the recorded housing deficiencies are individually contributing to health harms, nor on whether improvement of homes is leading to better health.

14.5.3 Multi-sectoral interventions

People who are homeless or live in poor housing are less healthy; yet it is less clear how far housing creates ill health. Some of the association between poor housing and poor health may be selection over the life course: more economically successful people, whose health is better than the average, will generally move into more affluent areas with better health levels, while more disadvantaged people will move to poorer housing. Intervention studies are a potential way round this confounding. Work by Thomson *et al.* (2003) identified reports of both benefits and adverse effects for physical illness, but generally improvements for mental health. Saegert *et al.* (2003) reaffirmed the findings of Fuller–Thompson and colleagues (2000) that studies commonly focus on single environmental exposures or specific conditions, most frequently lead poisoning, injury, or asthma. They considered that 'interventions that combine activities to make changes at several levels and examine multiple health outcomes will be more effective than those working at single levels'.

Two recent reports in England have sought to investigate this broader view of how housing improvement can affect health:

- ◆ Sheffield Healthy Cities provides an example of practical, committed action over the last 15 years to improve health in one deprived city ward through housing and regeneration (Saunders and Price 2003). The city was able to draw on both UK and European Union funds, initially for housing and, subsequently, for broader socio-economic development. There was community involvement and participation in decision making on the use of funds. There has also been a significant turnover in population, making it difficult to relate changes in housing to individual health. Housing has been greatly improved, and is more attractive to people to live in. Both deprivation indices and mortality rates have improved recently, but social problems, including drug misuse, have increased.

- ◆ In Wythenshawe, near Manchester, England, the mental health and quality of life of 2200 people was measured, before and afterwards, in an economic regeneration area and a comparison area (Huxley *et al.* 2002). Where most objective change occurred (in housing improvements), residents in the intervention area had greater satisfaction with physical health and living situation. However, mental health, and to a less extent, perceived quality of life, deteriorated in the intervention area. Qualitative interviews with a subsample of 200 indicated that improvements of infrastructure and economy did not meet residents' expectations. Mental ill health was particularly related to a feeling of 'entrapment' which the socio-economic programme did not address.

These studies reflect the need for broad study designs to investigate the impact of multi-sectoral interventions in housing and health. They also use various outcome measures, and combine ecological and direct approaches to evaluation.

14.6 Housing and neighbourhood quality and socio-economic position

Housing generally reflects, rather than creates, socio-economic gradients, and the particular contribution of housing to health gradients remains to be demonstrated (McCarthy 2002). Individual or household socio-economic position is also likely to determine the type of neighbourhood one lives in. It is possible that housing and neighbourhood quality are on the pathway linking socio-economic position to health. Whilst there is evidence to suggest that initiatives to improve neighbourhood and housing conditions might have benefits for health, we must also consider policies which will counteract the trend of increasing residential segregation by social position (Dorling and Rees 2003) and the widening social inequalities in housing conditions.

14.7 Policy implications

As we have seen, there are a number of area-based initiatives currently underway. Many of these are being under-utilized as sources of information which will contribute to the evidence base linking neighbourhood change to health improvement. Similarly, ongoing housing improvement initiatives, both national and local, could provide valuable information, but many of these are missed opportunities for understanding more about the relationship between housing and health.

Both objective and subjective measures of the residential environment are useful for evaluation studies. The relationship between perceived environmental quality and perceived health is subject to affect bias. Nevertheless, if recipients of an intervention do not perceive the objective change to be beneficial, it is possible that the expected health benefits will not materialize, as illustrated in the Wythenshawe example above.

We also need to broaden the scope of neighbourhood studies to consider the wider social and political processes that impact upon neighbourhoods and residents. In the US, Massey (1996) has described the close association between rising income inequality at a national level and rising concentrations of affluence and deprivation at the local level. Whilst the affluent are able to exercise their choice to move to more desirable neighbourhoods, poorer residents are less able to move, and so the rich and poor become spatially segregated. Increasing urbanization has focused this affluence and deprivation in the cities. The possible link between income inequality and neighbourhood deprivation or affluence has not been studied in countries outside the US, although associations between both the range and the absolute level of area deprivation with mortality have been shown using English data (Ben–Shlomo *et al.* 1996). Cross-country comparisons of income inequality and residential segregation by socioeconomic position could be undertaken, and these may highlight ways in which governments and societies might avoid escalating segregation and spiralling neighbourhood deterioration.

References

Anderson, L.M., St Charles, J., Fullilove, M.T., Scrimshaw, S.C., Fielding, J.E., Normand, J., *et al.* (2003). Providing affordable family housing and reducing residential segregation by income. *American Journal of Preventative Medicine*, **24**(3S), 47–67.

Balfour, J.L. and Kaplan, G.A. (2002). Neighborhood environment and loss of physical function in older adults: evidence from the Alameda County Study. *American Journal of Epidemiology*, **155**, 507–15.

Ben–Shlomo, Y., White, I.R., Marmot, M. (1996). Does the variation in the socioeconomic characteristics of an area affect mortality? *British Medical Journal*, **312**, 1013–14.

Blane, D., Mitchell, R., Bartley, M. (2000). The 'inverse housing law' and respiratory health. *Journal of Epidemiology and Community Health*, **54**, 745–9.

Bobak, M. and Leon, D.A. (1999). Pregnancy outcomes and outdoor air pollution: an ecological study in districts of the Czech Republic 1986–8. *Occupational and Environmental Medicine*, **56**:539–43.

Boreham, R., Stafford, M., Taylor, R. (2002). *Health Survey for England 2000: Social capital and health.* The Stationery Office, London.

Bosma, H., van de Mheen, H.D., Borsboom, G.J.J.M., Mackenbach, J.P. (2001). Neighbourhood socioeconomic status and all-cause mortality. *American Journal of Epidemiology*, **153**, 363–71.

Buka, S.L., Brennan, R.T., Rich–Edwards, J.W., Raudenbush, S.W., Earls, D. (2003). Neighbourhood support and the birth weight of urban infants. *American Journal of Epidemiology*, **3**, 157, 1–8.

Cabinet Office (2001). *A new commitment to neighbourhood renewal: a national strategy action plan.* Cabinet Office, London. Crown Copyright.

Campbell, C. and McLean, C. (2002). Ethnic identities, social capital and health inequalities: factors shaping African-Caribbean participation in local community networks in the UK. *Social Science and Medicine*, **55**, 643–57.

Carmon, N. and Baron, M. (1994). Reducing inequality by means of neighbourhood rehabilitation: an Israeli experiment and its lessons. *Urban Studies*, **31**, 1465–79.

Carstairs, V. and Morris, R. (1991). *Deprivation and health in Scotland.* Aberdeen University Press, Aberdeen.

Cattell, V. (2001). Poor people, poor places, and poor health: the mediating role of social networks and social capital. *Social Science and Medicine*, **52**, 1501–16.

Cattell, V. and Herring, R. (2002). Social capital, generations and health in East London. In: *Social Capital for health. Insights from qualitative research* (ed. C Swann and A Morgan). Health Development Agency, London.

Cubbin, C., LeClere, F.B., Smith, G.S. (2000). Socioeconomic status and injury mortality: individual and neighbourhood determinants. *Journal of Epidemiology and Community Health*, **54**, 517–24.

Cummins, S., Macintyre, S., Davidson, S., Ellaway, A. (2005*a*). Measuring neighbourhood social and material context: generation and interpretation of ecological data from routine and non-routine sources. *Health and Place*, **11**, 249–60.

Cummins, S., Stafford, M., Macintyre, S., Marmot, M., Ellaway, A. (2005*b*). Neighbourhood environment and its association with self-rated health: evidence from Scotland and England. *Journal of Epidemiology and Community Health*, **59**, 207–13.

Curtis, S., Cave, B., Coutts, A. (2002). Is urban regeneration good for health? Perceptions and theories of the health impacts of urban change. *Environment and Planning C*, **20**, 517–34.

Cutrona, C.E., Russell, D.W., Hessling, R.M., Brown, P.A., Murry, V. (2000). Direct and moderating effects of community context on the psychological well-being of African American women. *Journal of Personality and Social Psychology*, **79**, 1088–101.

Dayal, H., Chiu, C.Y., Sharrar, R., *et al* (1984). Ecologic correlates of cancer mortality patterns in an industrialized urban population. *Journal of the National Cancer Institute*, **73**, 565–74.

Department for Environment, Food, and Rural Affairs (2004). *Achieving a better quality of life: review of progress towards sustainable development. Government Annual Report 2003.* Department for Environment, Food, and Rural Affairs, London.

Diez–Roux, A., Merkin, S.S., Arnett, D., *et al.* (2001). Neighbourhood of residence and incidence of coronary heart disease. *New England Journal of Medicine*, **345**, 99–106.

Diez–Roux, A.V., Nieto, F.J., Muntaner, C., *et al.* (1997). Neighborhood environments and coronary heart disease: a multilevel analysis. *American Journal of Epidemiology*, **146**, 48–63.

Dorling, D. and Rees, P. (2003). A nation still dividing: the British census and social polarisation 1971–2001. *Environment and Planning A*, **35**, 1287–1313.

Duncan, C., Jones, K., Moon, G. (1993). Do places matter? A multi-level analysis of regional variations in health-related behaviour in Britain. *Social Science and Medicine*, **37**, 725–33.

Duncan, C., Jones, K., Moon, G. (1995). Psychiatric morbidity: a multilevel approach to regional variations in the UK. *Journal of Epidemiology and Community Health*, **49**, 290–5.

Duncan, C., Jones, K., Moon, G. (1999). Smoking and deprivation: are there neighbourhood effects? *Social Science and Medicine*, **48**, 497–505.

Finkelstein, M.M., Jerrett, M., DeLuca, P., *et al.* (2003). Relation between income, air pollution and mortality: a cohort study. *Canadian Medical Association Journal*, **169**, 397–402.

Fox, A.J., Jones, D.R., Goldblatt, P.O. (1984). Approaches to studying the effect of socio-economic circumstances on geographic differences in mortality in England and Wales. *British Medical Bulletin*, **40**, 309–14.

Fuller–Thomson, E., Hulchanski, J.D., Hwang, S. (2000). The housing/health relationship: what do we know? *Reviews in Environmental Health*, **15**, 109–33.

Giles–Corti, B. and Donovan, R.J. (2003). Relative influences of individual, social environmental, and physical environmental correlates of walking. *American Journal of Public Health*, **93**, 1583–9.

Ginn, J. and Arber, S. (2004). Gender and the relationship between social capital and health. In: *Social capital for health. Issues of definition, measurement and links to health* (ed. A Morgan and C Swann). Health Development Agency, London.

Gordon, D. (2003). Area-based deprivation measures—a U.K. perspective. In: *Neighbourhoods and health* (ed. I Kawachi and L Berkman). Oxford University Press, New York.

Haan, M., Kaplan, G.A., Camacho, T. (1987). Poverty and health: prospective evidence from the Alameda County study. *American Journal of Epidemiology*, **125**, 989–98.

Humpel, N., Owen, N., Leslie, E. (2002). Environmental factors associated with adults' participation in physical activity. A review. *American Journal of Preventative Medicine*, **22**, 188–99.

Humphreys, K. and Carr–Hill, R. (1991). Area variations in health outcomes: artefact or ecology. *International Journal of Epidemiology*, **20**, 251–8.

Huxley, P., Evans, S., Gately, C., Rogers, A. (2002). *Urban regeneration and mental health: evaluating an urban regeneration initiative as a mental health promotion strategy*. XXVIIth Congress of the International Academy of Law and Mental Health, Amsterdam 2002. *http://www.ialmh.org/amsterdam2002/11.07/mentalhealth.htm*

Janssen, N.A. *et al.* (2002). Air conditioning and source-specific particles as modifiers of the effect of PM10 on hospital admissions for heart and lung disease. *Environmental Health Perspectives*, **110**, 43–9.

Jencks, C. and Mayer, S. (1990). The social consequences of growing up in a poor neighbourhood. In: *Innter-city poverty in the United States* (ed. L Lynn Jr and M McGreary). National Academic Science Press, Washington DC.

Jones, K., Gould, M.I., Duncan C. (2000). Death and deprivation: an exploratory analysis of deaths in the Health and Lifestyle Survey. *Social Science and Medicine*, **50**, 1059–79.

Kawachi, I., Kennedy, B.P., Lochner, K., Prothrow–Stith, D. (1997). Social capital, income inequality and mortality. *American Journal of Public Health*, **87**, 1491–8.

Krieger, N. (1992). Overcoming the absence of socioeconomic data in medical records: validation and application of a census-based methodology. *American Journal of Public Health*, **82**, 703–10.

Leventhal, T. and Brooks–Gunn, J. (2003). Moving to opportunity: an experimental study of neighbourhood effects on mental health. *American Journal of Public Health*, **93**, 1576–82.

Leyden, K.M. (2003). Social capital and the built environment: the importance of walkable neighborhoods. *American Journal of Public Health*, **93**:1546–51.

Lochner, K.A., Kawachi, I., Brennan, R.T., Buka, S.L. (2003). Social capital and neighbourhood mortality rates in Chicago. *Social Science and Medicine*, **56**, 1797–805.

Macintyre, S. and Ellaway, A. (2003). Neighbourhoods and health: an overview. In: *Neighbourhoods and health* (ed. I Kawachi and L Berkman). Oxford University Press, New York.

Macintyre, S., Maciver, S., Sooman, A. (1993). Area, class and health: should we be focusing on places or people? *Journal of Social Policy*, **22**, 213–34.

Maheswaran, R. and Elliott, P. (2003). Stroke mortality associated with living near main roads in England and Wales. *Stroke*, **34**, 2776–80.

Martikainen, P., Kauppinen, T.M., Valkonen, T. (2003). Effects of the characteristics of neighbourhoods and the characteristics of people on cause specific mortality: a register-based follow-up study of 252,000 men. *Journal of Epidemiology and Community Health*, **57**, 210–17.

Massey, D.S. (1996). The age of extremes: concentrated affluence and poverty in the twenty-first century. *Demography*, **33**, 395–412.

McCarthy, M. (2002). Urban development and health inequalities. *Scandinavian Journal of Public Health*, **30** (suppl 59), 59–62.

Mitchell, R., Blane, D., Bartley, M. (2002). Elevated risk of high blood pressure: climate and the inverse housing law. *International Journal of Epidemiology*, **31**, 831–8.

Mohan, J., Barnard, S., Jones, K., Twigg, L. (2004). Social capital, geography and health: developing and applying small-area indicators of social capital in the explanation of health inequalities. In: *Social capital for health. Issues of definition, measurement and links to health* (ed. A Morgan and C Swann). Health Development Agency, London.

Morgan, M. and Chinn, S. (1983). ACORN group, social class, and child health. *Journal of Epidemiology and Community Health*, **37**, 196–203.

O'Campo, P., Xue, X., Wang, M.C., O'Brien Caughy, M. (1997). Neighborhood risk factors for low birthweight in Baltimore: a multilevel analysis. *American Journal of Public Health*, **87**, 1113–18.

Office of the Deputy Prime Minister (2004). *Housing Health and Safety Rating System (Version 2). Guidance.* Office of the Deputy Prime Minister, London. *http://www.odpm.gov.uk/stellent/groups/ odpm_housing/documents/page/odpm_house_603508.hcsp*

Pevalin, D. (2004). Intra-household differences in neighbourhood attachment and their associations with health. In: *Social capital for health. Issues of definition, measurement and links to health* (ed. A Morgan and C Swann). Health Development Agency, London.

Pevalin, D.J. and Rose, D. (2003). *Social capital for health. Investigating the links between social capital and health using the British Household Panel Survey. Research Report of the Health Development Agency.* Health Development Agency, London.

Pickett, K.E. and Pearl, M. (2001). Multilevel analyses of neighbourhood socioeconomic context and health outcomes: a critical review. *Journal of Epidemiology and Community Health*, **55**, 111–22.

Putnam, R.D. (1993). The prosperous community. Social capital and public life. *The American Prospect*, **Spring**, 35–42.

Roberts, E.M. (1997). Neighbourhood social environments and the distribution of low birthweight in Chicago. *American Journal of Public Health*, **87**, 597–603.

Saegert, S.C., Klitzman, S., Freudenberg, N., Cooperman–Mroczek, J., Nassar, S. (2003). Healthy housing: a structured review of published evaluations of US interventions to improve health by modifying housing in the United States 1999–2001. *American Journal of Public Health*, **93**, 1472–8.

Sampson, R.J. (1999). Systematic social observation of public spaces: a new look at disorder in urban neighbourhoods. *American Journal of Sociology*, **105**, 603–51.

Sampson, R.J., Morenoff, J.D., Earls, F. (1999). Beyond social capital: spatial dynamics of collective efficacy for children. *American Sociological Review*, **64**, 633–60.

Sampson, R.J., Morenoff, J.D., Gannon–Rowley, T. (2002). Assessing 'neighborhood effects': social processes and new directions in research. *Annual Review of Sociology*, **28**, 443–78.

Sampson, R.J., Raudenbush, S.W., Earls, F. (1997). Neighbourhoods and violent crime: a multilevel study of collective efficacy. *Science*, **277**, 918–24.

Saunders, J. and Price, C. (2003). *Regeneration and health in West Sheffield: narrowing the health gap—15 years of tackling health inequalities in the context of a healthy city.* Paper presented at the WHO Healthy Cities Conference, Belfast, 2003. *www.healthycitiesbelfast2003.com/FullPaperspdfs/Sunday19October/C4/JoannaSaunders352C4.pdf*

Schwartz, J. (1994). Air pollution and daily mortality: a review and meta analysis. *Environmental Research*, **64**, 36–52.

Semmenza, J.C. *et al.* (1995) Heat related deaths during the July 1995 heat wave in Chicago. *New England Journal of Medicine*, **335**, 84–90.

Shaw, M., Dorling, M., Brimblecombe, N. (1998). Changing the map: health in Britain 1951–91. *Sociology of Health and Illness*, **5**, 694–709.

Shaw, M., Tunstall, H., Dorling, D. (2005). Increasing inequalities in risk of murder in Britain: trends in the demographic and spatial distribution of murder, 1981–2000. *Health and Place*, **11**, 45–54

Shouls, S., Congdon, P., Curtis, S. (1996). Modelling inequality in reported long term illness in the UK: combining individual and area characteristics. *Journal of Epidemiology and Community Health*, **50**, 366–76.

Skjaeveland, O. and Garling, T. (1997). Effects of interactional space on neighbouring. *Journal of Environmental Psychology*, **17**, 181–98.

Sloggett, A. and Joshi, H. (1998) Deprivation indicators as predictors of life events, 1981–1992, based on the UK ONS longitudinal study. *Journal of Epidemiology and Community Health*, **52**, 228–33.

Stafford, M. and Marmot, M. (2003). Neighbourhood deprivation and health: does it affect us all equally? *International Journal of Epidemiology*, **32**, 357–66.

Stafford, M., Bartley, M., Boreham, R., Thomas, R., Wilkinson, R., Marmot, M. (2004). Neighbourhood social cohesion and health: investigating associations and possible mechanisms. In *Social capital for health. Issues of definition, measurement and links to health* (ed. A Morgan and C Swann). Health Development Agency, London.

Stafford, M., Cummins, S., Macintyre, S., Marmot, M. (2005). Gender differences in the health effects of neighbourhood infrastructure and social characteristics. *Social Science and Medicine*, **60**, 1681–92.

Subramanian, S.V., Jones, K., Duncan, C. (2003). Multilevel methods for public health research. In: *Neighbourhoods and health* (ed. I Kawachi and L Berkman). Oxford University Press, New York.

Takano, T., Nakamura, K., Watanabe, M. (2002). Urban residential environments and senior citizens' longevity in megacity areas: the importance of walkable green spaces. *Journal of Epidemiology and Community Health*, **56**, 913–18.

Thomson, H., Petticrew, M., Douglas, M. (2003). Health impact assessment of housing improvements: incorporating research evidence. *Journal of Epidemiology and Community Health*, **57**, 11–16.

Thomson, H., Petticrew, M., Morrison, M. (2001). Health effects of housing improvement: systematic review of intervention studies. *British Medical Journal*, **323**, 187–90.

Townsend, P. (1979). *Poverty in the United Kingdom*. Penguin, Harmondsworth.

US Department of Housing and Urban Development (2003). Moving to Opportunity for Fair Housing Program. US Department of Housing and Urban Development: Office of Policy Development and Research. Interim Impacts Evaluation. Available at: *http://www.huduser.org/ publications/fairhsg/ mtofinal.html*

Weich, S., Blanchard, M., Prince, M., Burton, E., Erens, B., Sproston, K. (2002). Mental health and the built environment: cross-sectional survey of individual and contextual risk factors for depression. *British Journal of Psychiatry*, **180**, 428–33.

Weitzman, E.R. and Kawachi, I. (2000). Giving means receiving: the protective effect of social capital on binge drinking on college campuses. *American Journal of Public Health*, **90**, 1936–9.

Wen, M., Browning, C.R., Cagney, K.A. (2003). Poverty, affluence, and income inequality: neighbourhood economic structure and its implications for health. *Social Science and Medicine*, **57**, 843–60.

Wiggins, R.D., Bartley, M., Gleave, S., Joshi, H., Lynch, K. (1998). Limiting long-term illness: a question of where you live or who you are? A multilevel analysis of the 1971–1991 ONS longitudinal study. *Risk Decision and Policy*, **3**, 181–98.

Wiggins, R.D., Joshi, H., Bartley, M., Gleave, S., Lynch, K., and Cullis, A. (2002). Place and personal circumstances in a multilevel account of women's long-term illness. *Social Science & Medicine*, **54**, 827–38.

Witten, K., McCreanor, T., Kearns, R., Ramasubramanian, L. (2001). The impacts of a school closure on neighbourhood social cohesion: narratives from Invercargill, New Zealand. *Health and Place*, **7**, 307–17.

Yen, I.H. and Kaplan, G.A. (1998). Poverty area residence and changes in physical activity level: evidence from the Alameda County Study. *American Journal of Public Health*, **88**, 1709–12.

Yen, I.H. and Kaplan, G.A. (1999). Poverty area residence and changes in depression and perceived health status: evidence from the Alameda County Study. *International Journal of Epidemiology*, **28**, 90–4.

Chapter 15

Social determinants, sexual behaviour, and sexual health

Anne M. Johnson, Catherine H. Mercer, and Jackie A. Cassell

15.1 Introduction

Over the past 20 years, there has been increasing attention paid to sexual health as an important public health issue, fuelled largely by the emergence of the human immuno-deficiency virus (HIV) pandemic. Underlying varying sexual health outcomes in individuals and populations are diverse patterns of human sexual behaviour. Globally, unsafe sex is a leading cause of disease burden, estimated to be greater than that caused by either high blood pressure, tobacco, or alcohol (Ezzati *et al.* 2002).

In this chapter, we discuss the complex relationship between social determinants, sexual behaviour, and sexual health. Our emphasis is on patterns of sexual health and behaviour in Britain in the context of changing social and economic conditions of the twentieth century, and of the emergence of HIV in its closing decades.

We go on to contrast the contemporary impact of HIV and sexually transmitted infections (STIs) in Britain with that in low-income countries where social and economic determinants interact with behavioural and biological factors to fuel the continuing spread of HIV, particularly in sub-Saharan Africa.

15.2 Why is sexual activity important to human health?

Sexual activity is an important component of human health and well being; a key component of the quality of adult partnerships and a prerequisite for natural conception and, thus, the survival of humankind.

Sex is an intrinsic part of most adult lives. In Britain in 2000, 95.6% of men and women had had sexual intercourse by their twenty-fifth birthday and 90% of men and women aged 16–44 had had sex within the past year (Johnson *et al.* 2001). The positive aspects of sexual activity are given scant attention in the biomedical literature, where concerns about adverse health outcomes dominate and focus on unplanned pregnancy, adverse outcomes of pregnancy, STIs, sexual violence, and infertility. Yet sexual relationships are an important and seldom studied element of the quality of human lives, which are highly valued by individuals.

In the last century, in the high-income nations, we have seen increasing dissociation between sexual behaviour and reproduction as a result of biomedical, technological, health service, and socio-economic developments. The relative importance of these various components is difficult to disentangle but there is little doubt that social and demographic change has had a major part to play. Perhaps most important amongst the social, biomedical, and legislative forces are those which have influenced the role of women in society. Until the mid twentieth century in Britain, the pleasures of sex were tempered by the dangers of poor health and social outcomes, particularly for women. Sex was potentially associated with unwanted pregnancy, including the social conse- quences of unmarried motherhood, and the risks of medically unsafe abortion, while planned pregnancies ran the risk of maternal mortality and morbidity and high infant mortality rates. But throughout the twentieth century, there were major improvements in reproductive health, themselves attendant upon improved living conditions, nutri- tion, hygiene, and medical care. Infant mortality declined from more than 80 per 1000 live births at the start of the century to less than 10 at the end of it, while completed family size fell from nearly four children to less than two in the 1980s (Coleman and Salt 1992). Following the introduction of penicillin in the 1940s, syphilis (previously a major cause of morbidity, mortality, and social exclusion for both adults and children) fell to extremely low rates (Adler 1980) (Fig. 15.1).

Notably, sex became safer for women. In addition to the improvements in maternal and child health, came major advances in contraception. The ability to control fertility through reliable contraception is an important contributor to changes in reproductive

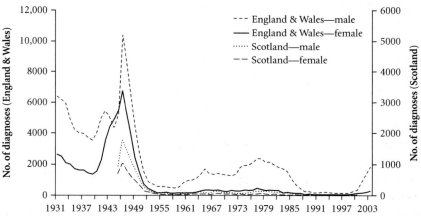

Fig 15.1 Diagnoses of syphilis (primary, secondary, and early latent) by sex; GUM clinics, England, Wales, and Scotland*, 1931–2003.

Source: KC60 statutory returns and ISD(D) 5 data; Health Protection Agency.

* Equivalent Scottish data are not available prior to 1945 and for 2001, 2002 and 2003. As N. Ireland data for 1931 to 2000 are incomplete, they have been excluded.

patterns. The movement to promote contraception knowledge, use, and development commenced with some of the pioneers of the early twentieth century and subsequent leaders of the women's movement (Stopes 1923). While technological developments have enabled social change, there is evidence that such advances are preceded by social and behavioural change that, in part, provides the impetus for technological solutions. Thus, for example, completed family size fell in parallel with infant mortality and some decades before the widespread availability of reliable contraception. The oral contraceptive pill, though developed by 1961, was not available to unmarried women until 1972, and widespread legal abortion was not available until the Abortion Law Reform Act of 1968. Since then, the legal abortion rate has slowly risen to reach 17 per 1000 women in England and Wales by 2001 (Office of National Statistics 2002), while sepsis and death due to illegal abortion has disappeared.

But safety is not limited to health concerns. As health outcomes improved, so social attitudes and expectations of sexual lifestyles changed. Pregnancy outside of marriage and single parenthood is no longer associated with the stigma and social exclusion of earlier decades. For 100 years from 1840 to 1940, the proportion of births outside marriage was around 4–7 %, but rose steeply from 1960 to reach 12% by 1980 and 40% by 2002 (Office of National Statistics 2004).

Marriage and fertility patterns have changed, with age at first marriage increasing markedly in the past 30 years to reach 30.6 years for men and 28.4 years for women in 2001; women's median age at first birth rose from 25.6 in 1950 to 29.7 in 2001. These demographic changes are influenced not only by the technical ability to control fertility but also by social factors. In twentieth century Britain, these can be traced back to the major social and legislative changes which include the enfranchisement of women in 1928, improvement in women's education, increasing financial independence of women and their increasing uptake of paid employment, particularly following the Second World War.

While the overall trends depict improving sexual and reproductive health in Britain, there have also been important negative outcomes, most notably the STI epidemic of the 1970s and emergence of the acquired immune deficiency syndrome (AIDS) pandemic in 1981. Figure 15.2 shows the curve for diagnosed cases of gonorrhoea in England and Wales from 1925 to 2003. This gives some clues to the sexual behavioural history of the century. A peak of gonorrhoea cases can be observed during the Second World War, when stable relationships were both disrupted and their formation inhibited and when both casual and commercial sex contacts likely increased (Adler 1980). Changing marriage patterns at the end of the war and the introduction of penicillin brought an initial decline in cases of gonorrhoea, but this was short-lived and, despite effective treatment and open-access health services, there was a major epidemic of gonorrhoea (and viral STIs) in the 1970s. In 1981 came the first intimation of what we now know to be the emerging HIV pandemic, with the description of the then fatal disease, AIDS, in homosexual men in the USA. At least in Britain there was a rapid

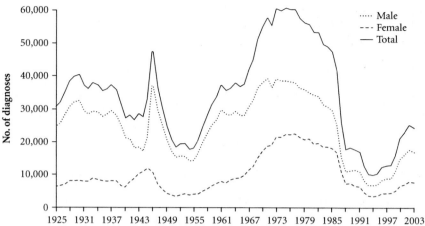

Fig 15.2 Diagnoses of gonorrhoea by sex; GUM clinics, England and Wales*, 1925–2003.

Source: KC60 statutory returns; Health Protection Agency.

* Scotland and N. Ireland data are excluded as they are incomplete from 1925 to 2003.

public health response from both voluntary and government agencies involving public education campaigns. Gonorrhoea diagnoses in homosexual and heterosexual communities plummeted, and the early 1990s saw the lowest count of cases ever recorded. The turn of the twenty-first century has, however, brought an upturn in diagnosis, to which we will return.

Underlying the remarkable variation in gonorrhoea diagnoses over the century are a combination of demographic, social, economic, biomedical, legislative, health service, and public health interventions (see Table 15.1) which combine forces in determining population patterns of sexual behaviour and their consequences. Despite major changes in sexual behaviour through the twentieth century, it was not until the emergence and threat of the HIV pandemic drew attention to the dearth of information on sexual behaviour in populations, that large-scale sexual behaviour studies were undertaken, with the explicit purpose of understanding the differential severity of the HIV pandemic in different groups and the likely rate of future spread (Johnson *et al.* 1992; Bajos *et al.* 1995; Cleland and Ferry 1995; Laumann *et al.* 1994). Studying sexual behaviour proved to be a controversial area for scientific enquiry and in many countries, including Britain, it was difficult to obtain funding for reliable large-scale studies. The first British National Survey of Sexual Attitudes and Lifestyles (Natsal) undertaken in 1990, was barred from public funding by the then Prime Minister, Margaret Thatcher, and rescued by funding from the charity, the Wellcome Trust (Johnson *et al.* 1994). This first study involved a national probability sample of nearly 19,000 adults, age 16–59, resident in Britain. In 2000, a second survey of over 12,000 adults aged 16–44 was funded by the Medical Research Council (Johnson *et al.* 2001). We will draw extensively on these two surveys here.

Table 15.1 Some interventions that may have influenced sexual behaviour and its outcomes in Britain in the twentieth century

	1900–1919	1920–1939	1940–1959	1960–1979	1980–1999
Treatment	Salvarsan for syphilis	Mass production of penicillin			Widespread introduction of antiretrovirals for HIV
Diagnosis	Wasserman test for syphilis described			Thayer–Martin medium introduced	HIV isolated; development of nucleic acid amplification methods
Prevention	Royal Commission recommends school sex education; First World War; chemical prophylaxis		Chemical prophylaxis and condoms		PSE; gay community campaign for HIV prevention; general media campaigns
Social and demographic factors/ legislation	Franchisement for women >21		Second World War; Beveridge report	Abortion Law Reform Act; legalization of homosexuality; introduction of 'the pill' to married women	

15.3 **What value do people place on sex?**

Much of the biomedical literature on sexual health actually focuses on sexual *ill health*. This includes sexually transmitted infections, unwanted pregnancy, sexual violence, abortion, and, more recently, sexual dysfunction (Mercer *et al.* 2003); and, in the developing world, maternal mortality and morbidity.

We take as our starting point, however, the value people place on sex as part of their lives. Sexual activity in human relationships and its pleasure and pitfalls are a visible component of modern popular culture. There has been an unprecedented increase in exposure to sexual imagery through film, video, and the printed media and, latterly, the internet. The methods for attracting partners are no longer limited to close social networks but have extended to dating agencies, printed media advertisements, and a growing internet market (Elford *et al.* 2001).

Sex is undeniably prominent in popular culture, but how important is it to individuals? Of those British men and women aged 16–44, interviewed in Natsal 2000, 96% considered happy sexual relationships to be 'very important' or 'quite important' for a happy and successful marriage (Natsal 2000, unpublished data); 10% of men and 13% of women who had experienced the break-up of at least one live-in partnership reported difficulties with their sex life as a reason for the break-up of that relationship. In the main, we enjoy our sexual relationships, with 97% of men and 93% of women reporting to enjoy sex always or most of the time (Natsal 2000, unpublished data). We are not, however, entirely satisfied with our sex lives, insofar as 53% of men and 40% of women in Natsal 2000, aged 16–44, said they would like sex 'much more often' or 'a bit more often' than currently—a significant gender difference. The frequency of sexual activity declines both with age and with duration of relationship within long-term relationships (Johnson *et al.* 1994). Overall, ageing is associated with significant increases in the proportion of sexually active men and women who report that they want more sexual activity.

Despite evidence of increasing sexual partner change, men and women retain relatively traditional long-term aspirations with respect to their sexual relationships: 83% of men and 88% of women interviewed in Natsal 2000 described their ideal lifestyle as 'married or cohabiting, with no other sex partners' in five years' time.

15.4 How is sexual behaviour related to health outcomes?

The relationship between behaviour and health outcomes may be modified at individual and population level by a number of influences including health service and biomedical interventions, while a range of socio-economic and demographic factors influence the behaviours themselves.

15.4.1 Sex and STIs/HIV

The most intensively studied relationships in sexual health have been those between sexual behaviours and STIs and HIV. STI transmission in populations depends upon the interaction between the biology of the organisms and the patterns of sexual behaviours in the population that transmit them. Specifically, the rate of partner change, the duration of infection of the organism, and the probability of transmission per partnership are key determinants (Yorke and Hethcote 1978). The duration of infection and probability of transmission of organisms can be modified by treatment programmes, while a range of socio-cultural, economic, and other factors, including educational interventions, influence behaviour patterns.

Epidemiological studies of individuals have clearly demonstrated the relationship between the number of sexual partners and the probability of STI acquisition (Fenton *et al.* 2004a; Hooper *et al.* 1978). Thus, in Natsal 2000, for example, fewer than 1% of men with one partner in the past five years reported an STI diagnosis, compared with 12% of those with ten or more partners (Fenton *et al.* 2005a) (Fig. 15.3).

However, it is more difficult to demonstrate how differential rates of partner acquisition are associated with differing STI transmission rates between different *populations*. There are few large, representative, probability sample surveys from different countries linked to population-based STI surveillance. Where these exist, methodologies and question formats (for example, even the definition of 'sexual partner') often vary, while socio-cultural factors may influence willingness to report socially censured behaviours.

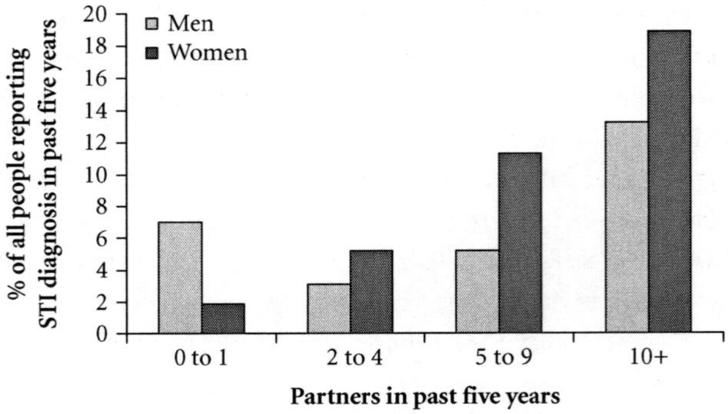

Fig 15.3 Percentage of respondents reporting an STI in the last five years and number of sexual partners. (**Base**: all respondents in Natsal 2000)

Thus, it is frequently difficult to make meaningful comparisons between different societies on the basic parameters that determine the spread of STIs.

In addition, the relationship between rates of partner acquisition and the probability of infection is, in different populations, a complex one. The risk of infection per partnership depends on the background prevalence of infection in that population—the higher the prevalence, the greater the chance of infection. Prevalence of infection, in turn, is likely to depend on the economic and health infrastructure available for treating STIs. There may also be interactions between different organisms, as for example the biological potentiation of HIV transmission by other STIs.

However, rates of partner change alone cannot fully explain transmission dynamics at population level. For example, factors such as condom use and circumcision rates have an essential role in influencing transmission probability, while the precise patterns of partnership formation are themselves important, a point we will now explore in detail. Crucial to the epidemiological effects of partnership formation patterns are: the extent of sexual mixing between different (high and low) activity classes; the nature of sexual networks; the relative contributions of serial and concurrent, casual and longer-term, partnerships (Rothenberg *et al.* 2000). This point is illustrated by a study of HIV transmission in four cities in Africa with varying HIV prevalence (Buve *et al.* 2001). Differences in sexual behaviour patterns alone could not explain these differences in HIV prevalence. Differences in behaviour were outweighed by other factors such as male circumcision and prevalence of genital ulcer disease, particularly genital herpes virus simplex infection. This study emphasized the interplay of complex behavioural and biological factors in determining HIV transmission, notwithstanding the methodological difficulties of obtaining valid data on sensitive behaviours.

15.4.2 The diversity of sexual behaviour and its role in sexual health outcomes

In recent years, there have been significant advances in the methods used to obtain reliable data on sexual behaviour (Fenton *et al.* 2001; Wellings *et al.* 1990). Research on the appropriate use of language, self-completion questionnaire formats, computerized self-interviews, and external and internal consistency checks have all contributed to improvement in the quality and validity of data in this field of scientific enquiry.

Recent studies of sexual lifestyle, using probability sampling and well-validated interview methods, demonstrate great diversity in behaviour both within individuals over the life course and between individuals in defined populations (Johnson et al. 1992; ACSF investigators 1992; Cleland and Ferry 1995). The population distribution of numbers of partners per unit time is positively skewed. In Natsal 2000, 50% of men aged 16–44 reported zero or one sexual partner in the past five years, 9% reported ten or more partners, while 1% reported more than fifty sexual partners (Johnson et al. 2001). This distribution means that a small proportion of the population, which has high rates of partner change, is at particularly high risk of STI acquisition and of subsequent transmission to others (see Fig. 15.3). Empirical data and data from mathematical models indicate that those in the upper tail of the distribution of partner change (sometimes referred to as the 'core group') (Yorke and Hethcote 1978) contribute disproportionately to the transmission of STIs in populations (Morris 1993).

The extent of sexual mixing between 'core' and 'non-core' groups in sexual partner choices is a key factor in explaining the relative containment of some STIs within the highest activity classes. Core groups typically include commercial sex workers and their clients, and, in North American and European populations, homosexual men who have high rates of partner change.

The disproportionate population burden of some STIs in certain population subgroups is evident from analyses of Natsal 2000. These demonstrate the increased rates of partner change and higher risk of STIs amongst men who have sex with men (Fenton et al. 2005a; Mercer et al. 2003). While only 2.6% of men reported male sex partners in the past five years in Natsal 2000, surveillance figures show that nearly 20% of gonorrhoea is homosexually acquired. Moreover, as STIs come under control and incidence declines, the transmission of infection becomes increasingly confined to core groups. Thus, for example, in the UK, where syphilis has become a rare disease with an incidence of around 5 per 100,000 male population, more than 50% of syphilis is homosexually acquired. In comparison, Chlamydia trachomatis, which is the most common curable STI, for which widespread testing has only recently become available, remains prevalent in both heterosexual and homosexual populations.

The sex industry (commercial sex workers and their clients) is a potential core group whose role in maintaining STI transmission varies markedly between different societies. This relationship is explored in greater detail later in the chapter.

At a population level, comparisons between industrialized countries demonstrate the striking fact that broadly similar patterns of sexual behaviour may not lead to similar STI/HIV outcomes. A comparison between British and French behaviour, for example, showed only small differences in sexual behaviours in the two countries, except that the reported prevalence of some 'risk indicators' (anal sex, sex with prostitutes) was somewhat higher in France. Yet France had an AIDS incidence three times higher than that of Britain in the early phase of the epidemic (Bajos *et al.* 1995). The authors conclude that earlier development of prevention policies in Britain combined with differences in the timing of entry of the virus to the population may have contributed to a marked difference between the epidemics in these two countries. This heterogeneity in HIV epidemics has been replicated throughout the world and emphasizes the complex interplay between behavioural and biological factors and interventions in STI control.

Comparison between US and British survey data shows that the US population had greater variability in sexual behaviour, a higher STI incidence, and lower condom usage. In both surveys, there was evidence of a strong association between number of partners and STI risk. However, in the US, there was a greater dispersion in the number of sexual partners (more people had one partner but a higher proportion had multiple partners). In the US, there was also a higher incidence of expressed unconditional opposition to certain sexual practices. This apparent disjuncture between public attitudes and private behaviours may have inhibited comprehensive effective public health action in the US, and thus enabled higher STI rates in the US (Michael *et al.* 1998).

15.4.3 **Sexual behaviour and pregnancy outcomes**

The relationship between individual sexual behaviour and pregnancy outcomes is less well described. However, the relationship between socio-economic development and fertility patterns has been well documented, and the patterns currently being played out in the developing world were those in evidence during the first half of the twentieth century in Britain. Overall, improvements in living conditions, hygiene, and some elements of medical care lead to a decline in maternal and infant mortality (Coleman and Salt 1992). Increasing population growth is then followed by increased fertility control and decline in birth rates as we have already described (see section 15.2).

In post-industrial societies, poor reproductive outcomes are no longer measured primarily in terms of maternal and infant mortality but in terms of unplanned pregnancy, abortion, and infertility. Britain has the highest teenage pregnancy rate in Europe (Department of Health Social Exclusion Unit 1999). Having intercourse before 16 is strongly linked to early motherhood; 31% of women in Natsal 2000 who reported having sex before 20 reported having a child before 18, compared with only 10% of those having sex for the first time after the age of 16 (Wellings *et al.* 2001). There are clear links between teenage pregnancy, antecedent social disadvantage, and subsequent social exclusion. Cross-sectional data from Natsal demonstrate that early sex (first intercourse before 16) and teenage pregnancy are linked to lower parental social class and social disadvantage but, most strongly, to poor educational attainment (Wellings *et al.* 2001). There is also a growing body of prospective data showing that poor educational attainment and aspiration is predictive of future teenage pregnancy (Bonell *et al.* 2003).

While the risk of undergoing termination of pregnancy is associated with increasing numbers of partners, it has little relationship with social class. Conversely, the risk of miscarriage and infertility shows no relationship with numbers of sexual partners (Johnson *et al.* 1994).

15.4.4 Sexual orientation and health outcomes

Men who have had sex with men are at increased risk of STIs and HIV infection as a result of both specific sexual practices (receptive anal sex) and high rates of partner change (Darrow *et al.* 1981). Research in gay men in the 1980s demonstrated the high levels of sexual activity associated with HIV infection and described the patterns of intense social and sexual mixing among men who have sex with men (Moss *et al.* 1987; Carne *et al.* 1987; Winkelstein *et al.* 1987).

Sex between men was a criminal offence in Britain until 1967 and subject to heavy penalties. Only in 1974 was it removed from the list of psychiatric disorders by the American Psychiatric Association. Natsal 1990 demonstrated that a relatively small proportion of men had male sexual partners, and that prevalence was higher in London, partly as a result of migration of men from outside London to an environment where homosexuality is more widely accepted (Johnson *et al.* 1994).

Homosexual behaviour, and indeed STIs and HIV, however, remain stigmatized. Fear, stigma, and prejudice are all elements which may delay a co-ordinated and open approach to STI control. Since 1990, there has, however, been a liberalization of social attitudes generally but, in particular, to male homosexuality. The proportion of men reporting that homosexuality was 'not wrong at all' increased from 21% in 1990 to 35% in 2000 and, among women, from 26% to 49%. Over the same time period in Britain, the proportion of men reporting homosexual partnerships in the past five years increased from 1.5% to 2.6%, as did the proportion of women reporting homosexual partnerships in the past five years (0.8% in 1990 to 2.6% in 2000) (Johnson *et al.* 2001).

Liberalization of the law and of social attitudes to homosexuality has led to less covert sexual activity and the ability of the gay community to mobilize around HIV prevention early in the epidemic. However, risk behaviour in the community has recently increased. Concern remains about the continuing incidence of new HIV infections and rising STI rates (Murphy *et al.* 2004).

There is a lack of reliable data on homosexual behaviour and partnerships in many developing countries, although homosexual transmission appears to be less frequent and the majority of HIV is transmitted heterosexually (Cleland and Ferry 1995).

15.5 How has sexual behaviour changed over time?

In section 15.2, we discussed the rapidly changing sexual and reproductive health outcomes in Britain in the twentieth century. But there are no reliable contemporary records documenting the changes in sexual behaviour that occurred. The studies of

Alfred Kinsey, undertaken in the US, were international bestsellers, attempting for the first time to report on the sexual behaviours of the general population (Kinsey *et al.* 1948, 1953). Though these studies were flawed by use of volunteer samples and their lack of representativeness, they were nevertheless a landmark in the history of sexual behaviour and sexual health research, opening the doors to wider discussion of sexual matters in the population.

The major changes in sexual behaviour over the last century have been captured by studies undertaken in the 1990s. In North America and Europe, these show a remarkably consistent pattern of declining age at first intercourse (Hubert *et al.* 1998) (Fig. 15.4) and an increasing number of sexual partners (Fig. 15.5). The circumstances of first intercourse also changed. Around half the women having first intercourse in Britain in the 1950s were married on that first occasion, but this proportion fell to less than 5% by the 1980s. However, the decline in age at first intercourse, and the increase in sex before marriage was already evident before the major technological and legislative changes of the 1960s which brought the contraceptive pill and legalized abortion. This again suggests that social and behavioural change provided the impetus for legal and technological change, rather than the reverse.

The gap between age at first intercourse and age at first live-in relationship has widened considerably over the past 50 years. While these two events were virtually

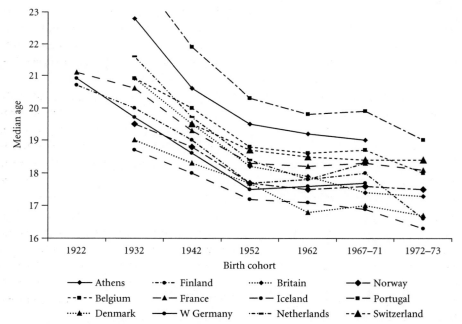

Fig 15.4 Age at first intercourse by generation; European women.

Source: Hubert *et al.* 1998.

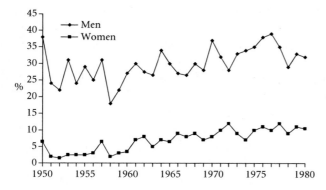

Fig 15.5 Percentage of respondents reporting 10 + heterosexual partners every by year of first sexual intercourse.

Source: Natsal 1990/91, Johnson *et al*. 1994, with permission from Blackwell Publishing Ltd.

coincident in the 1950s, there is now an average of four years for women and six years for men years between first intercourse and first live-in relationship—a time when young people enter a sexual market place with high rates of partner change (Natsal, unpublished data). In 2000, 53% of men and 39% of women aged 16–24 reported at least one new sexual partner in the past year (Johnson *et al*. 2001).

The increasing numbers of lifetime partners reported in the 1990 Natsal survey (Fig. 15.5) are consistent with the gonorrhoea epidemic of the 1960s and 1970s. The changes in the British survey were reflected in other studies in Europe and the US (Hubert *et al*. 1998; Laumann *et al*. 1994). It is likely that both increasing partnerships and the wider use of non-barrier contraceptive methods, particularly the oral contraceptive pill, may have contributed to these changes. However, further contribution to an increase in diagnoses may have been the wider availability of diagnostic services through a network of genito-urinary medicine clinics in Britain.

But sexual behaviour patterns were set to change rapidly in the 1980s in response to the new health threat of HIV/AIDS. In Britain, major public health education campaigns were implemented, first in the gay community and, subsequently, in the wider community, with the realization that HIV could be transmitted heterosexually. In the 1980s, gonorrhoea diagnoses declined precipitously, first in gay men and then in the general population (see Fig. 15.2) (Carne *et al*. 1987). Gonorrhoea figures provide a marker of the likely changes in behaviour at that time, and contemporary data in homosexual men recorded the declining rate of partner change and increased condom use in that community. In the heterosexual community, retrospective survey data record the rapid increase in condom use, particularly at first intercourse, and an apparent decline in numbers of sexual partners (Johnson *et al*. 1994). In the face of a substantial health threat, at least in Britain, remarkably rapid risk reduction was achieved, and Britain became a country with one of the lowest rates of HIV infection in Europe (UNAIDS 2004).

But this reduction in risk behaviour has proved difficult to sustain. Since 1995, most sexual health indicators in Britain have shown a reversal of trends, with an upturn in gonorrhoea and syphilis diagnoses (see Figs. 15.1 and 15.2), sustained high levels of teenage pregnancy, increasing risk behaviour among gay men, and sustained incidence of new infections in homosexual men (Dodds *et al.* 2004; Murphy *et al.* 2004). Similar trends have been observed in the US and other European countries. Data from the second Natsal survey undertaken in Britain in 2000 found a marked increase in the reporting of multiple sexual partnerships between 1990 and 2000 (see Fig. 15.5) as well as increasingly tolerant attitudes to sexual diversity (Johnson *et al.* 2001). Part of the measured change between 1990 and 2000 may be due to a greater willingness to report socially censured behaviour, as a result of changing social attitudes (Copas *et al.* 2002). However, the observed behavioural changes were co-incident both with corresponding increases in STI diagnoses and with demographic changes towards increasing population proportions of single and co-habiting individuals.

Increasing rates of risk behaviour may be attributable to a decline in the perceived threat of AIDS, partly as a result of the availability of antiretroviral therapy, as well as to a decline in public education about the threat of HIV. However, many other factors are likely to influence changing patterns of sexual behaviour. These include the rapidly changing market place for meeting sexual partners, the increased sexualization of media images, and continuing trends both towards greater involvement of women in the workplace and towards later childbirth and marriage.

In the industrialized countries, the twentieth century saw improving sexual and reproductive health for women, changing patterns of family formation, greater equality between the sexes in patterns of sexual behaviour, and greater control for women over their sexual, reproductive, and economic destiny. Government response to sexual health challenges and, latterly, to the HIV epidemic, though variable, was in general rapid, appropriate, and sustained. Despite recent upturns in poor sexual health outcomes, HIV epidemics in most of the industrialized world are a fraction of those in some of the hardest hit countries of sub-Saharan Africa. Globally, by 2003, 95% of the estimated 38.7 million people with HIV/AIDS live in low- or middle-income countries (UNAIDS 2004) (Fig. 15.6).

Many of the industrialized nations have managed, if not to eradicate, then at least to contain the HIV pandemic. This has been achieved, in part, because of antecedent factors that made the seed bed for HIV dissemination less fertile, but also through behaviour change as a result of national commitment to, and investment in, public education, needle exchange, STI control programmes, and, most recently, antiretroviral therapy.

As the pandemic has evolved in the industrialized nations, it has increasingly become one experienced by the socially marginalized and economically disadvantaged. STI and HIV rates are markedly higher in the US among the poor, ethnic minority groups, drug users, and gay men (Centers for Disease Control 2004). In Britain, while rates of heterosexually acquired infection are increasing, the majority of infections are acquired through sex abroad, particularly in sub-Saharan Africa (Public Health Laboratory Service, Communicable Disease Surveillance Centre 2002).

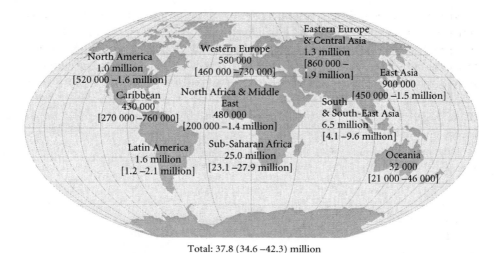

Total: 37.8 (34.6 –42.3) million

Fig 15.6 Adults and children estimated to be living with HIV as of end of 2003.
Source: UNAIDS.

15.6 **Sexual health in low-income countries**

In the areas of the world most affected by STIs/HIV (see Fig. 15.6), these patterns of containment of the HIV epidemic are seldom seen, and alarmingly high levels of HIV infection worldwide continue to increase to levels that are now having a major impact on life expectancy and socio-economic infrastructure (UNAIDS 2004). Unsafe sex is now estimated to be the second most important contributor to disease burden mortality worldwide (Ezzati *et al.* 2002).

In an excellent review, Buve *et al.* set out the complex interplay between social, economic, behavioural, and biological factors that have fuelled the spread if HIV infection in sub-Saharan Africa. There are important parallels between the factors contributing to sexual ill health in the developing world and those pertaining in the early part of the twentieth century in Britain (Buve *et al.* 2001).

Despite elements of modernization, urbanization, and education, women in many countries of sub-Saharan Africa retain a subordinate position to men, having little control over their own sex lives, or those of their husbands, and little control of their fertility. Reproductive health remains poor, as measured by high infant and maternal mortality rates. Age differences between spouses are often large with young women marrying older men and acquiring STIs/HIV from them at an early age (Gregson *et al.* 2002). Poverty lowers the priority of HIV in daily concerns; for women, this encourages the exchange of sex for money and goods. Urbanization and industrialization separate spouses and encourage high-risk sexual partnerships, normalizing the economic migration of young men from their birth communities. A decline in social and health services leads to poor control of STIs, which fuel the spread of HIV. Control over fertility is poor, access to condoms is often limited, and men are frequently reluctant to use them. Literacy levels are low, health education in many countries is limited and unco-ordinated, and, without political commitment at the highest level to HIV prevention, there are often fragmented HIV prevention programmes. There is also a history of misinformation relating to AIDS; for example, high-profile denial that HIV is the cause of AIDS or of the efficacy of condoms. With a few notable exceptions, such as Uganda, the picture is one of variable but increasing prevalence of infection throughout the region. HIV is now diminishing life expectancy and adversely affecting the economic infrastructure.

Buve *et al.* argue that:

> Populations in many parts of Africa are becoming trapped in a vicious circle as the HIV-1 epidemic leads to high mortality rates in young and economically productive age-groups, and thus leads to further impoverishment. Interventions to control HIV-1 should not only target individuals, but also aim to change those aspects of cultural and socio-economic context that increase the vulnerability to HIV-1 of people and communities. (Buve *et al.* 2001)

15.7 Demographic influences on sexual behaviour

We have already described the great diversity of sexual lifestyles evidenced by European and North American studies. In this section, we consider how sexual behaviour varies in relation to demographic factors.

The highest rates of partner change are seen among the young and unmarried (including those widowed, separated, and divorced) and those living in large cities (Johnson *et al.* 1994). However, beyond the effects of age, in Britain, rates of partner change do not vary greatly by social class but tend to be higher among the higher social classes, in contrast to other higher risk health behaviours which are frequently more prevalent among the most socio-economically disadvantaged. Similarly, studies in Africa suggest that the HIV epidemic first emerged among higher social class individuals in urban areas who had sufficient economic advantage to attract or pay for multiple sexual partnerships. It is only subsequently that HIV has become increasingly associated with economic disadvantage both in Africa and in the US, where STI rates are higher in African Americans and in socially disadvantaged groups. In contrast, in Britain, STI rates and use of services are remarkably similar across social classes. Recent evidence from Britain, however, suggests variation by ethnicity, with lowered risk among those from the Indian sub-continent and higher risk behaviours and poorer sexual health outcomes among African and Afro-Caribbean communities (Fenton *et al.* 2005*b*; Low *et al.* 1997).

There is ample evidence of the impact of social disruption and migration on sexual health; Fig. 15.2 clearly demonstrates the peak of gonorrhoea incidence in the Second World War. The relationship between war, sexual behaviour, and sexual health is well described (Adler 1980). Separation from spouses, and then inhibition of stable sexual relationships, encourages casual and commercial sex contacts. At the same time, the economic disruption of war frequently encourages women to exchange sex for money as a strategy for survival. Such women are at high risk of acquiring and transmitting STIs in the absence of condom use and STI control programmes, and such circumstances are a fertile seed bed for fuelling STI and HIV epidemics, creating a 'core group' of men and women at high risk of STI.

Onward transmission to individuals who have low rates of partner change is fuelled when those in the 'core group' have unprotected sex with their lower–risk regular partners, allowing diffusion of infection from the 'core' to the wider population. There is evidence that such epidemic dynamics have been important in the wide dissemination of HIV in Africa. For example, a classic study in Kenya in the 1980s demonstrated the rapidly rising prevalence of HIV in Nairobi sex workers and their clients and the subsequent diffusion of infection into the general population of women attending antenatal clinics (Quinn *et al.* 1986).

However, the economic aspects of demographic disruption appear to have contributed substantially to the development of the HIV epidemic in Africa—for example, through the migration associated with trucking and mining (Mabey and Mayaud 1997). In many countries, HIV has appeared first along truck routes, in trading towns, and in border areas where populations are highly mobile. Mobility itself has been identified as a risk factor for HIV, which spreads along migration routes. For example, HIV prevalence was particularly high at the border crossing points and along transport routes in mainland South-east Asia and along the heavily travelled corridor in West Africa between Cote D'Ivoire and Burkina Faso (UNAIDS 2001, 2004).

Migrants to urban areas are, typically, young single men who are at increased risk of engaging in high-risk behaviours with sex workers. Women too, are increasingly migrating from rural areas to cities. They often end up in low-paid jobs, relying on sex work for survival. Thus mobility, urban poverty, and industrialization, in the absence of an effective health infrastructure, contribute to the deterioration of sexual health and the transmission of STIs/HIV. The complex interplay of social, economic, behavioural, biological, and medical interventions result in the marked heterogeneity in patterns of sexual health and ill health across the world.

By contrast, in most of the countries of Western Europe and in the US, the period of economic prosperity and peace since the Second World War; well-established open-access health services, increasing participation of women in the workplace, and relative demographic stability have, overall, resulted in improved sexual health and relative containment of the HIV epidemic.

15.8 **The sex industry**

We have alluded throughout this chapter to the role of the sex industry in sexual health. We consider this in further detail here because of the clear social and economic considerations, which determine the extent and relative hazards of sex work and the highly variable role of the sex industry in different societies.

At the beginning of the twentieth century, in Britain, there was considerable concern about the high rates of gonorrhoea and syphilis, such that a Royal Commission on venereal diseases was established which reported in 1918. At that time, sex between clients and prostitutes was a substantial contributor to the spread of STIs (Sanger 1897). Women were frequently forced into prostitution by economic necessity, had little protection, no effective treatment, and suffered high rates of STIs. The economic origins of prostitution and its relationship to the subordination of women were well understood by the early feminists. Christabel Pankhurst, in her book *The Great Scourge and How to End It* (Pankhurst 1913) said of the economic origins of prostitution: 'Women, when they are politically free and economically strong, will not be purchasable for the base uses of vice.' And her solution?—'the cure briefly stated is votes for women and chastity for men'. The continuing debates about control of the sex industry and the protection of women from disease, violence, and exploitation are beyond the scope of this chapter.

However, contemporary data suggest that in Britain today, commercial partnerships constitute a small proportion of all sexual partnerships. In Natsal 2000, 9% of men aged 16–44 reported to have *ever* paid for sex, 1.3% of men reported paying for sex in the last year, and 19% of all partnerships reported were commercial partnerships (unpublished data). By contrast, across surveys of developing countries, a median of 9.7% of men report a commercial encounter in the past year (Cleland and Ferry 1995), and the proportion reporting commercial sex typically comprises 25–40% of men reporting non-regular sexual contact. Studies in Africa generally suggest a much higher proportion of men paying for sex than in Britain (Morison *et al.* 2001).

Women sex workers in Britain report high levels of condom use and have low rates of STIs and HIV compared with their counterparts in many low-income countries (Cleland and Ferry 1995; Ward *et al.* 2004). Women in developed countries are more able to negotiate safe sex, to achieve greater safety in the workplace, and to have access to health services for diagnosis and treatment of STIs. This is in stark contrast to the external economic necessities that forced women into prostitution in the nineteenth century. However, commercial sex is probably a much greater contributor to STI transmission in other parts of the world where, using the broader definition of giving or receiving 'any money, gifts or favour in return for sex', a median of 1.3% women report commercial sex, which included forms of exchange not covered by the Western, purely monetary concept of prostitution (Cleland and Ferry 1995).

In low-income countries more severely affected by the HIV epidemic, commercial sex workers have suffered high levels of infection, and commercial sex contributes substantially to HIV spread. Commercial sex work was an important source of HIV infection in Thailand, where the sexual initiation of men by a female sexual worker is common, and 24.2% of men in urban and 9.5% in rural areas reported paying for sex in the past year (Sittitrai *et al.* 1994). In Thailand, however, government commitment, early in the epidemic, led to implementation of the '100% condom' programme to promote condom use in brothels and other settings. The results of this well co-ordinated and funded approach led to very high levels of condom use (97% in brothels) and substantial control of the HIV epidemic (Mills *et al.* 1997). In many African countries, however, such focused, politically led and funded campaigns have been few, sex work is less highly organized, condom supplies are often poor, and levels of condom use have remained low (Morison *et al.* 2001; Williams *et al.* 2003).

It can be argued that with increasing socio-economic development and increasing emancipation, education, and economic independence of women, sex work becomes increasingly organized and safer, while the proportion of men paying for sex declines as greater equality in the sexual behaviour of men and women becomes the social norm.

15.9 Sexual health and the socio-economic environment

The devastating impact of the HIV epidemic in sub-Saharan Africa (where two-thirds of infections have occurred and up to 50% of the adult population are affected in the worst foci) can be attributed, in part, to the downstream consequences of income disparity, poverty, and adverse outcomes of elements of development programmes. In the context of HIV control, there is a growing understanding of the 'upstream' factors which lead to sexual ill health. Omran's concept of the 'epidemiological transition' (a transition from high to low mortality patterns which is associated with transformation in the age, cause, and sex structure of death) is important in helping us understand the determinants of sexual ill health amidst the AIDS pandemic (Omran 1971). With the 'epidemiological transition' come falls in death rates from infectious and parasitic diseases and in maternal mortality—which are accompanied by the demographic and behavioural changes already described in this chapter. The countries which have found it hardest to address and contain the threat of an AIDS epidemic have yet to go through the epidemiological transition. They are countries whose limited resources for HIV prevention have still to compete with immediate threats to life such as malaria, tuberculosis, maternal mortality, and diarrhoeal or vaccine-preventable disease in children.

The economic growth which should have contributed to the epidemiological transition in sub-Saharan Africa has slowed, with reversals of life expectancy in many countries. Spending on health, education, and social services has declined, partly as a result of structural adjustment programmes which imposed cuts in non-productive spending (Buve *et al.* 2001; Lurie *et al.* 1995).

Paradoxically, urbanization, modernization, and industrialization have created the demographic conditions which enhance migration, family instability, and casual sex; while the continuing low status of women fosters commercial sex work and disempowerment. Added to this is the impact of war and conflict which increase poverty, human rights abuses, sexual exploitation, and displacement. Yet in a climate of effective political leadership, greater equality of income distribution, financial investment, and established infastructure for education, legislation, and medical services, the adverse outcomes of sexual activity can be curtailed and the positive benefits of sex enjoyed, even in the era of HIV. It is hardly surprising if it is mainly in the resource-rich countries that prompt, well-resourced, and co-ordinated responses have achieved relative containment of HIV by comparison with resource-poor countries.

What can be done to reduce the growing threat of HIV in the countries most vulnerable to its effects on health, society, and the economy? Political commitment of the highest level appears important in HIV control. A World Bank research report suggested a range of social and economic interventions which should be delivered through governments. These are summarized in Table 15.2 (World Bank 1997). At least part of Uganda's relative success in controlling the HIV epidemic is related to early government recognition of the problem and early implementation of health education programmes and condom distribution (Mulder *et al.* 1995). Elsewhere, denial of the HIV problem and the competing views of government, church leaders and Non-governmental organizations, and donor agencies have often fragmented attempts to achieve a co-ordinated response. More recently, greater investment has been made through the Global Fund on AIDS, although there has been criticism both of the level of funding contributed by donor agencies and restrictions placed on use of funding.

However, the contribution of socio-cultural factors in determining HIV transmission raises social issues well beyond the scope of health care interventions. Income inequality within a society, low GNP per capita, and a high ratio of resident males to females aged 20–39 in urban populations are all significantly associated with increasing prevalence of HIV infection, as are the male–female literacy gap and the proportion of military personnel within urban populations (Over 1997). Poverty, income inequality, and gender inequality all facilitate the spread of AIDS, by increasing the proportion of the population who engage in or are directly affected by the consequences of high-risk sexual behaviour.

The improvement of sexual health cannot be viewed outside its socio-cultural and political context, particularly now that HIV is having an extensive impact on societies

Table 15.2 Governmental strategies for the prevention of HIV at population level

Influencing individual choices
- Education and information aimed at improving knowledge of HIV/AIDS and its transmission
- Lowering the costs of condom use
- Lowering the costs of safe injecting behaviour

Addressing social constraints that reduce safe behaviour
- Altering social norms
- Improving the status of women
- Reducing poverty

Engagement of government
- Provision of public goods—the collection and production of information about the prevention and control of HIV
- Reduction of the negative consequences (externalities) of behaviour tending to spread HIV, through the provision of sexual health services accessible to those at risk
- Consideration of the impact and potential impact of HIV/AIDS on other aspects of national wellbeing
- These governmental roles should be a supplement to, not replacement for, other initiatives.

Adapted from: Confronting AIDS: Public priorities in a global epidemic. World Bank Research Report (1997), chapter 3.
The full report is available at http://www.worldbank.org/aids-econ/confront/confrontfull/aids.html

and economies across the world. This must be achieved in the broader context of reducing social and economic inequalities and building health, education, and social services—both within nations and across the international community.

15.10 **Policy implications**

Globally, unsafe sex is a leading cause of disease burden and mortality. The sexual health of populations results from the complex interplay of demographic, social, medical, legislative, health service, and public health interventions. It follows that the policy implications for improving sexual health globally must include interventions to influence socio-economic and cultural environments and not only biomedical interventions or programmes for individual behaviour change.

Globally, poor sexual health is worst amongst the socially marginalized and economically disadvantaged. Thus, interventions which aim to reduce economic inequalities, promote social and economic stability, reduce migration, promote peace, reduce gender inequalities, and, in particular, improve the health, education, economic status of women are all key elements in the improvement of sexual health. It is changes in these elements that are likely to promote the individual behaviour changes which reduce adverse health outcomes.

There is evidence that the sexual behaviour of populations can change over short timescales (2–3 years) in response both to social change and population health promotion efforts. Population interventions (such as widespread HIV information and condom programmes) require political will and leadership at the highest level and should be widely disseminated in the general population to achieve rapid change. Government, religious leaders, community leaders, and consumer organizations all have key roles to play in leading appropriate interventions. Achieving culturally appropriate, sustained interventions initially requires recognition and acceptance of health outcomes which are traditionally stigmatized. Political commitment and prioritization is frequently hampered by denial, stigmatization, prejudice, and disjuncture between dominant social attitudes (e.g. unconditional opposition to sexual behaviours) and actual behaviours. A sound evidence base on sexual health epidemiology and actual sexual behaviours is essential to counter inertia and target interventions.

Rapid responses are required in the face of emerging epidemics (especially HIV). Delaying intervention in explosive epidemics decreases the chances and increases the costs of achieving control. Resources are essential and need to be appropriately invested in evidence-based interventions, whether at individual or community level.

Socio-economic development programmes need to consider the health effects of policies to improve economic status which may have adverse health outcomes, both directly and through their impact on demographic structures and, consequently, behaviours.

Appropriate delivery systems and infrastructure are essential for biomedical (e.g. contraception, antibiotics) and behavioural (e.g.condoms) interventions. These are not limited to health services but include media, social marketing, commercial outlets, schools, and places of worship.

The control of epidemics requires raising population awareness and knowledge, while treatment programmes and focused interventions require targeting of resources specific to the reproductive health problem or organism and its epidemic phase (contained in the core group or widespread). Once appropriate interventions are in place, they need to be sustained and adapted for future generations in response to changing patterns and social determinants of sexual health outcomes.

References

ACSF Iinvestigators (1992) AIDS and sexual behaviour in France. *Nature*, **360**, 407–9.

Adler, M.W. (1980) The terrible peril: a historical perspective on the venereal diseases. *British Medical Journal*, **281**, 206–11.

Bajos, N., Wadsworth, J., Ducot, B., Johnson, A.M., Le Pont, F., Wellings, J., *et al.* (1995) Sexual behaviour and HIV epidemiology: comparative analysis between France and Britain. *AIDS*, **9(7)**, 735–43.

Bonell, C.P., Strange, V.J., Stephenson, J.M., Oakley, A.R., Copas, A.J., Forrest, S.P., *et al.* (2003) Effect of social exclusion on the risk of teenage pregnancy: development of hypotheses using baseline data from a randomised trial of sex education. *Journal of the Epidemiology of Community Health*, **57**, 871–6.

Buve, A., Carael M., Hayes R.J., *et al.* (2001) The multicentre study on factors determining differences in rate of spread of HIV in sub-Saharan Africa: summary and conclusion. *AIDS*, **15** (Suppl. 4), S127–S131.

Carne, C.A., Weller, I.V.D., Johnson, A.M., *et al.* (1987) Prevalence of antibodies to human immunodeficiency virus, gonorrhoea rates and changing sexual behaviour in homosexual men in London. *Lancet*, **i**, 656–8.

Centers for Disease Control (2004) *http://www.cdc.gov/*.

Cleland, J. and Ferry, B. (1995) *Sexual behaviour and AIDS in the developing world.* Taylor Francis, London.

Coleman, D.A. and Salt, J. (1992) *The British population patterns, trends and processes.* Oxford University Press, Oxford.

Copas, A.J., Wellings, K., Erens, B., Mercer, C., McManus, S., Fenton, K.A., *et al.* (2002) The accuracy of reported sensitive sexual behaviour in Britain: exploring the extent of change 1990–2000. *Sexually Tramitted Infections*, **358**, 1851–4.

Darrow, W.W., Barrett, D., Jay, K., and Young, A. (1981) The gay report on sexually transmitted diseases. *American Journal of Public Health*, **71(9)**, 1004–11.

Department of Health Social Exclusion Unit (1999) *Teenage pregnancy.* ODPM Publications, Wetherby.

Dodds, J., Mercey, D.E., Parry, J.V., and Johnson, A.M. (2004) Increasing prevalence of male homosexual partnerships and practices in Britain 1990–2000: evidence from national probability surveys., *Sexually Transmitted Infections*, **80(3)**, 236–40.

Elford, J., Bolding, G., and Sherr, L. (2001) Seeking sex on the Internet and sexual risk behaviour among gay men using London gyms. *AIDS*, **15**, 1409–15.

Ezzati, M., Lopez, A.D., Rodgers, A., Vander Hoorn, S., Murray, C.J.L., and the Comparative Risk Assessment Collaborating Group (2002) Selected major risk factors and global and regional burden of disease. *Lancet*, **360**, 1347–60.

Fenton, K.A., Johnson, A.M., McManus, S., and Erens, B. (2001) Measuring sexual behaviour: methodological challenges in survey research. *Sexually Transmitted Infections*, **77**, 84–92.

Fenton, K.A., Mercer, C.H., Johnson, A.M., Korovessis, C.J., McManus, S., Erens, B., *et al.* (2005*a*) Reported STD clinic attendance and sexually transmitted infections in Britain: prevalence, risk factors, and proportionate population burden. *Journal of Infectious Diseases*, **191**, 5127–5138.

Fenton, K.A., Mercer, C.H., McManus, S., Erens, B., Macdowall, W., Wellings, K., *et al.* (2005*b*) Sexual behaviour in Britain: ethnic variations in high-risk sexual behaviour and STI acquisition risk. *Lancet*, **365**, 1246–55.

Gregson, S., Nyamukapa, C.A., Garnett, G.P., Mason, P.R., Zhuwau, T., Carael, M., *et al.* (2002) Sexual mixing patterns and sex-differentials in teenage exposure to HIV infection in rural Zimbabwe. *Lancet*, **359**, 1896–903.

Hooper, R.R., Reynolds, G.H., Jones, O.G., Zaidi, A., Wiesner, P.J., Latimer Lester, A., *et al.* (1978) Cohort study of venereal disease. I: the risk of gonorrhoea transmission from infected women to men. *American Journal of Epidemiology*, **108(2)**, 136–44.

Hubert, M., Bajos, B., and Sandfort, T. (1998) *Sexual behaviour and HIV/AIDS in Europe*. UCL Press, London.

Johnson, A.M., Mercer, C.H., Erens, B., Copas, A.J., McManus, S., Wellings, K.F.K.A., *et al.* (2001) Sexual behaviour in Britain at the millennium: partnerships, practices and HIV risk behaviours. *Lancet*, **358**, 1835–42.

Johnson, A.M., Wadsworth, J., Wellings, K., Bradshaw, S., and Field, J. (1992) Sexual lifestyles and HIV risk. *Nature*, **360**, 410–12.

Johnson, A.M., Wadsworth, J., Wellings, K., and Field, J. (1994) *Sexual attitudes and lifestyles* Blackwell Scientific Press, Oxford.

Kinsey, A.C., Pomeroy, W.B., and Martin, C.E. (1948) *Sexual behaviour in the human male.* W.B. Saunders, Philadelphia.

Kinsey, A.C., Pomeroy, W.B., Martin, U., and Gebhard, C.H. (1953) *Sexual behaviour in the human female.* W.B. Saunders, Philadelphia.

Laumann, E.O., Gagnon, J.H., Michael, R.T., and Michaels, S. (1994) *The social organization of sexuality: sexual practices in the United States.* The University of Chicago Press, Chicago and London.

Low, N., Daker–White, G., Barlow, D., and Pozniak, A.L. (1997) Gonorrhoea in inner London: results of a cross sectional study. *British Medical Journal*, **314(7096)**, 1719–23.

Lurie, P., Hintzen, P., and Lowe, R.A. (1995) Socioeconomic obstacles to HIV prevention and treatment in developing countries: the roles of the International Monetary Fund and the World Bank. *AIDS*, **9(6)**, 539–46.

Mabey, D. and Mayaud, P. (1997) Sexually transmitted diseases in mobile populations. *Genitourinary Medicine*, **73**, 18–21.

Mercer, C.H., Fenton, K.A., Johnson, A.M., Wellings, K., Macdowall, W., McManus, S., *et al.* (2003) Sexual function problems and help seeking behaviour in Britain: national probability sample survey. *British Medical Journal*, **327**, 426–7.

Michael, R.T., Wadsworth, J., Feinleib, J., Johnson, A.M., Laumann, E.O., and Wellings, K. (1998) Private sexual behavior, public opinion, and public health policy related to sexually transmitted diseases: a US–British comparison. *American Journal of Public Health*, **88**, 749–54.

Mills, S., Benjarattanaporn, P., Bennett, A., *et al.* (1997) HIV risk behavioral surveillance in Bangkok, Thailand: sexual behavior trends among eight population groups. *AIDS*, **11**(Supp 1), S43–S51.

Morison, L., Weiss, H.A., Buve, A., *et al.* (2001) Commercial sex and the spread of HIV in four cities in sub-Saharan Africa. *AIDS*, **15**(Suppl 4), S61–S69.

Morris, M. (1993) Telling tails explain the discrepancy in sexual partner reports. *Nature*, **365**, 437–40.

Moss, A.R., Osmond, D., Bacchetti, P., *et al.* (1987) Risk factors for AIDS and HIV seropositivity in homosexual men. *American Journal of Epidemiology,* **125,** 1035–47.

Mulder, D., Nunn, A., Kamali, A., and Kengeya–Kayondro, J. (1995) Decreasing HIV-1 seroprevalence in young adults in a rural Ugandan cohort. *British Medical Journal,* **311(7009),** 833–6.

Murphy, C., Charlett, A., Jordon, L., Osner, N., Gill, N., and Parry, J.V. (2004) HIV incidence appears constant in men who have sex with men despite widespread use of effective antiretroviral therapy. *AIDS,* **18(2),** 265–72.

Office of National Statistics (2002) *Abortion statistics. Legal abortions carried out under the 1967 Abortion Act in England and Wales, 2001.* AB No 28.

Office of National Statistics (2004) *Average age at marriage and divorce.* Social trends 34.

Omran, A.R. (1971) The epidemiologicition trans: a theory of the epidemiology of population change. *Milbank Memorial Fund Quarterly,* **49,** 509–38.

Over, M. (1997) Societal determinants of urban HIV infection: an exploratory cross-country regression analysis. Background paper to 'Confronting AIDS', (World Bank 1997).

Pankhurst, C. (1913) *The great scourge and how to end it.* London.

Public Health Laboratory Service, Communicable Disease Surveillance Centre (2002) *HIV and AIDS in the UK in 2001.* London.

Quinn, T.C., Mann.J.M., Curran, J.W., and Piot, P. (1986) AIDS in Africa: an epidemiologic paradigm. *Science,* **234,** 955–63.

Rothenberg, R.B., Long, D.M., Sterk, C.E., Pach, A., Potterat, J.J., Muth, S., *et al.* (2000) The Atlanta Urban Network Study: a blueprint for endemic transmission. *AIDS,* **14,** 2191–200.

Sanger (1897) *The history of prostitution.* The Medical Publishing Company, New York.

Sittitrai, W., Phanuphak, P., Barry, J., and Brown, T. (1994) A survey of Thai sexual behaviour and risk of HIV infection. *International Journal of STD—AIDS,* **5,** 377.

Stopes, M.C. (1923) *Contraception. Its theory, history, and practice* John Bale Sons and Daniellson, London.

UNAIDS (2001) *Population mobility and AIDS.* Technical update, Geneva.

UNAIDS (2004) *UNAIDS 2004 report on the global AIDS epidemic.*

Ward, H., Day, S., Green, A., Cooper, K., and Weber, J. (2004) Declining prevalence of STI in the London sex industry, 1985–2002. *Sexually Transmitted Infections,* in press.

Wellings, K., Field, J., Wadsworth, J., Johnson, A.M., Anderson, R.M., and Bradshaw, S.A. (1990) Sexual lifestyles under scrutiny. *Nature,* **348,** 276–8.

Wellings, K., Nanchahal, K., Macdowall, W., McManus, S., Erens, B., Mercer, C.H., *et al.* (2001) Sexual behaviour in Britain: early heterosexual experience. *Lancet,* **358,** 1843–50.

Williams, B.G., Taljaard, D., Campbell, C.M., Gouws, E., Ndhlovu, L., van Dam, J., *et al.*(2003) Changing patterns of knowledge, reported behaviour and sexually transmitted infections in a South African gold mining community. *AIDS,* **17,** 2099–107.

Winkelstein, W., Lyman, D.M., Padian, N., Grant, R., Samuel, M., Wiley, J.A., *et al.* (1987) Sexual practices and risk of infection by the human immunodeficiency virus. *Journal of American AIDS,* **257,** 321–5.

World Bank (1997) *Confronting AIDS: public priorities in a global epidemic. World Bank Research Report 1997.* Oxford University Press for the World Bank, New York.

Yorke, J.A. and Hethcote, H.W. (1978) Dynamics and control of the transmission of gonorrhea. *Sexually Transmitted Diseases,* **5(2),** 51–6.

Chapter 16

Ourselves and others—for better or worse: social vulnerability and inequality

Richard G. Wilkinson

16.1 **Introduction**

This chapter is more speculative than others in this book. It attempts to pull together some of the material from earlier chapters to provide a clearer understanding of the connection between individual psychosocial risk factors and our sensitivity both to the immediate social environment and to the broader social structure of modern societies. Although still conjectural, the picture which emerges makes a deeper sense than the parts alone. It begins to suggest a coherent reality behind the statistics from which we can draw many useful inferences about how to improve both the quality and length of people's lives in different contexts.

16.2 **Psychosocial risk factors**

One of the most important changes in our understanding of the social determinants of health reflected in this book has been the growing recognition of the power of psychosocial risk factors. The most important can probably be grouped under three headings: social status (in which I include issues of control), social affiliations, and stress in early life.

16.2.1 **Social status**

Social status is linked to health not simply through the direct physical effects of exposure to better or worse material conditions. It is also a matter of position in the social hierarchy, people's experience of superior and dominant status versus inferior and subordinate status, coupled with processes of stigmatization and exclusion of those nearer the bottom of the hierarchy. Although there is a robust relationship between income and health *within* all developed societies, among the 25 to 30 richest countries, there is no relation between gross national product per capita (an indication of average living standards) and death rates (Marmot and Wilkinson 2001; Wilkinson 1997). The fact that income and health are related *within* developed societies but not *between* them suggests that health among the most affluent countries is a reflection of social position and relative income, rather than of exposure to differences in living standards alone.

This does not imply that material living standards are unimportant: it means that their effects are mediated by how they are tied to, and signify, social position. Material standards are so closely associated with social position because, among animals and humans alike, the allocation of scarce resources in ranking systems is based on differences in power. This makes it almost impossible to design studies capable of distinguishing, unambiguously, between the effects of social position and material wealth in human populations. However, experiments with non-human primates, in which social status is manipulated and high- and low-status animals get the same diet and live in the same compounds, have not only shown that there are clear stress effects of social position, but also that these effects are sensitive to the exact nature of the social structure (Shively and Clarkson 1994; Sapolsky 1999). Social gradients in a number of physiological risk factors observed among baboons and macaques under these conditions are, as we saw in chapter 2, remarkably similar to those found in human populations.

Control

Social status influences health through a wide range of psychosocial pathways including aspects of the social organization of work discussed in Chapter 6. Both the amount of control people have over their work and 'effort–reward imbalance' are closely associated with social status in the workplace. If you do not have much control over your work, it is often because you are being told what to do by a superior and so is a reflection of your subordinate status. Indeed, low control is commonly accompanied by feelings of hostility (Williams *et al.* 1997). Although we often think of the amount of control people have in different situations as if it were mainly a reflection of physical circumstances, natural limitations on what we can do (for instance our inability to fly or to walk through walls) are not experienced as limitations on our sense of control. The stressful limitations are limitations on personal autonomy which reflect our subordination to others. This is likely to be why low control at work explains a significant part of the social gradient in health in the Whitehall study: in effect, it provides the fine grain of social position.

16.2.2 **Social affiliations**

The second group of psychosocial risk factors are those connected with social affiliations and involvement. As we saw in Chapter 8, social affiliations of almost any kind are protective of health. Close 'confiding' relationships, social support, friendship networks, and involvement in wider community life, all seem beneficial. Apparently confirming these connections, hostility and 'negative' relationships have been shown to be harmful to health (Stansfeld *et al.* 1997).

16.2.3 **Early life**

The third important category of psychosocial influences on health were those occurring in early life. Discussed in Chapter 3, these include pre- and postnatal factors which influence health throughout later life. People who were smaller as babies are, for instance, more likely to suffer from heart disease, diabetes, and stroke in later life. Although low birth weight was initially thought to reflect poor nutrition in pregnancy, it now looks as if it is more likely—at least in the rich countries—to reflect the effect of maternal stress on the HPA axis in the developing foetus. This possibility is supported not only by the failure to find convincing evidence of an association in rich countries between birth weight and maternal nutrition during pregnancy (Mathews *et al.* 1999) but also by studies which show that mothers of low birth weight babies give histories of stressful pregnancy (Sable and Wilkinson 2000) and experimental evidence that shows that animals stressed during pregnancy are more likely to have a small offspring. Several biological mechanisms have been suggested and correlations have been observed between maternal and foetal cortisol levels (Gitau *et al.* 1998; Teixeira *et al.* 1999). In addition, it has been shown that birth weight is positively associated with basal cortisol levels in middle age (Phillips *et al.* 1998).

As Chapter 3 points out, there is also good evidence that stress and lack of stimulation in early childhood compromises future health. This is perhaps the biological side of what psychologists have always told us about the effects of early childhood experience on personality development. Although the biological mechanisms are clearly quite different, it would seem that both pre- and postnatal development may be part of an extended period of early sensitivity during which stress responses are differentially 'tuned' according to the stressfulness, first, of the maternal environment in pregnancy, and then of the child's own early experience. A more stressful start in life seems to be associated particularly with increased risks of coronary heart disease, stroke, diabetes, raised blood pressure, and central obesity. It also appears to be associated with slow growth and reduced chances of upward social mobility.

16.3 **Social vulnerability**

These three groups of psychosocial risk factors (social status, friendship, and early experience) have a major impact on population health because they combine frequent exposures with large differences in relative risk. Mortality and morbidity rates may be two, three, or even four times as high among poorer compared to richer people, or among people who are more socially isolated compared to people with strong social ties. Even if occupational exposure to some toxic material was found to raise death rates as dramatically as this, it would not exert a significant influence on population health because occupational exposures usually only affect a tiny proportion of the population. Much larger proportions of the population are exposed to the hazards of low social status, weak social affiliations, and stress in early life.

As we saw in Chapter 2, psychosocial factors affect health through their capacity to cause long or frequently recurring periods of stress. The physiological responses to stress and their implications for the cardiovascular and immune systems are described in that chapter. It looks as if, while the body is preparing for muscular activity to meet some threat or emergency, other processes which do not contribute to meeting the immediate challenge are downregulated. These include tissue maintenance and repair, reproductive functions, growth, digestion, and, if the stress lasts for more than about an hour, immunity as well. The result is that living with high levels of stress for long periods makes us more vulnerable to a wide range of diseases.

16.3.1 Ourselves and others

If it is correct to say that social status, social affiliations, and early life experience are among the most important psychosocial influences on population health in rich countries, and they affect health because they are sources of chronic stress, then what the epidemiology is surely telling us is that these are the most powerful sources of stress in modern societies. This is an important point. Although things like unserviced debt or unemployment are also important sources of stress for those who suffer them, they may have less influence on population health because, in most societies, they affect fewer people.

It is probably not an over-interpretation to suggest that our three groups of psychosocial risk factors are likely to be related to each other. As well as being intensely social risk factors, they are all related to the doubts and insecurities we have about whether or not we are liked and valued by others. The insecurities that can come from poor attachment and a difficult early childhood are not unlike the insecurities associated with low social status. It looks as if one can exacerbate—or offset—the effects of the other. This is shown not only by some of the data but also by accounts of personal experience. Bertrand Russell (1956) quoted Beatrice Webb as saying (c. 1910) 'If I ever felt inclined to be timid as I was going into a room full of people, I would say to myself, "You're the cleverest member of one of the cleverest families in the cleverest class of the cleverest nation in the world, why should you be frightened?" ' Someone from a disadvantaged background coming into the same room would no doubt feel that their low social status increased their misgivings and was another thing about themselves they would prefer people not to know.

Friendship fits easily into the same picture. You feel at ease with friends because they like you, find you interesting, attractive, good company: they feed back positive signals and make you feel more confident and valued. In contrast, not having friends or feeling excluded and unwelcome increases all our self-doubts and anxieties about how we are seen.

As reflexive beings, we constantly monitor how others react to us, so much so that we know ourselves partly through each other's eyes. No one is unaware of the worries we can have about whether we are liked or disliked, regarded as interesting, attractive, and intelligent, or unattractive, boring, and socially undesirable. As well as affecting our sense of security in relation to others, low social status, lack of friends, and a difficult start in life have all been found to be related to higher basal cortisol levels.

If this is indeed what the social epidemiology is telling us, then it fits well with what many of the great sociologists have identified as the basis of our sensitivity to the social environment. What makes us socially malleable and provides the basis for socialization and conformity is the importance of how we appear to others and our capacity for shame and embarrassment. Just as this is the gateway through which our behaviour is made susceptible to the external influence of the social world, so it is the route through which society gets under the skin to affect health. It is because we are so sensitive to the eyes of others that pride and shame, acceptance and rejection, social inclusion or exclusion have such powerful influences on stress.

A recent experiment using an MRI scanner has shown how deeply aversive social exclusion can be. It was found that the pain of social exclusion activates the same parts of the brain—the anterior cingulate cortex and right ventral prefrontal cortex—as physical pain does (Lieberman 2003). Instead of looking at the effects of pain caused by real social exclusion, by the stigma of poverty, or by the experience of being looked down on, a computer game was used to simulate a very mild experience of exclusion. People were asked to play a computer game of 'catch' with what they thought were two remote (and unseen) players using other computer terminals. The computer was programmed so that after a short time the two other 'virtual' players ceased passing the ball to the experimental subjects and passed it between each other instead. So the experience which looked on the MRI brain scan like physical pain resulted from nothing more than a computer programme which led you to believe that two people whom you had never met preferred to pass a ball between themselves rather than to you.

16.4 **The wider society**

With this view of the nature of our vulnerability to the social environment, we can now turn our attention to the features of the wider society which make us more or less vulnerable. Almost any social problem can be looked at from an individual or societal viewpoint. We could, for instance, find explanations of why some people are more likely than others to suffer unemployment or to become involved in drug abuse or violence. We would find at least part of the explanation lay in people's early childhood, in their family life, and school careers. But if we want to understand why one society has, say, 20% unemployed, while another has only 2%, we need to look at the working of the economic system. It will, of course, always be the most vulnerable 2% or 20% who are unemployed, in much the same way as we know that although a country's overall traffic accident rate will be determined by the condition of its roads, regulations, and the weather, young men will always have more than their share of accidents.

16.4.1 **Inequality and the social environment**

There are reasons for thinking that the scale of inequality in a society affects both the impact of social status differences and the nature of social affiliations—two of the three categories of psychosocial influences on health which we have discussed. How the extent of inequality affects social status differences is obvious enough: wider income differences are almost synonymous with increased relative deprivation and relative poverty. Where income differences are larger, people on smaller incomes will experience themselves as falling further behind the rest of society.

As for social affiliations, several kinds of evidence suggest that wider income differences between rich and poor are socially corrosive. First, evidence from numerous studies—at least 30, including a meta-analysis (Hsieh and Pugh 1993)—show that violence is reliably more common in more unequal societies. Figures 16.1 and 16.2 are examples of this relationship. Second, studies looking at levels of trust, internationally (Uslaner 2002) and among the 50 states of the USA (Kawachi *et al.* 1997), suggest that people are much less likely to trust each other where income differences are bigger. Thirdly, Putnam's work on social capital shows that people are much more likely to be involved in community life where income differences are smaller (Putnam *et al.* 1993; Putnam 2000). He found that among the 20 regions of Italy and the 50 states of the USA,

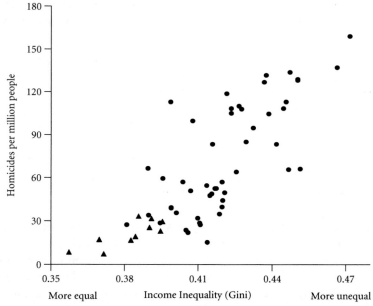

Fig. 16.1 Homicide rates in relation to income inequality among US states (circles) and Canadian provinces (triangles). Homicide is more common in more unequal US states and Canadian provinces.

Source: Daly *et al.* 2001.

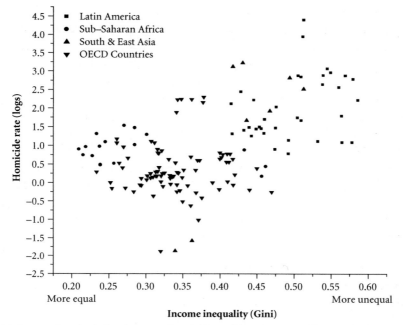

Fig. 16.2 International relation between homicide and income inequality. Homicide rates are higher in countries in which income differences are larger (shown to the right). Relationships like this have been demonstrated many times.

Source: Fajnzylber *et al.* 2002.

involvement in community life tended to be higher where income differences were smaller. As well as these strong cross-sectional associations, Putnam also drew attention to the remarkably similar time trends as social capital moved inversely with inequality during the twentieth century. He says that throughout the first two-thirds of the century, income inequalities narrowed and social capital strengthened. But, in the late 1960s, both reversed their direction and, in Putnam's words, 'America reversed course and started becoming both less just economically and less well connected socially and politically' (Putnam 2000, p.359).

What these findings seem to be telling us is that inequality is socially divisive. In a sense, the scale of material differences within a society serves as an indicator of social distances and, hence, of the importance of social hierarchy or class. The human tendency to choose friends from among our social equals suggests that inequality is a significant social barrier. In addition, the nature of social interaction up and down the social hierarchy is almost certainly different from what it is between equals. Issues to do with dominance and subordination, superiority and inferiority, respect and disrespect, are much more likely to intrude in 'vertical' relations, and may become more prominent in more unequal societies.

16.4.2 **Inequality and health**

If income inequality is indeed closely related to some of the most powerful influences on health, one would expect to find that health and income inequality were related. A large majority of the studies of this issue, both within societies and between them, have shown that this is indeed so. In a recent review of the literature—including studies of homicide and inequality—we found some 169 separate analyses in 155 papers (Wilkinson and Pickett, forthcoming). After including whatever control variables the authors thought fit, 132 of these found statistically significant associations between greater inequality and worse health. Only eight found significant associations the other way round. Others found no significant relationships either way. However, although the bulk of the evidence shows that more egalitarian societies tend to have higher standards of health and longevity, some remain unimpressed and believe that 'there is little support for the idea that income inequality is a major generalizable determinant of population health' (Lynch *et al.* 2004, p.5).

Much of the disagreement on the role of inequality hinges on what people think are the most plausible mechanisms linking it to health and what other influences should be separated off as extraneous and controlled out of the picture. To take an analogy, if we were looking at the effects of economic growth rather than at how unequal and hierarchical a society is, it would be a mistake to control for anything which is likely to be an aspect of economic growth itself—such as income, ownership of cars or other consumer durables, diet, central heating, proportion of the population employed in manufacturing rather than in agriculture, house size, urbanization, population density, or education. If we did control for them, we would be removing some of the effects of economic growth. The problem with social hierarchy, and so with inequality which serves as its marker, is that social stratification is perhaps the next most fundamental variable to economic development in determining the characteristics of a society. Although its affects are less well understood, they clearly involve the whole social structure and much social behaviour, presumably including anything which is patterned by social class. De Tocqueville chose to start his famous book *Democracy in America* with exactly this point. His opening paragraphs are:

> Among the new objects that attracted my attention during my stay in the United States, none struck me with greater force than the equality of conditions. I easily perceived the enormous influence that this primary fact exercises on the workings of the society. It gives a particular direction to the public mind, a particular turn to the laws, new maxims to those who govern, and particular habits to the governed.

> I soon recognized that this same fact extends its influence far beyond political mores and laws, and that its empire expands over civil society as well as government: it creates opinions, gives rise to sentiments, inspires customs, and modifies everything that it does not produce.

> In this way, then, as I studied American society, I saw more and more in the equality of conditions, the generative fact from which each particular fact seemed to flow, and I kept finding that fact before me again and again as a central point to which all of my observations were leading. (p.1)

Although income inequality is likely to be related to health because it reflects the scale of class differentiation in a society, research workers have tried to isolate some purer income inequality effect on health, and have variously chosen to control for poverty, individual income, differences in the provision of medical care, welfare transfers, female labour force participation, illiteracy, alcohol consumption, educational differences, marital status, smoking, household size, race, urbanization, segregation, unemployment, area deprivation, obesity, social capital, population density, diet, crime, physical activity, and blood pressure. While some of these might be legitimate, others are likely to be pathway, or mediating, variables. If our aim is to test for health effects of bigger class inequalities, then it is clearly not legitimate to control for factors which reflect the scale of those class inequalities.

The view that income inequality does indeed serve as a measure of class differentiation within a national class hierarchy, is supported by the fact that 80% of studies of larger areas—whole countries, regions, states, and cities—show inequality is related to poorer health. In contrast, only half the studies of inequalities in smaller areas (e.g. counties and local areas) provide support. The same tendency towards weaker

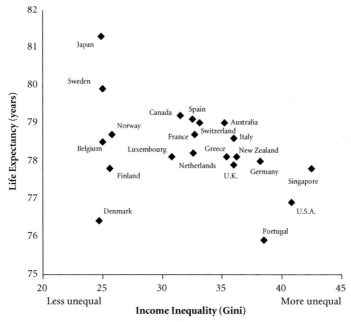

Fig. 16.3 Life expectancy and income distribution in the 21 richest countries. After being disrupted by rapid changes in inequality in the rich countries, the relation between income distribution and life expectancy apparent earlier, has re-emerged. More unequal countries (on the right) tend to have lower life expectancy. When controlled for GNP per capita and weighted by population size, the correlation coefficient $r = -0.86$.

Source: De Vogli *et al.* 2005.

associations in studies of smaller areas was also reported in the meta-analysis of studies of homicide and inequality (Hsieh and Pugh 1993).

Figures 16.3, 16.4, and 16.5 provide different indications of the relationship between health and inequality. Figure 16.3 shows the international relation between inequality and life expectancy in the richest developed countries. Figure 16.4 shows data for 528 cities in five different rich countries: USA, Australia, Canada, Sweden, and Britain. Although there is a very clear relationship between inequality and death rates across all these cities, if we look at each country on its own, we find that it is only the American and British cities which are ordered by inequality. So, although the cities of other countries clearly fit into the overall distribution, inequality does not tell us why one Australian or Swedish city is healthier than another. There are several possible explanations for this pattern. It might be that social classes are defined more exclusively within a national rather than a local frame of reference in those countries, so that it is national rather than local inequality which matters. It could also be something to do with the fact that there is more inequality in the USA and Britain than in the other countries.

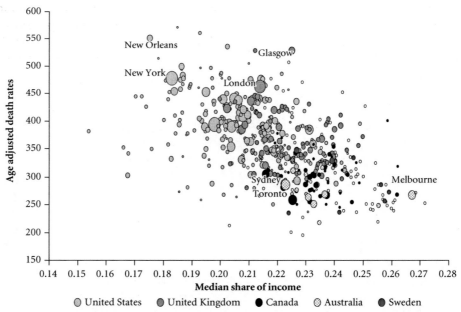

Fig. 16.4 Income inequality and death rates among working-age men in 528 cities in five countries. Graph shows that cities in which income differences are smaller tend to have lower death rates. The measure of income distribution used here is the proportion of society's income going to the poorest half of the population, so the more equal cities are to the right. At the most unequal end of the distribution is New Orleans; the opposite end, with much lower death rates, is Melbourne.

Source: Ross *et al.* 2005.

Lastly, it might reflect the way inequality is measured. Despite initial impressions to the contrary (Ross *et al.* 2000), health has now been shown to be ordered by inequality in Canadian cities if the inequalities are measured in 'market incomes'—that is, income before adjustment for the effects of taxes paid and benefits received (Sanmartin *et al.* 2003).

Lastly, Fig. 16.5 shows how the effects of inequality fit into the broader pattern of economic development. It shows infant mortality rates in rich and poor countries: the three parallel curves show infant mortality for countries with high, medium, and low inequality. We can see that infant mortality rates fall fast as very poor countries get richer, but the richer they get, the smaller any further reductions in infant mortality become. There are sharply diminishing returns of declining mortality to increasing income. In contrast, inequality appears to make an important difference at all stages in economic development.

At this point we could simply end with a summary of the evidence we saw earlier that the quality of social relations (trust, violence, involvement in community life) is poorer where income differences are greater; we could note that problems of low social status are likely to be increased by greater inequality, and reminding ourselves of the three powerful psychosocial influences on health from which we started. Together, this would lead us to expect the relation between health and the scale of inequality which so many papers have now demonstrated. But the story is a good deal more interesting than that.

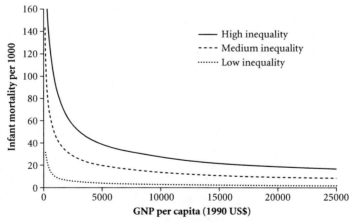

Fig. 16.5 National infant mortality rates in relation to GNP per head and income distribution. Graph is based on national data from both rich and poor countries. It shows that infant mortality rates decline rapidly as poor countries become richer, but then continue to decline very slowly as countries become much richer. The top curve shows that more unequal countries tend to have higher infant mortality rates at each stage of economic development. The curves below it are for medium- and low-inequality countries.

Source: Hales *et al.* 1999.

16.5 **Why social status and friendship?**

Issues to do with social status and friendship seem to form a double act: they crop up together in different scenes like a duo playing opposite parts to each other. At the beginning of this chapter, we saw them as powerful psychosocial factors affecting the health of each of us. Later, we saw them again as societal variables which moved inversely in relation to each other: where social status differences are greater, the quality of social relations deteriorates. And we also noted that we choose our friends from among our social equals. Why is it that they appear together, both as risk factors affecting individual health and as they move inversely in society?

The answer seems to be that they are the two opposite ways in which human beings can associate. What human social stratification, animal dominance hierarchies, and pecking orders have in common is that they are all ranking systems based on the use of power to gain preferential access to scarce resources. Except between kin, access to resources is based on power and coercion, regardless of the needs of others. At the extreme, might is right and the strongest gets the lion's share. In contrast, friendship is almost the opposite of that. It is marked by sharing, mutuality, reciprocity, and a recognition of each other's needs. Gifts and food sharing are such potent symbols of friendship because they are a demonstration of mutuality and a rejection of competition for scarce resources.

In essence then, it looks as if social stratification and friendship represent the two opposite ways in which human beings can associate. Either we compete for resources and the most powerful wins, or we agree not to. But why do social status and friendship figure so prominently as psychosocial influences on health, even in modern populations where high living standards mean that the vast majority of the population are not going to be deprived of the necessities of life? Why is it that these contrasting relationships are such powerful influences on stress and anxiety?

16.5.1 **Within species competition . . . or co-operation**

The explanation is perhaps that, among most animal species, including our prehuman ancestors, the main potential competition for resources comes, not from other species, but from members of the same species. Because members of the same species have all the same needs, they are also the greatest potential threat to each other's well being. So, everything a low-status baboon might find and enjoy, from a morsel of food to a place to lie in the shade, can be—and often is—taken by a baboon higher in the dominance hierarchy.

Various systems, such as territoriality, have developed to reduce the ever-present danger of conflict between members of the same species. As human beings, we have the potential to compete with each other not only for food, but also for clothing, jobs, sexual partners, housing, and everything else. However, as well as the potential to be each other's worst rivals, we also have the potential to be each other's best source of co-operation, assistance, care, support, learning, and love. In other words, the nature of our relationships determines whether other people are the worst threat, striking fear into our hearts, or best source of help, making us feel secure and at ease. Because other people can be the best or the worst, getting our social relationships right has always been crucial to well being.

Writing in the seventeenth century, Thomas Hobbes (1651) made the same danger of 'the competition of each against all' for access to scarce resources, the basis of his political philosophy. Because he thought conflict could only be avoided if there was a government with the power to keep the peace, he assumed that, in earlier forms of society without it, living in a 'state of nature', life would be 'nasty, brutish and short'. However, we now know that the way prehistoric hunting and gathering societies actually tried to reduce the danger of conflict was through systems of food sharing and gift exchange. As Sahlins (1974) suggested, it was because of the potential for conflict that people kept relations sweet by making huge investments in each other. As a result, these societies were highly egalitarian: they avoided the dangers inherent in some going short while others had plenty.

The potential for conflict over access to resources provides three reasons why low social status has become deeply aversive. First, in animal dominance hierarchies, lower-status males have fewer reproductive opportunities: dominant males try to monopolize access to females as a scarce 'resource'. Second, when food and other necessities are scarce, low-status animals will be the first to go without and suffer the consequences. And thirdly, unless low-status animals show submission responses and avoid any challenge to dominants, they risk attack.

16.5.2 **Social strategies and early life**

Social relationships range from antagonistic and adversarial to affiliative and affectionate. Inequality carries connotations of the adversarial basis of dominance hierarchies, while equality suggests more affiliative relationships. One is associated with social tension, anxiety, and keeping one's guard up, while the other is associated with relaxation, mutual support, and safety. We have separate social strategies for affiliative and dominance relationships. Affiliative relations involve making social investments in people, empathy, mutual aid, reciprocity, and a capacity for affection. In contrast, strategies for coping with dominance hierarchies involve competing for social rank, showing deference and obsequiousness to superiors, social prejudice, and snobbery against inferiors, while using put-downs and occasional aggression to defend against usurpers.

Where the balance between these two social strategies is struck varies from one species to another, and within the same species, over time, as conditions of feast or famine come and go. Although equally closely related to us, chimpanzees and bonobos are quite different in this respect. Bonobos are much more egalitarian and less hierarchical than chimps (de Waal and Lanting 1997). Human social organization shows that we have the capacity for both extremes of social organization and everything in between. Before agriculture (that is, for over 90% of our existence as 'anatomically modern' human beings), the evidence suggests that we lived in very egalitarian societies (Erdal and Whiten 1996; Boehm 1999). But in our recent historical past as agriculturalists, we have lived in more or less hierarchical, and sometimes tyrannical societies. It might seem easy enough to have a social repertoire which allowed us to choose the appropriate balance between affiliative behavioural strategies on the one hand, and the mixtures of aggression, timidity, and fear appropriate to ranking systems for any given society on the other. But, as Kemper pointed out, 'It is important that power-status outcomes, emotions, and neurophysiological and autonomic systems are firmly bound together' (Kemper 1988, p.308). How can this be achieved if the variation in forms of social organization among our human and prehuman ancestors is so great? How can the neurophysiology be set up to support such different kinds of social relations and behaviour?

In this situation, it seems likely that the period of early sensitivity, during which the HPA axis and stress responses seem to be 'tuned' or 'programmed', allows the hormonal influences on social behaviour to be adjusted in the light of early experience. Why else should early experience have consequences for health and behaviour which last for the rest of life? Although in modern societies people have often regarded children with poor attachment, who have had less early stimulation and little close interaction, as if they were permanently damaged, it may well be that their stress responses are prepared for less affiliative and more conflictual social relations. Whilst early social experience in modern nuclear families may be a poor guide to the nature of social life in the wider society, in small nomadic hunting and gathering bands, children would not have grown up in a nuclear family clearly distinguished from the rest of society. Their early experience of relationships and the quality of care in the foraging band may have provided a good guide to the kind of social relations they were likely to have to deal with in adult life.

16.6 Liberty, equality, fraternity

In bringing together some of the threads from earlier chapters, we have suggested a picture of our individual vulnerability to our social environment, and then used it to explain why population health is sensitive to particular dimensions of the wider social structure and environment. (A fuller discussion of all these issues can be found elsewhere; see Wilkinson 2005.) But in an important sense, the picture which emerges is not new. Rather, it is a reminder of what people once recognized intuitively. In the French Revolution, the crowds demanded 'liberty, equality, fraternity'. By liberty, they meant not being subservient to the landed aristocracy and feudal nobility. The demand for liberty was a demand not to be beholden to anyone—in effect, a demand for autonomy. The link between this and the problems of low social status, subordination, and lack of control which are so damaging to health are clear.

In more gender neutral terms, fraternity is clearly about friendship, more affiliative social relations, and community life. It expresses a desire for a more sociable society, which we know leads to better health. Equality comes into this picture as a precondition for the other two: with large socio-economic inequalities, societies will have bigger problems of low social status, feelings of inferiority, and subordination; with larger inequalities, the quality of social relations will deteriorate, leading to increases in violence and reductions in both trust and involvement in community life.

As economic growth lifts the populations of the developed countries into a post-scarcity era, the importance of social relations to human well being is recognized increasingly widely (Layard 2003; Putnam 2000). But it is odd that a picture of the socially corrosive effects of inequality, which was once intuitively obvious to many, now has to be pieced together from research.

In terms of the progress which has been made in understanding the determinants of population health over the last couple of decades, what is striking is not only the recognition of the power of psychosocial influences on health, but also how *intensely* social the most powerful sources of stress seem to be. As Lassner *et al.* (1994) remarked, in a paper comparing cardiovascular reactivity to social and asocial sources of stress, 'it appears that conflicts and tensions with other people are by far the most distressing events in daily life in terms of both initial and enduring effects on emotional wellbeing' (p.69).

Perhaps the key to understanding why social relations are so important to us is to recognize what a powerful selective force the social environment has been in human evolution. So much so that, as Dunbar has demonstrated (2001), there is a very strong relation among primate species between the typical size of each species' social group and the ratio of the size of the neocortex in relation to the rest of the brain. As Fig. 16.6

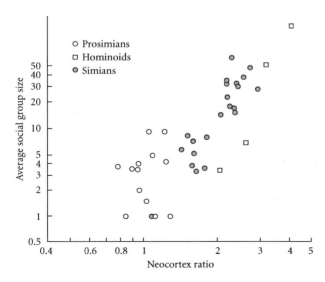

Fig. 16.6 The social brain: the size of the neocortex in relation to the rest of the brain is related to the average size of the social group among species of primates.

Source: Dunbar 2001.

shows, the bigger the typical social group size of a primate species, the larger the neocortex ratio. This suggests that much of the growth of the human brain served to equip us with the ability to handle the complexities of social life. But, just as we saw that the distinction between friendship and dominance relations grew out of contrasting ways of dealing with the problem of access to scarce resources, so we must remember that the quality of social relations in modern societies is built on material foundations.

References

Boehm C (1999). *Hierarchy in the forest: the evolution of egalitarian behaviour*. Harvard University Press.

Daly M, Wilson M, Vasdev S (2001). Income inequality and homicide rates in Canada and the United States. *Canadian Journal of Criminology*; **43**:219–36.

De Vogli R, Mistry R, Gnesotto R, Cornia GA (2005). Has the relation between income inequality and life expectancy disappeared? *Journal of Epidemiology and Community Health*; **59**:158–62.

de Waal FBM, Lanting F (1997). *Bonobo: the forgotten ape*. University of California Press, Berkeley.

Dunbar RIM (2001). Brains on two legs: group size and the evolution of intelligence. In: *Tree of origin: what primate behavior can tell us about human social evolution* (ed. Frans B.M. de Waal). Harvard University Press.

Erdal D, Whiten A (1996). Egalitarianism and Machiavellian intelligence in human evolution. In: *Modelling the early human mind* (ed. P. Mellars, K. Gibson). McDonald Institute Monographs, pp. 139–60. Cambridge University Press.

Fajnzylber P, Lederman D, Loayza N (2002). Inequality and violent crime. *Journal of Law and Economics*; **45(1)**:1–40.

Gitau R, Cameron A, Fisk NM, Glover V (1998). Fetal exposure to maternal cortisol. *Lancet*; **352**:707–8.

Hales S, Howden–Chapman P, Salmond C, Woodward A, Mackenbach J (1999). *Lancet*; **354**:2047.

Hobbes T (1651/1996) *Leviathan* (ed. Richard Tuck.) Cambridge University Press, Cambridge.

Hsieh CC, Pugh MD (1993). Poverty, income inequality, and violent crime: a meta-analysis of recent aggregate data studies. *Criminal Justice Review*; **18**:182–202.

Kawachi I, Kennedy BP, Lochner K, Prothrow–Stith D (1997). Social capital, income inequality and mortality. *American Journal of Public Health*; **87**:1491–8.

Lassner JB, Matthews KA, Stoney CM (1994). Are cardiovascular reactors to asocial stress also reactors to social stress? *Journal of Personality and Social Psychology*; **66(1)**:69–77.

Layard R (2005). *Happiness*. Allen Lane, York.

Marmot M, Wilkinson RG (2001). Psychosocial and material pathways in the relation between income and health: a response to Lynch et al. *British Medical Journal*; **322**:1233–6.

Mathews F, Yudkin P, Neil A (1999). Influence of maternal nutrition on outcome of pregnancy: prospective cohort study. *British Medical Journal*; **319**:339–43.

Phillips DIW, Barker DJP, Fall CHD, Seckl JR, Whorwood CB, Wood PJ, *et al.* (1998). Elevated plasma cortisol concentrations: a link between low birth weight and the insulin resistance syndrome? *Journal of Clinical Endocrinology and Metabolism*; **83(3)**:757–60.

Putnam RD (2000). *Bowling alone: collapse and revival of American community*. Simon and Schuster, New York.

Putnam RD, Leonardi R, Nanetti RY (1993). *Making democracy work: civic traditions in modern Italy*. Princeton University Press, Princeton.

Ross N, Dorling D, Dunn JR, Hendricksson G, Glover J, Lynch J (2005). Metropolitan income inequality and working age mortality: a five country analysis using comparable data. Journal of Urban Health; **82(1)**:101–10.

Ross NA, Wolfson MC, Dunn JR, Berthelot JM, Kaplan GA, Lynch JW. (2000). Relation between income inequality and mortality in Canada and in the United States: cross sectional assessment using census data and vital statistics. *British Medical Journal*; **320**:898–902.

Russell B (1956). *Portraits from memory, and other essays*. Allen & Unwin, London.

Sable MR, Wilkinson DS. (2000). Impact of perceived stress, major life events and pregnancy attitudes on low birth weight. *Family Planning Perspectives*; **32(6)**:288–94.

Sahlins M (1974). *Stone age economics*. Tavistock, London.

Sapolsky RM (1999). Hormonal correlates of personality and social contexts: from non-human to human primates. In: *Hormones, health, and behavior: a socio-ecological and lifespan perspective* (ed. C. Panter–Brick, C.M. Worthman). Cambridge University Press, New York.

Shively CA, Clarkson TB (1994). Social status and coronary artery atherosclerosis in female monkeys. *Arteriosclerosis and Thrombosis*; **14**:721–6.

Stansfeld SA, Rael EGS, Head J, Shipley M, Marmot M (1997). Social support and psychiatric sickness absence: a prospective study of British civil servants. *Psychological Medicine*; **27**:35–48.

Teixeira JMA, Fisk NM, Glover V (1999). Association between maternal anxiety in pregnancy and increased uterine artery resistance index: cohort based study. *British Medical Journal*; **318**:153–7.

Uslaner E (2002). *The moral foundations of trust*. Cambridge University Press.

Wilkinson RG (1997). Health inequalities: relative or absolute material standards? *British Medical Journal*; **314**:591–5.

Wilkinson RG (2005). *The impact of inequality: how to make sick societies healthier*. New Press, New York.

Wilkinson RG, Pickett KE (in press). Income inequality and health: a review and explanation of the evidence. *Social Science and Medicine*.

Williams RB, Barefoot JC, Blumenthal JA, *et al.* (1997). Psychosocial correlation of job strain in a sample of working women. *Archives of General Psychiatry*; **54(6)**:543–8.

Index

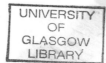